GLOBAL PERSPECTIVE ON DIABETIC FOOT ULCERATIONS

Edited by **Thanh Dinh**

Global Perspective on Diabetic Foot Ulcerations
Edited by Thanh Dinh

Published by InTech

Janeza Trdine 9, 51000 Rijeka, Croatia

Publishing Process Manager Mirna Cvijic

Technical Editor Teodora Smiljanic

Cover Designer InTech Design Team

Additional hard copies can be obtained from orders@intechopen.com

Global Perspective on Diabetic Foot Ulcerations, Edited by Thanh Dinh
p. cm.
ISBN 978-953-307-727-7

For EU product safety concerns:
IN TECH d.o.o., Prolaz Marije Krucifikse Kozulić 3, 51000 Rijeka, Croatia,
info@intechopen.com or visit our website at intechopen.com.

Meet the editor

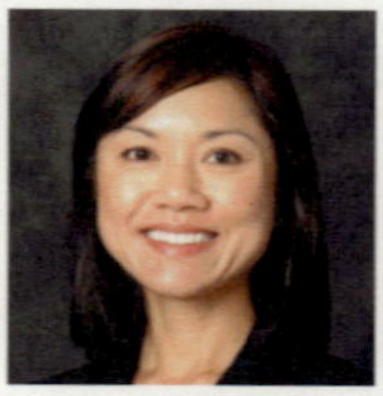

Dr. Thanh Dinh is currently an Assistant Professor in Surgery at Harvard Medical School and an Attending Podiatric Surgeon at Beth Israel Deaconess Medical Center in Boston, MA. Her clinical and research interests include Diabetic Foot Complications and Diabetic Microcirculation. She has published original research and scientific reviews in several prominent scientific journals, contributed to a number of textbooks covering Diabetes Mellitus, and serves as a reviewer for the International Journal of Lower Extremity Wounds. She is a currently a co-investigator on an NIDDK grant, Mechanisms of Neuropeptides Action in Diabetes, and an NIH grant, Impaired Wound Healing in Diabetic Foot Ulceration. In addition to her research activities, Dr. Dinh serves as the Assistant Director of Residency Training of the Podiatric Surgical Program at BIDMC as well as the Director of Externship Education.

Contents

Preface

Over the last decade, it is becoming increasingly clear that diabetes mellitus is a global epidemic. The influence of diabetes is most readily apparent in its manifestation in foot complications across cultures and continents. In this unique collaboration of global specialists, we examine the explosion of foot disease in locations that must quickly grapple with both mobilizing medical expertise and shaping public policy to best prevent and treat these serious complications.

In other areas of the world where diabetic foot complications have unfortunately been all too common, diagnostic testing and advanced treatments have been developed in response. The bulk of this book is devoted to examining the newest developments in basic and clinical research on the diabetic foot. It is hoped that as our understanding of the pathophysiologic process expands, the devastating impact of diabetic foot complications can be minimized on a global scale.

Dr. Thanh Dinh
Assistant Professor, Surgery, Harvard Medical School
Podiatric Surgeon, Beth Israel Deaconess Medical Center
Boston,
USA

Part 1

Global Impact of Diabetic Foot Complications

1

Possible Diabetic-Foot Complications in Sub-Saharan Africa

Ezera Agwu[1], Ephraim O. Dafiewhare[2] and Peter E. Ekanem[3]
[1]*Department of Microbiology;*
[2]*Department of Internal Medicine;*
[3]*Department of Anatomy*
Kampala International University, Western Campus,
Uganda

1. Introduction

In Sub-Saharan Africa, fast uncontrolled urbanization and changes in standard of living are responsible for the rising epidemic of diabetes mellitus and the observed increase presents a substantial public health and socioeconomic burden in the face of scarce resources (Mbanya et al., 2010). Ten to fifteen percent of diabetic patients develop foot ulcers at some stage of their lives and nearly fifty percent of all diabetes-related admissions are due to diabetic foot problems (Kumar and Clark, 2009). The epidemiology of Ketosis-prone atypical diabetes in Africans is not well understood because of scarce data for pathogenesis and subtypes of diabetes. The prevalence of undiagnosed diabetes mellitus is high in most countries of sub-Saharan Africa, and individuals who are unaware they have the disorder are at very high risk of chronic complications. Therefore, the prevalence of diabetes-related morbidity and mortality could grow substantially

Causes of amputation in sub-Saharan Africa vary between and within countries (Ephraim *et al.*, 2003, Thanni and Tade 2007) depending on ethnic background and socio-economic status (Leggetter *et al,* 2002, Rucker-Whitaker *et al.,* 2003). In sub-Saharan Africa, tumours and trauma are the leading causes of lower extremities amputation (Abbas and Musa, 2007, Thanni and Tade 2007), with increasing incidence of cardiovascular risk factors (Akinboboye et al., 2003).

In Kenya, rates of vascular amputations vary between 25% and 56% with Muyembe and Muhinga (1999) reporting that the leading indications of lower extremities amputation were trauma, tumours and complications of diabetes mellitus, each accounting for 26.5% of the amputations done. Another Kenya study recorded seven years later by Awori and Atinga, (2007) reported that 17.5% of patients who underwent amputation were due to diabetes-related gangrene. Two years later in 2009, diabetic vasculopathy accounted for 11.4% of the amputations and 69.6% of the non vascular cases while other causes of amputation included: 35.7% trauma, 20% congenital defects, 14% infection and 12.8% tumours respectively (Ogeng'o et al., 2009).

Kidmas et al., (2004) in Nigeria reported 26.4% diabetic foot sepsis as one of the main indications for lower limb amputations while Sié Essoh *et al.*, (2009) from Ivory Coast (Cote D'Ivoire) reported 46.9% below knee diabetes related amputation and 11.2% below elbow diabetes-related amputations as common procedures performed. However, in Zimbabwe, Sibanda et al., (2009) reported 9% diabetes related lower limb amputation rate among 100 patients evaluated. Thus, different regions of Africa reported decreasing trend in diabetes related amputations.

Non-diabetes related lower extremities amputation have also been well documented. Obalum and Okeke, (2009) in Nigeria reported 61.8% trauma as the most common indication of lower limb amputation with motorcycle related accidents accounting for 61.9% of the trauma related cases. This was followed by 19.0% lower limb amputations due to pedestrians involved in road traffic accidents. Again, Abbas and Musa (2007) reported 42.8% trauma related lower extremities amputation and 18.4% lower extremities amputations due to other malignancies. Below knee amputation was the commonest amputation carried out constituting 62.8% of the 35 lower limb amputations. A Nigerian study by Kidmas *et al.*, (2004) also found that trauma and malignant conditions of the limb were the main indications for lower limb amputations in 29.9% and 23% patients respectively. According to Awori and Atinga, (2007) in a study done in Kenya, 24.3% had tumours, 16.2% of which were mainly osteogenic sarcoma while trauma accounted for 18.9%. Fifty five per cent of the amputations were above-the-knee, 24 (31%) below-the-knee, four (5%) hip disarticulations and seven (9%) were foot amputations.

The prominence of diabetic foot among debilitating tropical diseases which influences the duration of patients hospital admission is noteworthy. Diabetic foot is a important health issue in sub-Saharan Africa, where it must compete for resources with other prevalent non-communicable diseases. One of the reasons for the poor outcome of diabetic foot complications in developing countries is the lack of patient education and inadequate medical supervision. Thus, health education tailored to the individual's risk status, which promotes self-care and addresses misconceptions and medical supervision are needed to effectively contain the multi-factorial pathology of diabetic foot ulcerations.

Though the risk factors for developing diabetic foot ulcers are manageable, poor outcomes of foot complications may be due to: poor awareness among patients and some cadre of health care providers, poor and delayed access to health care, poor referrals for specialist treatment, lack of team approach for the treatment of the complicated diabetic foot, absence of refresher training programmes for health care providers and lack of quality assurance programmes.

Diabetic foot infection is the most common soft tissue infection associated with diabetes mellitus, with disease-related peripheral neuropathy and peripheral vascular disease playing major roles in this complication of diabetes. More serious complications include failure of ulcers to heal and gangrene which may lead to osteomyelitis, amputation, and death. Diabetic foot ulcers may begin after minor trauma, become infected and may progress to cellulitis, soft tissue necrosis, and extension into bone. Exploration of the ulcer is crucial to determine its depth (the palpable bone strongly suggests osteomyelitis). It is also important to determine the presence of sinus tracts and to obtain a culture. Involved organisms include group A *Streptococcus* and *S aureus,* as well as aerobic gram-positive cocci, gram-negative rods, and anaerobes. It is highly promising to know that organism's involed in delayed healing diabetic foot complications in Nigeria including Staphylococcus and Pseudomonas species were susceptible to Quinolones (Agwu et al., 2010). If this information is confirmed in other parts of Africa, it will offer health care workers the scenario to design an intervention that will help reduce the incidences of diabetic foot complications and chances of lower linb amputations to barest minimum.

To reduce the incidence of Diabetes mellitus related amputation, medical supervision and patient education on prevention of diabetic foot complication are recommended. The predominant risk factors for foot complications are underlying peripheral neuropathy, peripheral vascular disease (Abbas and Archibald., 2007) and infection. Gangrene is a more serious complication of **diabetic foot disease** that causes long-standing disability, loss of income, amputation or death. Reasons for poor outcomes of **foot complications** in various less-developed countries include: lack of awareness of **foot** care issues among patients and health care providers alike; very few professionals with an interest in the **diabetic foot** or trained to provide specialist treatment; non-existent podiatry services; long distances for patients to travel to the clinic; delay among patients in seeking timely medical care, or among untrained health care providers in referring patients with serious **complications** for specialist opinion; lack of the concept of a team approach; absence of refresher training programs for health care professionals; and finally lack of surveillance activities (Abbas and Archibald., 2007). Other important factors include use of ill-fitting foot-wears and complete absence of foot wears (Krasner et al., 2007).

Abbas and Archibald., (2007) suggested the following ways of improving **diabetic foot** disease outcomes that do not require exorbitant outlay of financial resources: implementation of sustainable training programmes for health care professionals, focusing on the management of the complicated **diabetic foot** and educational programmes that include dissemination of information to other health care professionals and patients; sustenance of working environments that inculcate commitment by individual physicians and nurses through self growth; rational optimal use of existing microbiology facilities and prescribing through epidemiologically directed empiricism, where appropriate; and using sentinel hospitals for surveillance activities.

In Uganda and indeed many other African countries, little has been documented about diabetes care and far fewer data exist for diabetic foot among the diabetics. The worst scenario is the high prevalence of unknown cases in where people only discover they are diabetic when they can no longer contain the associated complications. Lack of diabetes clinic in major hospitals and at the grass root could explain the poor education of diabetic foot patients on what to do and how to manage the situation. Evaluation of diabetic foot complications in this region is a study designed to fill the knowledge gap, sensitize the appropriate authorities to intervene and remind the diabetics on the need to participate in an integrated community directed efforts to reduce the impact of diabetic foot to the barest minimum. The situational analysis of diabetic foot epidemic, prevention and control in South Western Uganda is very necessary. The objective of this manuscript is therefore to outline the current prevalence and impact of diabetic foot and its associated complications among the diabetics in South Western Uganda

2. Methods

This was a biphasic study made up of a prospective stake-holders descriptive survey and a retrospective cross sectional health-point survey of diabetic foot and its associated complications among diabetic patients attending randomly selected hospitals in Bushenyi, Sheema, Rubirizi and Mbarara districts of South Western Uganda. Hospital records of diabetic patients attending clinics at Mbarara metropolis made available for this assessment are those which fulfilled our data inclusion criteria which states that clinical data must be confirmed by laboratory investigation and laboratory data must be confirmed by clinical observation.

For reasons not explained by participating hospitals but which may include difficulty in information storage and retrieval, occasioned by changing hospital policies which allow patients to go home with their case files, the only data made available for this study were data generated in the year 2005. For retrospective data, Mbarara Regional Referral Hospital was selected based on: 1) presence of diabetes clinic, 2) possession of a side laboratory for rapid tests for diabetes, 3) being a referral hospital which covers referral cases from district hospitals and 4) having medical and surgical records which might include data on diabetic foot.

Pre-tested data collection tool was used to obtain socio-demographic information from the case-files of diabetic patients in Mbarara region of Uganda and also diabetes and diabetic foot associated disease complications as contained in patient's case-files.

To get a glimpse of the current diabetic management situation in an environment with few diabetic clinics, structured questionnaires were self-administered to randomly selected diabetes stakeholders such as Clinicians, Medical Laboratory Scientists, diabetic patients and nursing officers working in hospitals located in South-Western Uganda and its environs. Criteria for diabetes stakeholders' selection include: having worked in- or being in-charge of clinical chemistry laboratories, Medical and Surgical wards of hospitals located in Mbarara and its environs. Mbarara and environs were defined as hospitals located in a nearby Bushenyi district such as Kampala International University Teaching Hospital (KIUTH), Comboni Hospital, Kitagata Hospital and Lugazi Health Center IV. Information obtained from the officers included comments on the overall routine approaches in diabetic care including existence of diabetic clinic, inspection of the feet of diabetics (during ward round and out-patients consultations), diabetes education, surveillance, and complications of diabetic foot.

At random, five clinicians and two senior nursing officers at KIUTH; two diabetic patients two clinicians and one nursing officer at Lugazi Health Center IV; one nursing officer at Kitagata hospital and one clinician at Comboni hospital were interviewed. The retrospective data included in this study were from patients clinically diagnosed with diabetes mellitus and subsequently confirmed with standard clinical chemistry methods in the side laboratories of the participating hospitals. Clinical data not confirmed in the laboratory and laboratory data not confirmed by the clinical records were excluded from the study. The Research and Ethics Board of Kampala International University Uganda approved this study.

3. Results

The 233 data reviewed were from 104 (44.6%) males and 129 (55.4%) females aged from 10 years old to 60 years and above with a mean age of 40 years (Table 1). According to our data source, there were no routine diabetic clinics in most hospitals in the year 2005 when the retrospective data of the study population were reviewed. Known diabetic patients were cared for at the Medical and Surgical departments of the hospital. The hospital records evaluated did not distinguish between insulin dependent and non-insulin dependent diabetes making it difficult to determine the impact of diabetes types on disease establishment and progression (Table 1). The complications and co-morbidities reported in this study (Table 2) were obtained from the records of medical out- and in- patient departments of the clinic.

Consequently 233 diabetic patients presented 32 different diabetes associated co-morbidities and complications with peripheral nephropathy (22.8%) being the most prevalent complications followed by infection (9.5%) (vaginal candidiasis, Urinary tract infection, skin infection; and 1.7% obesity. Others listed in the table are co-morbidities found among the diabetic patients seen during the period. Other unclassified disease conditions accounted for 4% of the total complications/co-morbidities recorded (Table 2).

Interestingly there were no clear records of diabetic foot among the reported 32 complications and co-morbidities outlined above (Table 2). This unique and conspicuous absence of diabetic foot in the record of 233 diabetic patients prompted a prospective descriptive study involving stakeholders of diabetes disease and its management in Mbarara district and its environs.

Age (years)	No (%) prevalence	
	Male	Female
<10	0 (0.0)	0 (0.0)
11-20	6 (2.6)	2 (2.6)
21-30	20 (8.6)	14 (6.0)
31-40	25 (10.7)	23 (10.0)
41-50	14 (6.0)	25 (10.7)
51-60	18 (7.7)	32 (13.7)
>60	21 (9.0)	29 (12.4)
Total	104 (44.6)	129 (55.4)

n=233

Table 1. Age and sex distribution of 233 dependent diabetic patients attending clinics in Mbarara district of Uganda

Stake-holders opinion clearly indicated that in Mbarara and environs with no diabetes clinics, foot inspection is not done routinely during ward-round even among known diabetics. Also there were inadequate diabetes education and surveillance. The main assistance rendered to the known diabetics include monitoring and control of blood glucose level and care for any major complaints they may have. Stakeholders also outlined the fact that most patients do not even know they have diabetic foot because of loss of sense of touch due to peripheral neuropathy. The diabetic foot complications reported by stakeholders include: peripheral neuropathy (sensory, motor and/or autonomic), chronic leg ulcers and gangrene. The clinicians reported that many foot lesions treated among diabetic patients were not documented as part of the final diagnosis for these patients. That may account for the absence of diabetic foot in previous hospital records retrieved for the retrospective study

complication/co-morbidity	No (%) positive	
Peripheral Neuropathy*	53	(22.8)
Esophagitis	20	(8.6)
HIV/ AIDS	18	(7.7)
Cataract*	16	(6.9)
Renal disease	14	(6.0)
Peptic ulcer disease	9	(3.9)
Malaria	9	(3.9)
Oral thrush	9	(3.9)
Vaginal candidiasis*	7	(3.0)
Diarrhea	6	(2.6)
Urinary tract infection*	10	(4.3)
Tuberculosis	6	(2.6)
Herpes zoster	5	(2.2)
Psychosis	5	(2.1)
Hypertension	4	(1.7)
Obesity*	4	(1.7)
Pancreatitis	4	(1.7)
Skin infections*	3	(1.3)
Asthma 1	3	(1.3)
Arthritis	3	(1.3)
Pneumonia	2	(0.9)
Parkinsonism	2	(0.9)
Dental carries	2	(0.9)
Anemia	2	(0.9)
Sepses*	2	(0.9)
Testicular swelling	1	(0.4)
Spontaneous Abortion	1	(0.4)
Road traffic accidents	1	(0.4)
Phimosis	1	(0.4)
Epilepsy	1	(0.4)
Others	10	(4.0)

n= 233
NOTE: The items with * are absolute or relative complications of diabetes mellitus

Table 2. Complications and co-morbidities found among diabetic patients attending clinic at Mbarara Regional Referral Hospitals in 2005.

4. Discussion

Damage to the nervous system, is one of the serious complications of diabetes. A person with diabetes may not be able to feel his or her feet properly. Normal sweat secretion and oil production that lubricates the skin of the foot is impaired. These factors together can lead to abnormal pressure on the skin, bones, and joints of the foot during walking and can lead to breakdown of the skin of the foot. Sores may develop. Damage to blood vessels and impairment of the immune system from diabetes make it difficult for wounds to heal. Bacterial infection of the skin, connective tissues, muscles, and bones can then occur. These infections can develop into gangrene, because of the poor blood flow. If the infection spreads to the bloodstream, this process can become life-threatening.

The relative absence of diabetes clinics in the participating hospitals at the time of this investigation may highlight the observed apparent absence of diabetic foot in the data obtained in retrospect from the hospital records of the 233 diabetic patients. We could not confirm zero prevalence of diabetic foot among the records of the diabetic patients reviewed because information obtained from the prospective survey suggests that the foot findings may not have been documented as part of the diagnoses (since it has never been part of the routine practice during ward rounds and at the Out-patient department clinics). Stakeholders report of patients not knowing about foot infection points to lack of diabetes education in the society. The non-inclusion of foot inspection in the non-diabetic clinics has made it difficult to determine the prevalence of diabetic foot among the diabetics in the studied area. In this study, we could not confirm the prevalence of diabetic foot among the studied population and we also have no result to compare with the reported percentage prevalence of diabetic foot all over Africa.

Such reports include but not limited to: 15% by Boulton, (2000); 63.9% reported by Monabeka and Nsakala-Kibangou (2001); 24% reported by Nouedoui *et al.*, (2003); 13% reported by (Ndip et al., 2006, Tchakonté *et al.*, 2005, Kengne *et al.*, 2009); 16.7% by Amoussou-Guenou et al., (2006); 53% by Ogbera et al., (2006); 13.4 by Ahmed et al., (2009); 33% reported by Mugambi-Nturibi et al., (2009);

The majority of the reported complications were similar to reported diabetic foot complications elsewhere in Africa. Notable among the reported complications is 22.8% peripheral neuropathy reported in this study. This is lower than: 68% old Nigerian report by Akanji and Adetuyidi (1990) and slightly lower than 27.3% reported by Ndip *et al.*, (2006) in Cameroon. However, it is similar to 22.7% reported by Ahmed et al., (2009) in Khartoum, Sudan.

Akanji and Adetuyidi (1990) reported a 68% prevalence of neuropathy, 54% foot ischaemia 42% hypertension, 38% chronic osteomyelitis 35% soft tissue changes. Sixty per cent were anaemic at presentation. Mixed bacterial organisms were cultured in 70% of the cases and 20% nephropathy in Nigerian diabetics with foot lesions. The initiating factors were observed to be predominantly trivial trauma and "spontaneous" blisters. Allied with the golden rules of prevention (i.e. maintenance of glycemic control to prevent peripheral neuropathy, regular feet inspection, making an effort not to walk barefooted or cut **foot** callosities with razors or knives at home and avoidance of delays in presenting to hospital at the earliest onset of a **foot** lesion), reductions in the occurrence of adverse events associated with the **diabetic foot** is feasible in less-developed settings.

Other possible complications associated with diabetic foot in Africa

There are few reports relating the level of research in Africa showing different possible disease complications which may be associated with diabetic foot. These reports are impressive but definitely not enough to represent the true picture of the situation in Africa largely because many African countries either do not presently have any report on diabetic foot or the incidence are under-reported.

The prevalence of active **foot** ulceration was reported by Boulton, (2000) to vary from about 1% in Europe and North America to more than 11% in reports from some African countries. Monabeka and Nsakala-Kibangou (2001) reported 2.8% trophic disorders and 1.2% mal perforant with total of 22.6% mortality rate before surgical intervention was high (22.6%). The complications reported by Nouedoui *et al.,* (2003) in Yaunde, Cameroon, included: 4.39% gangrenous lesion while 89% have various un-identified infections in young patients with short history of diabetes and poor education about diabetes. Bouguerra *et al.,* 2004 reported a high prevalence of mycotic infection among **diabetic** patients compared to their non-**diabetic** colleagues. Tchakonté *et al.,* 2005 reported a strong correlation between an history of **foot** ulcer, a neuropathy and **foot** deformations and the evidence of a **diabetic foot**. Ndip et al., (2006) reported high prevalence of diabetic foot lesions and associated complications. Specific observations include: 21.3% ischemia and 17.3% deformity, 12.3% had a previous history of foot lesions, 47% had a risky nail-trimming habit and 22% wore ill-fitting shoes.

According to Feleke et al., (2007), infection is the most serious complication of diabetes and recognized as leading cause of morbidity while cardiovascular diseases were the leading cause of mortality. However, **Diabetic foot** ulcers were the major cause of infection followed by tuberculosis, skin infection, subcutaneous infections, Pneumonia. *S. aureus from wound infection and E. coli from urinary tract infection were the common pathogens.* Muthuuri (2007), found that post-amputation mortality was 28% and the mortality was found to be associated with high co-morbidity, mainly due to: 100% uncontrolled diabetes mellitus, 75% Sepsis, 42% ischaemic heart disease, 25% uncontrolled hypertension and renal insufficiency. The mortality associated with **diabetic foot** ulcer disease may be predicted by measurable characteristics such as high blood sugars, raised White blood cell count, high creatinine, high serum lipids, abnormal ECG and abnormal arterial Doppler scans (Muthuuri, 2007). These parameters point to conditions that are themselves **complications** of diabetes mellitus and whose management will reduce mortality. The management of **diabetic foot** is therefore, multidisciplinary.

Abbas et al., (2009) characterised the role of ethnicity in the occurrence of diabetic **foot** ulcer disease in persons with diabetes in Tanzania and found that: ethnic Africans were more likely to: present with gangrene ($P < 0.01$) and have intrinsic **complications** such as neuro-ischaemia or macrovascular disease which delays ulcer healing while Indians were more likely to be obese ($P < 0.001$), have large vessel disease ($P < 0.001$) and mode of intervention such as sloughectomy or glycaemic control with insulin or oral agents seams to determine the same outcome like in African counterparts. Peripheral vascular disease and gangrene are playing a larger role in ulcer pathogenesis and outcomes for both ethnic groups than was previously thought (Abbas et al., 2009). In a study by Obalum and Okeke 2009 in Nigeria, 61% trauma found was the most common followed by below knee amputation was done in 51 (75.0%) of cases, stump wound infection was found in 26.5% while three (4.7%) patients died. Ahmed et al., 2009 could not identify the causative agents of 48.7% patients with hand sepsis while 42.9% prevalence was due to trauma; 36.1% cellulitis, 29.5% deep seated abscess, 14.3% digits amputation and 1.7% of patients were unavoidably hand-amputated.

Kengne *et al.,* 2009 in reviewing the changing pattern of diabetic foot with time found **foot** ulcer to be associated with 115% more bed use and a nonsignificantly lower risk of death or dropout.

Bahebeck et al., (2010), in an effort to identify clinical patterns and outcomes related to the treatment of these diabetic foot infections reported that life-threatening hand and **foot** infections in **diabetic** patients account for a large proportion of amputations and a substantial number of deaths and concluded that 7 patterns of serious limb- or life-threatening infection were identified and, in the absence of vascular surgical intervention, mortality can be reduced at the expense of more amputations. The seven pattern of limb infections were as follows: 30.36% of the patients studied had necrotizing cellulitis, 21.43% had wet gangrene, 16.07% had acute extensive osteomyelitis, 8.93% had dry gangrene, 8.93% had gas gangrene, 7.14% had necrotizing fasciitis, and 7.14% had diffuse hand infections. Mani et al., 2011 reported that since some 15% of the population with diabetes develop **foot complications**, the reported observations of venous incompetence in patients with diabetes but not **foot** disease offer hope of alleviating symptoms if not preventing ulcers.

Tsimerman et all 2011 found that circulating micro-particle characteristics are related to the specific type of vascular **complications** and may serve as a bio-marker for the pro-coagulant state and vascular pathology in patients with Type 2 Diabetes Mellitus. Shapoval et al., 2011 defined surgical tactics based on concrete **complications** of the diabetic foot syndrome, frames conditions for the unification and uniform registration of the form and severity of the disease and volume of the surgical treatment. Ragunatha et al., 2011. Suggested that well-controlled diabetes decreases the prevalence of diabetic mellitus specific cutaneous disorders associated with chronic hyperglycemia. Oguejiofor *et al.,* 2010. Long duration of diabetes mellitus and peripheral neuropathy are risk factors for **foot** complication in Nigerians with diabetes mellitus. Asumanu et al., 2010, in Ghana reported surgical complications which included foot infections, cellulitis, and abscesses.

There is an adage that says "prevention is better than cure" Therefore, this discussion will be incomplete without noting the principles of diabetic foot care which include: daily feet inspection; early reporting of any foot injury among diabetic patients; checking shoes inside and outside for sharp bodies/areas before wearing; use of lace-up shoes with adequate room for the toes; keeping feet away from sources of heat; and checking bath temperature before stepping in (Kumar & Clark). According to the stakeholders, the use of advocacy and health education by health care providers in prevention and control of diabetic foot complications is yielding good results as it is now common to see diabetic patients talking about how to avoid risky behavious such as avoiding certain food as a way of prevention and control of diabetes.

5. Conclusion

Africa and South Western Uganda have contributed to the knowledge about possible foot complications as outlined above. Relative absence of diabetic foot in the retrospective data of South Western Uganda was confirmed prospectively as due to lack of specialized diabetic foot clinic in the studied population, absence of specialised diabetes clinics, poor education and various complications influenced diabetic foot in South Western Uganda region of Africa.

Examination of the diabetic foot and appropriate documentation of findings among the diagnosis should be encouraged among healthcare workers, especially clinicians. Also refresher courses on care of diabetics should be encouraged among all healthcare workers. Diabetes clinics should be included in all health centres IVs and above OR major health centres in African countries. Another important thing is adequate and relevant health education for patients with diabetes mellitus in health care institutions, the media and diabetes associations. These measures will help reduce the morbity and mortality associated with the diabetic foot among diabetic patients.

Finally, it is recommended that further local studies should be done in order to be able to document the true prevalence of diabetic foot ulcers among diabetics in the community. These shall lead to deeper studies that will help identify the causes of those ulcers and determination of ways of preventing or minimizing those causes, thereby giving the diabetics a better overall quality of life.

6. Acknowledgment

We wish to acknowledge: Ms Boretor Lucy who collected the data from Mbarara hospital; Management and staff of Mbarara Regional Referral hospital, for making the 2005 retrospective data on diabetes available for this investigation; all stake-holders who assisted in generating the prospective data for this manuscript

7. References

Abbas, A.D. & Musa, A.M. (2007). Changing pattern of extremity amputations in University of Naiduguri Teaching Hospital, Nigeria. Niger J Med. 16:330–333.

Abbas, Z.G. & Archibald, L.K. (2007). Challenges for management of the diabetic foot in Africa: doing more with less. Int Wound J. Dec;4(4):305-13. Epub 2007 Oct 24.

Abbas, Z.G.; Lutale, J.K. & Archibald LK. (2009). Diabetic foot ulcers and ethnicity in Tanzania: a contrast between African and Asian populations. *Int Wound J. Apr;* 6 (2) :124-31. Epub 2009 Apr 2.

Agwu E., Ihongbe, J.C. & Inyang N.J. (2010). Prevalence of Quinolone susceptible *Pseudomonas aeruginosa* and *Staphylococcus aureus* in delayed-healing diabetic foot ulcers in Ekpoma Nigeria. *Wounds.* 4: 100-105.

Ahmed, M.E.; Mahmoud, S.M.; Mahadi; S.I.; Widatalla, A.H.; Shawir, M.A. & Ahmed, M.E. (2009). Hand sepsis in patients with diabetes mellitus. *Saudi Med J.* 30 (11) : 1454-8.

Akanji, A.O. & Adetuyidi, A. (1990). The pattern of presentation of foot lesions in Nigerian diabetic patients. *West Afr J Med.* 9(1):1-5.

Akinboboye, O.; Idris, O.; Akinboboye, O.; Akinkugbe, O. (2003). Trends in coronary artery disease and associated risk factors in sub-Saharan Africa. *J Hum Hyperten.* 17:381–387

Amoussou-Guenou, K.D.; Zannou, D.M.; Ade, G.; Djrolo, F.; Avimadje, M.; Bigot, A.; Koffi-Tessio, A. & Houngbe; F. (2006). Morbidity of diabetic foot in Internal Medicine CNHU HKM, Cotonou *Mali Med.* 21(4):4-7.

Asumanu, E.; Ametepi, R. & Koney, C.T. (2010). Audit of diabetic soft tissue infection and foot disease in Accra. *West Afr J Med.* Mar-Apr;29(2):86-90.

Awori, K.O. & Ating'a, J.E.O. (2007). Lower limb amputations at the Kenyatta National Hospital, Nairobi. *East Afr Med J.* 84:121–126.

Bahebeck, J.; Sobgui, E.; Loic, F.;, Nonga, B.N.; Mbanya, J.C. & Sosso, M. (2010). Limb-threatening and life-threatening diabetic extremities: clinical patterns and outcomes in 56 patients. *J Foot Ankle Surg.* 2010 Jan-Feb;49(1):43-6.

Bouguerra, R.; Essaïs, O.; Sebaï, N.; Ben-Salem, L.; Amari, H.; Kammoun, M.R.; Chaker, E.; Zidi, B. & Ben-Slama C. [Prevalence and clinical aspects of superficial mycosis in hospitalized diabetic patients in Tunisia. *Med Mal Infect.* 2004 May ; 34 (5):201-5.

Boulton, A.J. (2000). The diabetic foot: a global view. *Diabetes Metab Res Rev.* Sep-Oct;16 Suppl 1:S2-5.-UK

Diouri, A.; Slaoui, Z.; Chadli, A.; El-Ghomari, H.; Kebbou, M.; Marouan, F.; Farouqi, A. & Ababou, M.R. (2002). Incidence of factors favoring recurrent foot ulcers in diabetic patients. *Ann Endocrinol (Paris) Dec;63(6 Pt 1):491-6.*

Ephraim, P.L.; Dillingham, T.R.; Sector, M., Pezzin, L.E. & Mackenzie, E.J. (2003). Epidemiology of limb loss and congenital limb deficiency: a review of the literature. *Arch Phys Med Rehabil.* 84(5):747–761.

Feleke, Y. Mengistu Y. & Enquselassie F. (2007). Diabetic infections: clinical and bacteriological study at Tikur Anbessa Specialized University Hospital, Addis Ababa, Ethiopia. *Ethiop Med J.* Apr; 45 (2):171-9.

Kengne, A.P.; Choukem S.P.; Dehayem, Y.M.; Simo, N.L.; Fezeu, L.L. & Mbanya, J.C. (2006). Diabetic foot ulcers in Cameroon: can microflora prevalence inform probabilistic antibiotic treatment? J Wound Care. 2006 Sep;15(8):363-6.

Kengne, A.P.; Djouogo, C.F., Dehayem MY, Fezeu L, Sobngwi E, Lekoubou A, Mbanya JC. (2009). Admission trends over 8 years for diabetic foot ulceration in a specialized diabetes unit in cameroon. Int *J Low Extrem Wounds.* 2009 Dec;8(4):180-6.

Kengne, A.P.; Dzudie, A.I.; Fezeu, L.L. & Mbanya, J.C.. (2006). Impact of secondary foot complications on the inpatient department of the diabetes unit of Yaounde Central Hospital. Int J Low Extrem Wounds. 2006 Mar;5(1):64-8.

Kidmas, A.T.; Nwadiaro, C.H. & Igun, G.O. (2004). Lower limb amputation in Jos, Nigeria. *East Afr Med J.* 81(8):427-9.

Leggetter, S.; Chaturvedi, N.; Fuller, J.; Edmonds, M.E. (2002). Ethnicity and risk of diabetes-related lower extremity amputation. *Arch Intern Med.* 162:73–78.

Mani, R.; Yarde, S. & Edmonds, M. (2011). Prevalence of deep venous incompetence and microvascular abnormalities in patients with diabetes mellitus. *Int J Low Extrem Wounds.* Jun;10(2):75-9.

Mbanya, J.C.N.; Motala, A.A.; MD, Sobngwi, E.; Assah, F.K. & Enoru ST. (2010). Diabetes in sub-Saharan Africa. The Lancet, Volume 375, Issue 9733, Pages 2254 - 2266, 26 June

Monabeka, H.G. & Nsakala-Kibangou, N. (2001)Epidemiological and clinical aspects of the diabetic foot at the Central University Hospital of Brazzaville. Bull Soc Pathol Exot. Aug;94(3):246-8.

Mugambi-Nturibi, E.; Otieno, C.F.; Kwasa T.O.; Oyoo, G.O. & Acharya, K. (2009) Stratification of persons with diabetes into risk categories for foot ulceration. East Afr Med J. 86(5):233-9.

Muthuuri, J.M. (2007). Characteristics of patients with diabetic foot in Mombasa, Kenya. East Afr Med J. Jun;84(6):251-8.

Muyembe, V.M. & Muhinga, M.N. (1999). Major limb amputation at a provincial general hospital in Kenya. *East Afr Med J.* 1999;76:163–166.

Ndip, E.A.; Tchakonte, B. & Mbanya, J.C. (2006). A study of the prevalence and risk factors of foot problems in a population of diabetic patients in cameroon. Int J Low Extrem Wounds. Jun;5(2):83-8.

Nouedoui, C.; Teyang, A. & Djoumessi, S. (2003). Epidemiologic profile and treatment of diabetic foot at the National Diabetic Center of Yaounde-Cameroon. Tunis Med. Jan;81(1):20-5.

Obalum, D.C. & Okeke; G.C. (2009). Lower limb amputations at a Nigerian private tertiary hospital. *West Afr J Med.* Jan; 28(1):24-7.

Ogbera, A.O.; Fasanmade, O.; Ohwovoriole, A.E. & Adediran, O. (2006). An assessment of the disease burden of foot ulcers in patients with diabetes mellitus attending a teaching hospital in Lagos, Nigeria. Int J Low Extrem Wounds. Dec;5(4):244-9.

Ogeng'o, J.A.; Obimbo, M.M. & King'ori J. (2009). Pattern of limb amputation in a Kenyan rural hospital. *Int Orthop.* 33(5): 1449–1453.

Oguejiofor, O.C.; Odenigbo, C.U.; Oguejiofor, C.B. (2010). Evaluation of the effect of duration of diabetes mellitus on peripheral neuropathy using the United Kingdom screening test scoring system, bio-thesiometry and aesthesiometry. Sep;13(3):240-7.

Ragunatha, S.; Anitha, B.; Inamadar. A.C.; Palit, A. & Devarmani, S.S. (2011). Cutaneous disorders in 500 diabetic patients attending diabetic clinic Indian J Dermatol. Mar;56(2):160-4.

Rucker-Whitaker, C.; Feinglass, J.; Pearce, W.H. (2003). Explaining racial variation in lower extremity amputation. A 5 year retrospective claims data and medical record review at an urban teaching hospital. *Arch Surg.* 138:1347–1351.

Shapoval, S.D.; Riazanov, D.I.; Savon, I.L.; Zinich, E.L. & Smirnova, D.A. (2011). The attempt of clinical classification of the complicated diabetic foot syndrome iKhirurgiia (Mosk). (6):70-74.

Sibanda, M.; Sibanda, E. & Jönsson, K. (2009). A prospective evaluation of lower extremity ulcers in a Zimbabwean population. Int Wound J. 2009 Oct; 6(5):361-6.

Sié Essoh, J.B.; Kodo, M.; Djè Bi Djè, V. & Lambin, Y. (2009). Limb amputations in adults in an Ivorian teaching hospital. *Niger J Clin Pract.* 12 (3):245-7.

Tchakonté, B.; Ndip, A.; Aubry, P.' Malvy, D.;, Mbanya, J.C. (2005). The diabetic foot in Cameroon. Bull Soc Pathol Exot. Jun;98(2):94-8.

Thanni, L.O.; Tade, A.O. (2007). Extremity amputation in Nigeria—a review of indications and mortality. *Surgeon.* 5:213–217.

Tsimerman, G.; Roguin, A.; Bachar, A.; Melamed, E.; Brenner, B. & Aharon, A. (2011). Involvement of microparticles in diabetic vascular complications. Thromb Haemost. 2011 Jun 28;106(2).

World Health Organization. The World Health Report (1997). Conquering, suffering, enriching humanity. Geneva: WHO;

2

Reducing Diabetic Foot Problems and Limb Amputation: An Experience from India

Sharad Pendsey
Diabetes Clinic & Research Centre
"Shreeniwas", Opp. Dhantoli Park
Nagpur
India

1. Introduction

India has a dubious distinction of having largest number of persons with diabetes in the world. Type 2 diabetes has become the most common metabolic disorder. Its prevalence is growing more rapidly among people in the developing world, primarily due to marked demographic and socioeconomic changes in these regions. India currently leads the world with an estimated 41 million people with diabetes; this figure is predicted to increase to 66 million by 2025. The diabetes epidemic is more pronounced in urban areas in India, where prevalence rates of diabetes are roughly double than those in rural areas. Diabetic foot is one of the most devastating chronic complications of diabetes and is the leading cause of lower limb amputation.

Although population based data are not available, rough estimates indicate that in India approximately 45,000 legs are amputated every year, and the numbers are increasing each year. Almost 75 % of these amputations are carried out in neuropathic feet with secondary infection, which are potentially preventable. Certain factors like bare - foot walking, illiteracy, low socioeconomic status, late presentation by patients, ignorance about diabetic foot care among primary care physicians and belief in alternative systems of medicine contribute to this high prevalence. Lack of trained professionals in diabetes foot care in India and the profession of podiatry being non - existent compound the problem further. The novel project "Step - by - Step Improving Diabetes Foot care in the developing world" was initiated in India. The goal was to train healthcare professionals in basic foot care, improve their educational skills, and provide them hand on experience in treatment of trivial foot lesions. The aim was to encourage them to set up minimum model diabetic foot clinics where they would be able to prevent trivial foot lesions becoming catastrophe.

This carefully designed and executed project to improve diabetic foot care in the developing world turned out to be a major success. The strength of the Step by Step project was that it consisted of basic and an advanced course to be attended by the same delegates. In all, 100 teams of doctors & nurses were selected for training in diabetes foot care. The participants selected were specifically from smaller cities and towns, and had no previous training in diabetes foot care. They were offered a 2 day Basic Course in 2004 followed by a 2 day

Advanced Course in 2005. The courses were held in the 4 metros of India (New Delhi, Mumbai, Chennai, Kolkata), with 25 teams participating in each metro. Each team was given educational material, books on diabetic foot, video and CDs (patient education and education for healthcare professionals) and special diagnostic and therapeutic instruments kits. A national and international faculty of experienced educators in the field was responsible for teaching and chaired the practical sessions.

2. Diabetic foot Indian scenario

Type 2 diabetes has become the most common metabolic disorder. Its prevalence is growing more rapidly among people in the developing world, primarily due to marked demographic and socioeconomic changes in these regions. India currently leads the world with an estimated 41 million people with diabetes; this figure is predicted to increase to 66 million by 2025. The diabetes epidemic is more pronounced in urban areas in India, where prevalence rates of diabetes are roughly double than those in rural areas. (Mohan et al., 2007).

Diabetic foot is one of the most devastating chronic complications of diabetes and is the leading cause of lower limb amputation. (Boulton et.al., 2005). It is often an inching, painless surprise that holds in its dark portals a soon rising flood of complications. It is a quiet dread of disability, long stretches of hospitalization, mounting impossible expenses with the ever dangling end result of an amputated limb. The phantom limb plays its own cruel joke on the already demoralized psyche. The diabetic foot, no wonder is one of the most feared complications of diabetes.

From the 41 million population of diabetic persons in India, 90% do not even see a specialist in their life time. Majority are treated either by primary care physicians or by practitioners of alternative medicine while some buy and follow treatment exclusively on the basis of advertisements published in lay press which assure guaranteed success in cure for diabetes. (Pendsey, 2010).

As the number of diabetics worldwide increase, there will be more diabetic foot problems. The escalating number of foot problems is due not only to the increasing diabetic population but to the fact that they are now living long enough to develop foot complications. Many healthcare professionals involved in managing persons with diabetes show little interest in diabetic foot problems, furthermore the diabetic foot is frequently regarded with hopelessness as if progression down the road to major amputation is inevitable once ulceration has developed. (Pendsey, 2010).

Although population based data are not available, rough estimates indicate that in India approximately 45,000 legs are amputated every year, and the numbers are increasing each year. Almost 75 % of these amputations are carried out in neuropathic feet with secondary infection, which are potentially preventable. In India clinical profile of diabetic foot differs because of several factors such as practice of walking barefoot, wearing inappropriate footwear like Hawaiian slippers, illiteracy, low socioeconomic status, late presentation by patients, faith in alternative system of medicine and lack of awareness among primary care physicians about diabetic foot and its consequences. (Pendsey, 2010).

Lack of trained professionals in diabetes foot care in India and the profession of podiatry being non - existent compound the problem further. (Pendsey ,2007).

In India neuropathic lesions are dominant and account for 80% of foot ulcers and the remaining 20% being neuroischaemic. Among the causative factors, extrinsic factors like injuries due to sharp objects ,inappropriate footwear and thermal injuries account for 70% of neuropathic foot ulcerations. Intrinsic factors which are indicators of long standing polyneuropathy such as foot deformities, limited joint mobility, bony prominences and neuroarthropathy account for remaining30% of neuropathic foot ulcerations.

Peripheral vascular disease (PVD) has been reported to be low among Asians (Pendsey 1998) ranging between 3 - 6% as against 25 - 45% in Western world. (Marinelli et al.,1979; Migdalis et al., 1992; Walters et al., 1992). The prevalence of PVD increases with advancing age and is 3.2% below 50 years of age and rises to 55% in those above 80 years of age. Similarly it also increases with increased duration of diabetes, 15% at 10 years and 45% after 40 years (Janka,et al., 1980). In India the number of diabetic patients above the age of 80 years or with the duration of diabetes of more than 30 years is extremely low, thus explaining the low prevalence of PVD in Indian diabetics. (Pendsey 1998).

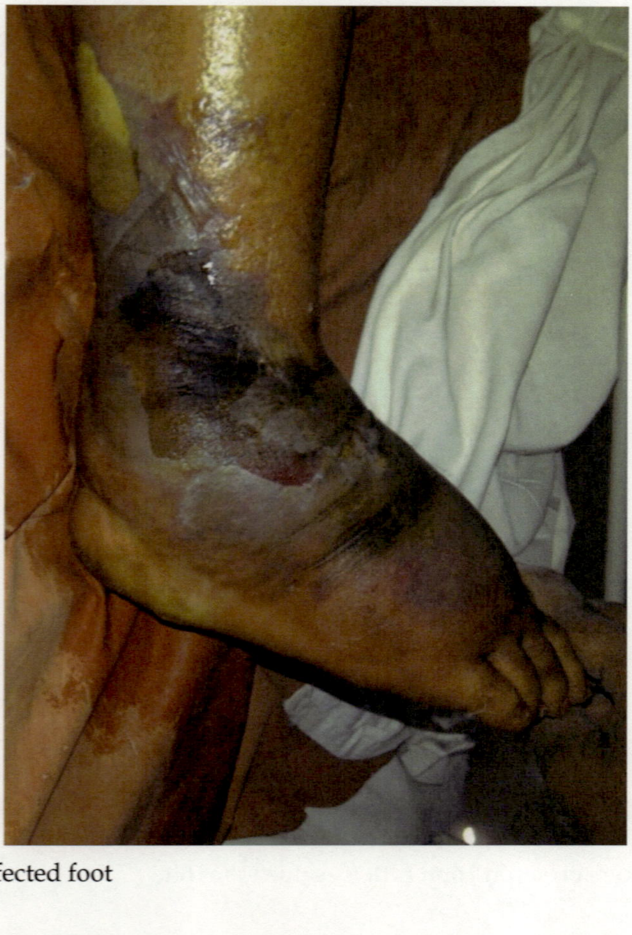

Fig. 1. Severely infected foot

Severely infected foot is the hallmark of Indian diabetic foot. It is not uncommon to see a patient with foul smelling, oedematous and severely infected foot with moribund general condition. Such patients have life threatening infection and therefore invariably require primary limb amputation. (Pendsey 2010).

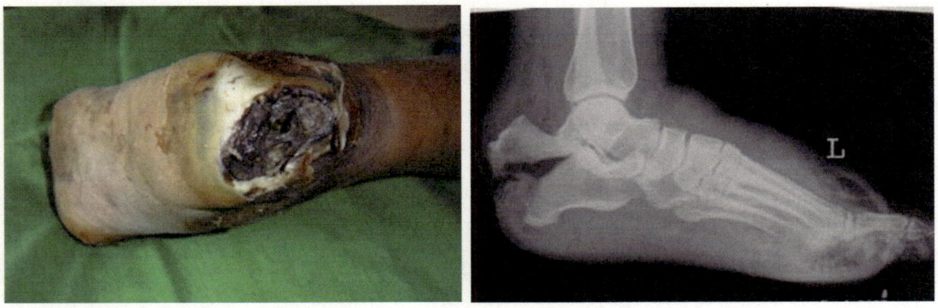

(a) (b)

Fig. 2. (a). Infected heel with necrosis of the soft tissue (b). Radiograph showing osteomyelitis of calcaneum, soft tissue swelling with gas shadow in the area of forefoot.

Certain atypical presentations are seen because of socio economic and cultural factors prevalent in India. Patients with neuropathy and consequent loss of protective sensations,

who sleep on the floor are invariably bitten by house rats who nibble toes creating deep foot ulcerations. Patients notice the ulcers on waking up to find blood stained bed linen, in the morning.Patients notice the ulcers on waking up to find blood stained bed linen, in the morning.

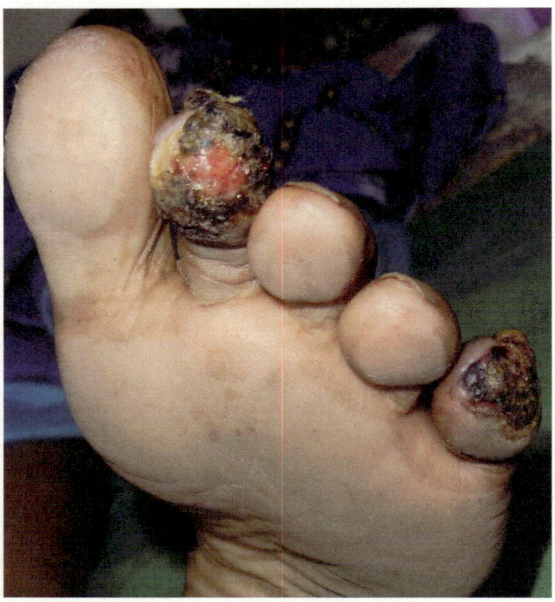

Fig. 3. Showing ulcers on second and fifth toes due to rat bite

Patients with neuropathy who visit religious places (temples) during summer months when the day temperature ranges between 43 and 47 degrees Celsius, develop severe thermal injuries . They are compelled to walk barefoot as religion does not permit wearing shoes.

Indians are known for sitting cross legged for long hours at work and during worship. Repeated and prolonged pressure over lateral malleolar areas lead to formation of bursae. Such bursae over lateral malleoli are dark and hypertrophied but are usually harmless in non neuropathic individuals. In diabetics with neuropathy, these bursae get ulcerated and often secondarily infected, creating a surgical emergency. Indian women wear metal (silver being commonest) toe rings in one or more toes of both feet, which is part of tradition. In neuropathic feet with deformities of toes, these toe rings often cause strangulation in presence of swelling of the feet. In tropical climate due to excessive sweating, fungal infection quickly sets-in, in web spaces. In diabetics with neuropathy these macerated ulceration often gets secondarily infected and find their way, quickly, to deep plantar compartments creating a limb threatening situation. (Pendsey 2010).

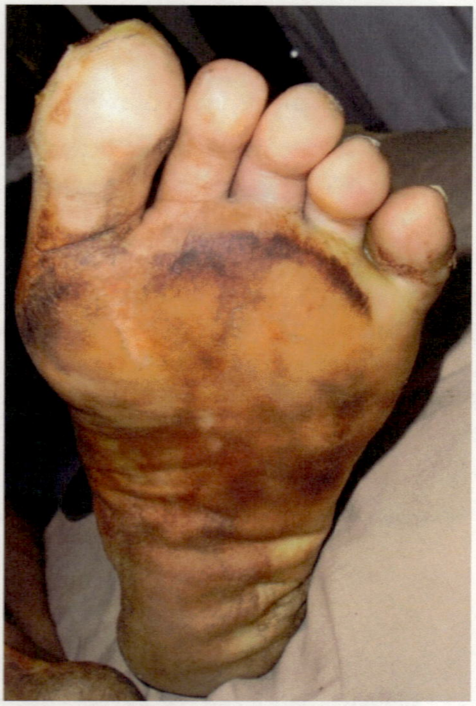

Fig. 4. Showing thermal injury on the plantar area of right foot.

3. Step by step diabetic foot care project in India

In view of the magnitude of the problem of diabetic foot, it was felt that there was an urgent need for training of doctors and nurses in diabetic foot care, in the Indian sub continent. Trivial foot lesions precede 85 % of leg amputations. Training of doctors and nurses will help them to take care of such trivial lesions and prevent the majority of leg amputations and simultaneously offer preventive foot care and advice about proper footwear.

The Step - by - Step project was hence conceived with a common objective of improving diabetes foot care in the developing world. (Bakker,et al.,2006; Pendsey, 2007a, 2010b). The Project Committee consisted of SharadPendsey, India (Chairman), Karel Bakker, The Netherlands, Althea Foster, United Kingdom, Zulfiqarali G. Abbas, Tanzania, Vijay Vishwanathan, India. It had academic support from International Diabetes Federation (IDF) , Diabetic Foot Society of India (DFSI), Muhimbili University college of health sciences (MUHS) and International working group on Diabetic Foot (IWGDF) . The project received financial grant from World Diabetes Foundation (WDF).

3.1 Goals

To create more awareness of diabetic foot problems

To provide sustainable training of health care professionals in the management of diabetic foot

To facilitate the cascading of information from health care professionals who have undergone training to other health care professionals and thus export expertise

To reduce the risk of lower limb complications in people with diabetes

To empower people with diabetes to care for their feet better, detect problems earlier and seek timely help when problems arise.

3.2 Methods

Special foot care education materials, both visual and audio-visual, were designed specifically for people with diabetes in developing countries.Foot care education materials, visual and audio-visual, were also designed for healthcare professionals working with people with diabetes in developing countries. Kits of diagnostic instruments (10gm monofilament, tuning fork, etc) were distributed to participants.

Therapeutic instruments' kits (Bard Parker handle with surgical blades, nail clipper, nail files, artery and tooth forceps, scoop, probe, and scissors) were also distributed to the participants.

3.3 Project at a glance

In all, 100 teams of doctors & nurses - India (94), Bangladesh (3), Sri Lanka (2), Nepal (1) were selected for training in diabetes foot care. The participants selected were specifically from smaller cities and towns, and had no previous training in diabetes foot care. They were offered a 2 day Basic Course in 2004 followed by a 2 day Advanced Course in 2005. The courses were held in the 4 metros of India (New Delhi, Mumbai, Chennai, Kolkata), with 25 teams participating in each metro. Each team was given educational material, books on diabetic foot, video and CDs (patient education and education for healthcare professionals) and special diagnostic and therapeutic instruments kits (Pendsey 2007).

A national and international faculty of experienced educators in the field was responsible for teaching and chaired the practical sessions.

3.4 Basic course

In this 2 - day practical training programme, according to a step - by - step approach, participants were taught to take a history, perform physical examination, screen for neuropathy and ischaemia, and classify and stage the foot. Having identified feet at risk, they were taught to organize appropriate foot care education and take timely action in cases of ulceration or advanced foot problems. Referral pathways were discussed and adapted to local circumstances. The training sessions for the basic course were designed to be interactive and informal with practical workshops. The formal lecturing was kept to a minimum. Participants were expected to educate their patients and cascade their acquired knowledge and skills to colleagues in their regions in order to create a spin - off effect and perpetuate and sustain achievements of the project.

To practice the techniques for debridement and cutting undermined edges of ulcers, the participants were provided with sweet limes as 'guinea pigs' to imitate diabetic feet. The delegates were taught some quite elaborate procedures with the help of these sweet limes - trimming calluses, probing ulcers and cutting out undermined edges using a forceps.

All participants had been requested not to cut their nails for one month prior to the training, so that they could practice nail cutting on each other using nail clipper provided by the project. This particular session worked as a great icebreaker and helped develop a friendly and collaborative atmosphere (Bakker et al., 2006).

Patients with diabetic foot problems were presented and the faculty discussed them and demonstrated the practical skills of callus removal and nail trimming. Appropriate educational material designed for doctors, nurses and in particular for people with diabetes in developing countries, was discussed. In view of the many different languages and dialects that exist in the Indian subcontinent and considering the levels of literacy, a special emphasis on easy to understand audiovisual materials and pictures were given.

In the last session, delegates were divided up into smaller discussion groups and brainstormed ideas and plans for implementing the Step - by - Step Project. Then each group reported back to the whole group. Delegates were thus equipped to educate and examine patients, to record what they find and what action they take, to use the written material to improve their knowledge of the diabetic foot, and to gradually build their own diabetic foot programme. The delegates left the basic course, well equipped, to start a minimum model diabetic foot clinic in their respective regions. (Bakker et al., 2006;.Pendsey ,2007)

3.5 Advanced course

As a prerequisite for participation in the basic course, attendees agreed to attend an advanced course within one year. At the advanced course, they were given a specially prepared patient education video and another video for training health care professionals in their regions, thus spreading awareness about diabetic foot disease and its prevention and management.

Advanced subjects - such as the management of vascular disease, biomechanics, neuropathic osteoarthropathy (Charcot Foot), imaging modalities of the diabetic foot, indications for amputations, newer treatments and effective techniques of education - were taught. An important part of the advanced course was also reporting of the achievements in the first year. Delegates presented their activities as posters. It was gratifying to see how the teams were working in their respective centers. The majority had started practicing what they had learnt, e.g. educational activities, screening for high risk feet, use of a stepwise algorithm to analyse and investigate diabetic foot cases and management of trivial lesions (callus removal, nail trimming, deroofing of bullae, etc). Most posters were very good and showed high levels of effort and interest amongst the participants. All teams submitted cases for presentation and five were selected to make oral presentation. The cases were discussed in detail by the faculty with active participation by the delegates. To enhance participation, a quiz on foot care was also arranged. Paramedics were encouraged to show their skills on preventive foot care. They actually worked on patients removing calluses, cutting difficult nails, dressing wounds etc. The participation in this activity was spontaneous and all paramedics participated. From the way they did the job in the presence of a large number of people and in front of a live camera, it was quite clear that the practical skills they had learned during the basic course had been effectively used and frequently applied. All faculty members appreciated the dexterity and confidence shown by the paramedics. In summary, the attending delegates were adequately trained in preventative diabetic foot care. The delegates scored significantly higher on a questionnaire on foot care knowledge at the end of each course than they had done at the beginning.

Characteristics	1st year	2nd year	Increase (%)
Patients screened for high risk feet	**45,000**	**82,761**	**83.92**
Patients who received foot care education	**45,000**	**79,399**	**76.44**
Patients with high risk feet	**15,000**	**38,082**	**153.88**
Patients receiving treatment for trivial foot lesions	**4500**	**9716**	**115.91**
Referral to tertiary Centre	**350**	**388**	**10.85**
Limbs salvaged	**900**	**1943**	**115.88**

Table 1. Showing the overview of the work by the delegates.

3.6 Impact

100 foot care clinics (minimum model) were started. It is anticipated that they will cascade information to large numbers of persons with diabetes, and also to other healthcare professionals, including paramedics, physicians, educators, healthcare policymakers and lay people. The formal training is expected to reduce the amputation rate among these patients

by about 50% .There will be a long-term network of all the participants to ensure percolation of knowledge throughout the country.

3.7 Results

The data was collected by a questionnaire sent to all participating delegates and results of 1st year after the basic course and 2nd year after the advanced course were evaluated 85 teams, from India, responded to the questionnaire for both years. From the overview of the work carried out by the delegates it was apparent that there was a significant increase in every activity they conducted in the second year, over the first year. In the absence of any formal training in diabetes foot care, about 20% of patients with trivial foot lesions would be expected to have lower extremity amputation.(Muller et al., 2002; Ramsey et al., 1999;).

Thus, in the 1st year, at least 900 lower limbs and in the 2nd year 1943 limbs were salvaged. (Pendsey 2007).

4. Conclusion

This carefully designed and executed project to improve diabetic foot care in the developing world turned out to be a major success. The strength of the Step by Step programme is that the project consists of a two-year set up: a basic and an advanced course to be attended by the same delegates. The prerequisite to participate in the first course was to agree to follow the second course. The attendees were supplied with a free full set of clinic equipment. Combined with the education and teaching materials, and the acquired knowledge, the participants could immediately start to improve the local foot care management. The lively and interactive exchange of thoughts through the presentation of case reports by the delegates made them more alert to common pitfalls. The delegates realised the possibility of improving management by means of rather simple and affordable care, including education of patients. Another strength of the project was the interaction of both doctors and nurses or paramedics in the teams. The faculty felt that the enthusiasm of the participants to do even better in the future was amazing and many showed commitment to roll out the learning to others in the region. The clinical profile of diabetes differs across the world on account of differences in social, economic and cultural factors. The burden of diabetes as well as its complications like the diabetic foot increasing. Every small step taken to improve diabetic foot care will be a step in right direction in preventing this dreaded complication of diabetic foot.

5. Acknowledgement

The author acknowledges World Diabetes Foundation for providing Financial Grant for the Step-by-Step Foot care project.

6. References

Bakker, K.; Abbas, ZG. & Pendsey, SP. (2006). Step by step, improving diabetic foot care in the developing world. A pilot study for India, Bangladesh, Sri Lanka and Tanzania. *Pract Diab Int*, 23:365-369.

Boulton, AJ.; Vileikyte, L.; Ragnarson-Tennvall G., et al., (2005). The global burden of diabeticfoot Disease. *Lancet*, 366:1678-1679.

Janka , HU.; Standl, E. & Mehnert ,H. (1980). Peripheral vascular disease in diabetes mellitus and its relation to cardiovascular risk factors: Screening with Doppler ultrasonic technique. *Diabetes care*, 3:207-213.

Marinelli, MR.; Beach, KW.; Glass, MJ., et al., (1979). Non - invasive testing vs. clinical evaluation of arterial disease : a prospective study. *JAMA*, 241:2031-2034.

Mohan, V.; Premlatha, G. & Sastry, NG. (1995). Peripheral Vascular Disease in non insulin Dependent diabetes mellitus in South India. *Diabetes Res Clin Pract* , 27:235–240.

Mohan, V.; Sandeep, S.; Deepa, R.; Shah, B. & Varghese, C. (2007). Epidemiology of type 2 diabetes: Indian scenario. *Indian J Med Res.*, 125:217-230.

Migdalis, IN.; Kourti, A.; Zachariadis, D. & Samartizis, M. (1992). Peripheral Vascular Disease in newly diagnosed non-insulin-dependent diabetes. *Int Angiol* ,11:230–232.

Muller, IS.; de Grauw, WJ.; Van Gerwen, WH., et al., (2002). Foot ulceration and lower limb Amputation in type 2 diabetic patients in Dutch primary health care. *Diabetes care* 25:570-574.

Pendsey, SP. (1998). Peripheral Vascular disease: an Indian scenario, *Diabetologia Croatica* 27-4:153-156

Pendsey, SP. (2005). Step-by-step project on diabetic foot to help reduce leg amputation by 50%. *Asian J Diabetol*, 7-3:48-50.

Pendsey, SP. (2007) & Abbas, ZG. (2007). The Step–by–Step Program for reducing diabetic foot problems . A model for the developing world, *Current Diabetes Reports*, 7:425–428.

Pendsey, SP. (2010). Clinical Profile of Diabetic Foot in India, *The International Journal of Lower Extremity wounds* , 9(4):180-184.

Ramsey, SD.; Newton, K.; Blough D., et al.(1999). Incidence, outcomes, and cost of foot ulcers in patients with diabetes. *Diabetes Care* , 22:382-387.

Walters, DP.; Gatling, W., Mullee, MA. & Hill, RD.(1992). The prevalence, detection and epidemiological correlates of peripheral vascular disease : a comparison of diabetic and non - diabetic and non - diabetic subjects in an English Community, *Diab Med*.9:710–715.

Part 2

Diagnostic Considerations in Diabetic Foot Complications

3

Screening of Foot Inflammation in Diabetic Patients by Non-Invasive Imaging Modalities

Takashi Nagase[1], Hiromi Sanada[1], Makoto Oe[1], Kimie Takehara[1], Kaoru Nishide[2] and Takashi Kadowaki[3]

[1]*Department of Gerontological Nursing/Wound Care Management Graduate School of Medicine, The University of Tokyo*

[2]*Department of Nursing, St. Marianna Medical University Hospital*

[3]*Department of Metabolic Diseases, Graduate School of Medicine, The University of Tokyo*

Japan

1. Introduction

Diabetic foot is defined as infection, ulceration and/or destruction of deep tissues associated with neurological abnormalities and various degrees of peripheral vascular disease in the lower limb of the patients with diabetes mellitus (DM) (the International Working Group on the Diabetic Foot, 1999). Foot disorders are among the most serious and costly complications of DM (Apelqvist et al., 2008). When uncontrolled, diabetic foot can result in ulcer formation and subsequent amputation of the lower limb. Foot ulcers occur in 12 to 25 % of DM patients, and precede 84 % of all nontraumatic amputations in the growing DM population (Brem et al., 2006). It is thus quite urgently needed to prevent diabetic ulcer formation in the "at risk" foot by multi-disciplinary team approach (Apelqvist et al., 2008).

How can we identify "at risk" foot in the DM patients? According to the guidelines by the International Working Group of the Diabetic Foot, "at risk" foot should be identified by inspection and examination according to symptoms such as non-sensory or sensory neuropathy, foot deformities, bony prominences, signs of peripheral ischemia, previous ulcer or amputation (Apelqvist et al., 2008). The patients are categorized according to the risk classification system. Based mainly on Lavery et al. (Lavery et al., 1998), these categories include the following: no sensory neuropathy (category 0); sensory neuropathy (category 1); sensory neuropathy and signs of peripheral vascular disease (PAD) and/or foot deformities (category 2); and previous ulcer (category 3) (the International Working Group on the Diabetic Foot, 1999). Clinical effectiveness of this risk classification system was indeed substantiated by Peters et al. (Peters & Lavery, 2001), where ulceration occurred in 5.1, 14.3, 18.8, and 55.8% of the patients in categories 0, 1, 2, and 3, respectively during three years of follow-up. More recently, the International Working Group on the Diabetic Foot revised the risk classification system more focusing on the associated PAD (Lavery et al., 2008). However, we consider that there should be some limitatons in these approaches of risk assessment only based on conventional clinical examination. Although the report by Peter et al. (Peters & Lavery, 2001) showed clinical effectiveness of these approaches, occurrence rate of ulcers was unacceptably high in the higher categories. This fact may indicate necessity of more advanced approaches to detect the pre-ulceration status in the "at risk" foot in the more timely manner.

We consider that the screening of latent inflammation should be a key strategy for the assessment of pre-ulceration of the at risk foot. It should be kept in mind that DM patients may occasionally be insensitive to inflammatory pain in minor traumas caused by ill-fitting shoes, walking barefoot or callus formation, because of their sensory disturbances. If the patients continue walking, the overlooked inflammation may result in subsequent ulceration (Apelqvist et al., 2000; Apelqvist et al., 2008). Temperature elevation and edema should be accompanied by such latent inflammation. Recent advances of non-invasive imaging modalities such as thermography and ultrasonography may provide us with visual information of tissue temperature changes and edema associated with inflammation.

In our previous publications, we used thermography and ultrasonography for assessing wound status of pressure ulcers, confirming their clinical versatility for detecting inflammation. Delayed healing of pressure ulcers due to latent inflammation could be prospectively evaluated by high temperature of wound bed visualized by thermography (Nakagami et al., 2010). Also, the subcutaneous tissue damages such as edema or the discontinuous fascia could be clearly visualized by ultrasonography in the patients with pressure ulcers of the deep tissue injury type (Aoi et al., 2009; Nagase et al., 2007; Yabunaka et al., 2009).

Based on these experiences on pressure ulcers, we have introduced use of thermography and ultrasonography into the management of diabetic foot. In this chapter, we first mention variation of thermographic finding of the diabetic foot according to our own new classification system (Nagase et al., 2011). Furthermore, we describe our clinical research on the thermographic and ultrasonographic screening for the latent inflammation in the diabetic foot callus (Nishide et al., 2009).

2. Variations of thermographic morphological patterns in diabetic foot

2.1 Thermometry of diabetic foot: An overview

Thermometry of the diabetic foot has been established as an effective way for detecting inflammation and for assessing risks of ulceration (Bharara et al., 2006). Acute increase of the plantar temperature is regarded as a predisposing sign for pre-ulcer inflammation, requiring urgent intervention. For example, Armstrong et al. (Armstrong et al., 2007) and Lavery et al. (Lavery et al., 2004; Lavery et al., 2007) showed that foot temperature monitoring can reduce the ulceration rate in the "at risk" foot (category 2 or 3). In their randomized controlled studies, the DM patients in the intervention groups were guided to monitor temperatures of the several landmark points of their feet at home using a digital handheld thermometer. When the skin temperature was elevated compared with the contralateral side (>2.2°C), the patients were instructed to contact the research nurses and to reduce their activities until the temperatures normalized. Rates of ulceration were significantly reduced in the intervention groups than in the non-intervention control groups.

It has been already known that chronic temperature elevation may be observed in the neuropathic diabetic feet, mainly due to increased arteriovenous (A-V) shunt flow (Brem et al., 2006; Chan et al., 1991; Flynn & Tooke, 1995; Sun et al., 2005; Sun et al., 2008). Chronic temperature decrease implies association of PAD (Benbow et al., 1994; Brem et al., 2006). Unstable skin temperature due to impairment of thermoregulation is also noted in the neuropathic diabetic feet (Kang et al., 2003; Rutkove et al., 2005). Bharara et al. (Bharara et al., 2008a, b) demonstrated that foot temperature recovery after cold or warm immersion showed different trends between in the DM patients with and without neuropathy.

2.2 Use of thermography for assessing diabetic foot: Unsolved problems

Thermography is regarded as an imaging modality of thermometry. Thermography can estimate circulation and vascular patency by visualizing temperature distribution (Bharara et al., 2006; Nagase et al., 1996), and thus, it may be a potentially ideal tool for assessing inflammation and vascular stenosis of diabetic foot. We are using infrared (IR) thermography (Nagase et al., 2011; Nishide et al., 2009), which were also used in some of the abovementioned studies of diabetic foot thermometry (Sun et al., 2005; Sun et al., 2008; Sun et al., 2006) and in the more recent report evaluating healing tendency of the diabetic foot ulcer (Bharara et al., 2010). Liquid crystal (LC) thermography was conventionally used in the papers published in 1980's and 90's (Benbow et al., 1994; Chan et al., 1991; Stess et al., 1986). Interestingly, LC thermography has been now reappraised by many recent researchers (Bharara et al., 2008a, b; Frykberg et al., 2009; Roback et al., 2009). IR thermography can visualize thermal patterns without direct contact to the skin or wounds. LC thermography requires direct contact, and thus IR thermography may be better for detecting temperature of the non-contact area (such as the medial arch and the dorsal part of the feet) or the area colonized by pathogens such as the skin with tinea pedis or the infected wounds (Nagase et al., 2011). On the other hand, LC thermography has advantages because it is inexpensive, easy to use even in home-care setting, and appropriate for assessment of plantar temperatures under the influence of load (Bharara et al., 2008a, b; Frykberg et al., 2009). LC thermography costs approximately $ 1,800, whereas IR thermography costs approximately $ 25,000, and this fact is one of the factors at present which might prohibit mass production of IR thermography for patient use at home.

In either type, we consider that thermography has an outstanding advantage compared with the conventional pinpoint thermometry: thermography enables visualization of morphological patterns of temperature. A whole image of the plantar temperature distribution can be obtained only by thermography. However, this advantage has not been fully appreciated in most of the previous studies. Temperatures of several anatomical landmark points or areas were measured and analyzed in such papers. For example, Sun et al. (Sun et al., 2005; Sun et al., 2006) indicated that the temperature of the medial plantar arch was the highest and that of the lesser toes was the lowest in the normal and in some of the DM population. We consider, however, that this type of measurement can be accomplished also by the conventional thermometry, as Armstrong et al. (Armstrong et al., 2007) and Lavery et al. (Lavery et al., 2004; Lavery et al., 2007) did in the clinical settings.

Morphological thermographic patterns of the plantar temperature were previously described in a very limited number of articles. Using LC thermography, Chan et al. (Chan et al., 1991) designated temperature distribution in normal subjects as a "symmetrical butterfly pattern" in which the medial arch showed the highest temperature as reported by Sun et al. (Sun et al., 2005; Sun et al., 2006). However, Stess et al. (Stess et al., 1986) indicated that such a typical symmetrical pattern was observed in only nine out of the 16 normal subjects (56%). They described other atypical thermographic patterns, including those of DM patients, simply as "mottling and discrete areas of color variation." Wang et al. (Wang et al., 2004) also mentioned possible variation of thermographic patterns in the normal subjects, by showing data of the only three healthy volunteers..

We consider that there may be three reasons why interpretation of the plantar thermographic patterns has been so difficult and insufficient. (1) There is an absolute lack of the information of thermographic patterns of the normal subjects. Any interpretation is impossible without a normal control as a reference. (2) It is quite reasonable to consider that the plantar thermographic patterns can be affected by the vascular anatomy and circulatory status of the foot. No previous reports mention this point. (3) There has been no classification system of the plantar thermographic patterns, which enables more detailed description of the individual variations.

2.3 Possible patterns of plantar thermography and the vascular anatomy: A concept of "angiosome"

We have concluded that the new classification system of the thermographic patterns should be established based on the vascular anatomy of the foot. However, the vascular anatomy of the foot is very complicated with considerable individual anomalies (Adachi, 1928; Attinger et al., 1997; Yamada et al., 1993). The lower limb is supplied by the three main arteries: the anterior tibial artery, the posterior tibial artery, and the peroneal artery. The dorsal foot is supplied by the dorsalis pedis artery, which is derived from the anterior tibial artery. The plantar forefoot area is supplied by the two branches of the posterior tibial artery, the medial and lateral plantar arteries. These two arteries are connected to each other by the superficial and deep plantar arches. The medial plantar artery has the superficial and deep branches. The dorsalis pedis artery descends near the first metatarsal bone, making anastomosis with the deep plantar arch. The heel is supplied by the medial and lateral calcaneal arteries, derived from the posterior tibial artery and the peroneal artery, respectively. The concomitant veins run together with the main arteries. There are also the superficial subcutaneous venous networks. How and to what extent should this complex vascular anatomy be reflected to our novel thermographic classification?

A key word is "angiosome." What is angiosome? Angiosome is a concept in the field of plastic surgery, and is defined by Taylor and Palmer (Taylor & Palmer, 1987) as the "composite unit of skin and underlying deep tissue, supplied by a source artery." This "unit" can be considered as a possible tissue flap which can be transplanted to other places of the body by maintaining the vessel circulation, for example, through the microscopic anastomoses of the artery and vein in case of "free" flaps (Harii et al., 1974). It is noteworthy that the neighboring angiosomes are linked by "choke vessels", which act as a safety valve, if the main source artery is damaged (Taylor & Palmer, 1987).

Attinger et al. (Attinger et al., 2006) proposed four angiosomes in the plantar area: the medial plantar artery (MPA) angiosome, the lateral plantar artery (LPA) angiosome, the medial calcaneal artery (MCA) angiosome and the lateral calcaneal artery (LCA) angiosome (Fig.1A). The dorsal foot is composed of the single dorsalis pedis artery (DPA) angiosome. Therefore, it is quite reasonable to consider that the abnormal "mottling" patterns in DM patients are possibly caused by vessel stenosis or A-V shunts, and thus may well correspond to the territories of the plantar angiosomes.

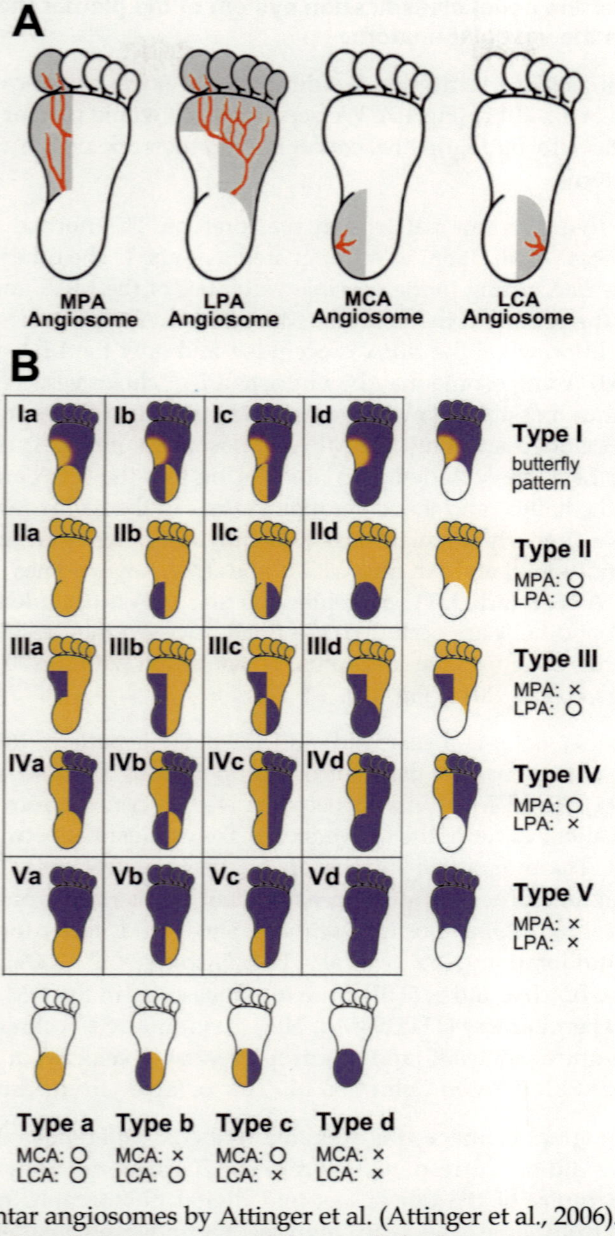

Fig. 1. (A) Four plantar angiosomes by Attinger et al. (Attinger et al., 2006). MPA: medial plantar artery, LPA: lateral plantar artery, MCA: medial calcaneal artery, LCA: lateral calcaneal artery. (B) Conceptual classification of the thermographic patterns with 20 different categories. Orange and blue colors indicate higher and lower temperatures, respectively. Reprinted from Journal of Plastic, Reconstructive & Aesthetic Surgery, Vol. 64 No.7. Nagase, T. et al. Variations of plantar thermographic patterns in normal controls and non-ulcer diabetic patients: Novel classification using angiosome concept. p.860-866, 2011. with permission from Elsevier.

2.4 Development of the novel classification system of the plantar thermographic patterns based on the vascular anatomy

According to the angiosome territories, we developed a novel classification of 20 different categories (Nagase et al., 2011) (Fig.1B). We separated the whole plantar area into the distal forefoot and the heel to build up the conceptual framework of the classification of the thermographic patterns.

We distinguished five different patterns in the forefoot. The normal "butterfly pattern" (Chan et al., 1991; Stess et al., 1986) was designated as Type I. The other four patterns were conceptually defined according to the possible viabilities of the MPA and LPA angiosomes. Type II represents the condition that both the MPA and LPA angiosomes are intact. Type III represents the condition when the MPA is occluded and only the LPA angiosome is intact. (In this type, the MPA angiosome may be nourished by "choke vessels" from the adjacent angiosomes, and, thus, possibly shows lower temperature.) Type IV represents the condition when the LPA is occluded and only the MPA angiosome is intact. Type V represents that both the MPA and LPA are occluded. It is noteworthy that the MPA and LPA angiosomes are overlapped in the hallux, and the lower temperature in the hallux may be observed only in type I and V. We similarly distinguished four different patterns in the heel area. Type a represents the condition that both the MCA and LCA angiosomes are intact. Type b represents that MCA is occluded. Type c represents that LCA is occluded. Type d represents that both the MCA and LCA are occluded. We finally crossed the five forefoot patterns and the four heel patterns, obtaining the conceptual classification with the 20 different categories from Ia to Vd (Nagase et al., 2011)(Fig. 1B).

32 healthy volunteers (36.8 ± 11.8 years old) and 129 diabetic patients (67.2 ± 10.5 years old) were included in our survey as the control group and as the DM group, respectively (Nagase et al., 2011). The DM group participants were recruited from the patients at the Diabetic Foot Outpatient Clinic at the University of Tokyo Hospital between November 2008 and October 2009. Thermographic images of the bilateral feet were taken from the all participants. At the time of temperature measurement by thermography, the subjects were guided to keep resting supine position without shoes and socks for 15 minites before measurement as equilibration (Nagase et al., 2011; Nishide et al., 2009). The ankle brachial index (ABI) and toe brachial index (TBI) were also measured in the DM group. We used an IR thermography Thermotracer (TH5108ME, NEC Avio Infrared Technology Co.Ltd.Tokyo, Japan) for temperature analysis, and Form pulse-wave velocity/ankle brachial index (PWV/ABI) BP-203RPEII (Omron Colin Co.Ltd., Tokyo, Japan) for measuring ABI and TBI.

Each plantar thermographic image was allocated to the 20 different categories as described above. If the images did not correspond to any of the 20 categories, they were designated as "atypical."Thermography of the dorsal feet and digital photographs of the skin surfaces were also obtained from some cases with "atypical "thermographic patterns.

2.5 Variations of plantar thermographic patterns in the normal controls

Of 64 feet from the 32 normal controls, 48 feet (75%) were allocated to the seven categories from the 20 categories (Nagase et al., 2011)(Fig.2A). Notably, the typical "butterfly pattern" (Id) was observed in 30 feet (46.9%). The next frequent category was IIa (13 feet, 20.3%). The other five categories were occupied by only one foot for each.

We can consider that the categories Id and IIa may be the normal thermographic patterns. We also consider that these data from the normal subjects should be regarded as a reference for evaluating thermographic patterns of DM population. As stated before, Stess et al. (Stess et al., 1986) described that the "butterfly patterns" was observed in about a half of the normal subjects in their study with the smaller sample size. We confirmed their findings in our larger study. In other words, the normal patterns (Id and IIa) were observed in only about 70% of the normal subjects in our study. This fact should be kept in mind when we interpret the data of plantar thermometry in the normal subjects and in the DM patients.

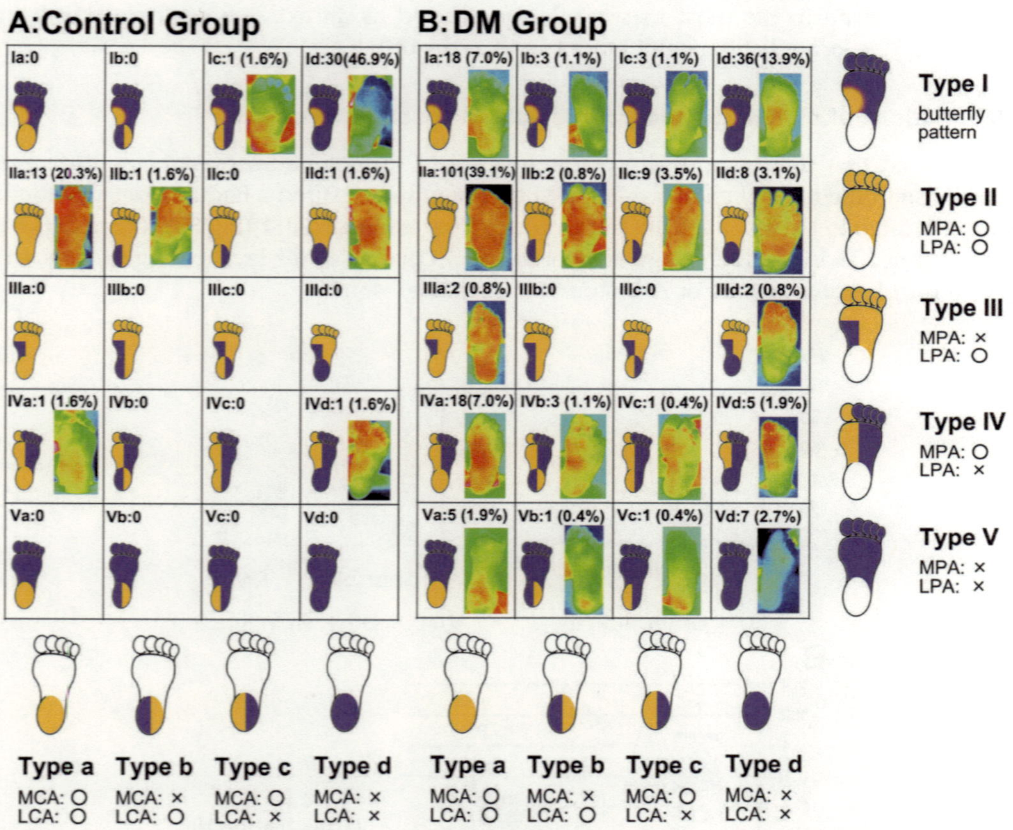

Fig. 2. Variations of the plantar thermographic patterns in the normal control group (A) and in the DM group (B). Representative thermographic images are included in the chart. Note that Id and IIa are the two main categories in the controls. Variations are broader in the DM group than in the control group. Reprinted from Journal of Plastic, Reconstructive & Aesthetic Surgery, Vol. 64 No.7. Nagase, T. et al. Variations of plantar thermographic patterns in normal controls and non-ulcer diabetic patients: Novel classification using angiosome concept. p.860-866, 2011. with permission from Elsevier.

There were 16 "atypical" feet (15.0%) which could not be allocated to any of the 20 categories (data not shown). We consider that 8 feet out of these cases are due to the anatomical variation of the arteries. Four feet from the two participants were characterized by high temperature in the hallux only. We consider that, from their IR themographic data of the dorsal feet, the hallux is directly supplied by the DPA in these cases, as described by Attinger et al. (Attinger et al., 2006). High temperature was observed in the most toes in the other four feet. We interpreted these cases as follows: As stated above, the vertical descending branch of the DPA reaches the plantar arterial arch and the LPA (Attinger et al., 2006), as the most important "choke vessel." Adachi (Adachi, 1928) indicated that there is a "watershed" which divides the plantar arterial arch into the DPA dominant territory and the LPA dominant territory. The location of the "watershed" varies among individual, determining to what extent the lesser toes are mainly supplied by the DPA. The cases with high temperature in the most toes can be interpreted as an extreme example where the "watershed" is located at the point more lateral to the fifth toe.

2.6 Variations of plantar thermographic patterns in the DM patients

We revealed that thermographic patterns in the DM groups had a remarkable difference from those in the normal controls: The DM thermographic patterns had a wider variations, being allocated to the 18 out of the 20 categories (Nagase et al., 2011)(Fig.2B). These data can be interpreted as individual irregularity of blood circulation at the level of angiosomes, that is, stenosis of source arteries or A-V shunt between angiosomes.

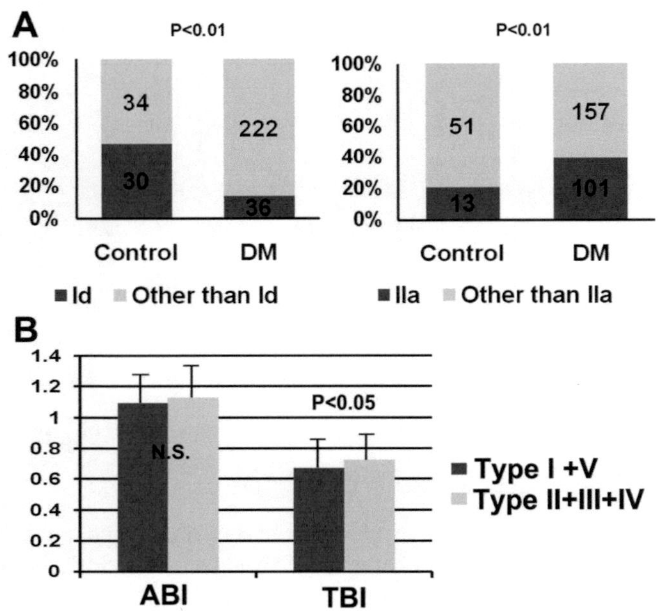

Fig. 3. (A) Comparison of the ratio of Id and IIa feet between the control and the DM groups. By chi-square test. (B) Comparison of ABI and TBI values between the type I + V subgroup and the type II + III + IV subgroups within the DM group. N.S.: not significant. By Student's *t* test. Reprinted from Journal of Plastic, Reconstructive & Aesthetic Surgery, Vol. 64 No.7. Nagase, T. et al. Variations of plantar thermographic patterns in normal controls and non-ulcer diabetic patients: Novel classification using angiosome concept. p.860-866, 2011. with permission from Elsevier.

Although the two most frequent categories were the same, Id and IIa, the frequency was reversed: Statistical analyses confirmed that feet ratio in the Id category was significantly lower and that in the IIa category was significantly higher in the DM group than in the control group (Nagase et al., 2011)(Fig.3A). We consider that the reversal may reflect chronic temperature elevation in the diabetic neuropathic feet (Brem et al., 2006; Chan et al., 1991; Flynn & Tooke, 1995; Sun et al., 2005; Sun et al., 2008). It is also noteworthy that a considerable percentage of the DM feet belonged to type IV (27 feet, 10.5%) and type V (14 feet, 5.4%) (Nagase et al., 2011). These two types suggest stenosis of the LPA or the more proximal artery (such as the posterior tibial artery). We consider that intensive foot care for prevention of ulceration associated with PAD should be required for these two types.

There were 33 "atypical "feet (12.8%) in the DM group (data not shown). An impressive pattern with high temperature only in the hallux and the fifth toe was observed in 5 feet in 4 cases. We consider that this phenomenon may be due to lateral compression by the ill-fitting shoes. Impaired thermoregulation by neuropathy may cause this pattern even after 15 minutes of equilibration.

ABI and TBI are clinical gold standards for estimating blood flow of the lower leg and the toe, respectively. To validate that thermographic patterns really reflect circulatory status, we further compared values of ABI and TBI between the subgroups of the DM group: the type I + V subgroup (in which the hallux temperature should be relatively low) and the type II + III + IV subgroup (in which the hallux temperature should be relatively high). ABI did not show statistically significant difference between these subgroups. However, TBI was significantly lower in the type I + V subgroup than in the type II + III + IV subgroup (Nagase et al., 2011)(Fig.3B). These findings may support our idea that the thermograpohic pattern with lower temperature in the toes reflects decreased blood supply in that region.

2.7 Discussion and future perspectives: Significance of "atypical" patterns

We newly established the novel classification system of the planter thermographic patterns, by which the morphological evaluation of the whole images is possible. Our paper was a first study clearly demonstrating the more remarkable variation of the plantar thermographic patterns in the DM patients compared with those in the normal controls (Nagase et al., 2011).

Our findings described above can be summarized as follows. (1) Id and IIa categories can be regarded as normal patterns, which can be observed in about 70% of the normal subjects. (2) DM patients showed a remarkably wider variation compared with the normal controls, possibly reflecting stenosis of source arteries or A-V shunts. (3) Ratio of Id was lower and that of IIa was higher in the DM group than in the control group, possibly suggesting neuropathic temperature elevation. (4) Type IV and V seen in the DM group may reflect compromised circulation of the LPA, requiring interventions.

There were several limitations in our study which should be reexamined in future. There was a bias between the control group and the DM group, especially in age and sex. Precise evaluation of the circulatory status by angiography or meticulous examination using a Doppler probe (Attinger et al., 2006) should be needed to substantiate relationship between thermographic patterns and circulation more thoroughly. Relationship between neuropathy and thermographic patterns should also be investigated in future. Our classification with the

20 different categories might be too complicated in clinical use. We consider that the distinction of only type I – V may be reasonable in the usual diabetic foot care.

Here, we come to the point where the story should be returned to the Introduction. How can we detect latent inflammation in the at risk diabetic foot by thermography? We only briefly mentioned cases with "atypical" thermographic patterns. However, such atypical findings should be of particular clinical importance for detecting inflammation. The irregular focal elevation of the temperature should be a sign of latent inflammation. In our study, four feet from the four cases among the 16 "atypical" feet in the normal control group exhibited such hot spots of the temperature, which were associated with the ingrown toenails or the callus formation. Also, 19 feet from the 15 cases among the 33 atypical feet in the DM group exhibited similar hot spots associated with the callus, the ingrown nails or tinea pedis, all of which might be potential causal factors of ulceration.

In the next chapter, we further describe our other study of screening for latent inflammation in the diabetic foot by thermography and ultrasonography, focusing on the callus (Nishide et al., 2009). However, it is very reasonable to consider that, in any fields of medicine, the abnormalities cannot be sufficiently evaluated unless the normal findings are well described. In conclusion, we again emphasize that the information described in this chapter should be a basic reference for analyzing the foot thermographic patterns.

3. Thermographic and ultrasonographic screening for latent inflammation in diabetic foot callus

3.1 Callus formation in diabetic foot

Callus is defined a "localized hyperplasia of the horny layer of the epidermis due to pressure or friction" (Dorland's medical dictionary). Callus is a quite common phenomenon frequently seen in the healthy people. However, callus formation is of particular clinical importance in the DM patients by the following reasons.

First, callus is one of the most frequent among changes in foot structures in the diabetic foot. Foot structure abnormalities which are common in, or specific for, the diabetic population include excessive callus formation, limited joint mobility, foot deformity, and soft-tissue modifications not showing as bony deformity. Bus (Bus, 2008) indicated that callus formation (prevalence 51-59%) and prominent metatarsal heads (65%) are the most common, followed by claw/hammer toe deformity (32-49%), hallux valgus (33%) and limited joint mobility (23-35%).

Second, pathophysiology of callus formation is very complicated and clinically relevant in DM patients. Peripheral neuropathy is associated with atrophy of the intrinsic foot muscles, hyperextension of the metatarsophalangeal joints, clawing of the toes, and distal displacement of the protective sub-metatarsal head fat pads, contributing to an increase in plantar pressures (Abouaesha et al., 2001; Bus, 2008; Pavicic & Korting, 2006). Autonomic neuropathy causes dry skin with fissures and tears more susceptible to pressure, and motor neuropathy also contributes to gait changes further resulting in pressure increase (Pavicic & Korting, 2006). Once callus is formed, abnormal loading is further increased forming vicious cycle (Apelqvist et al., 2008). Pataky et al. (Pataky et al., 2002) indicated that peak plantar pressure and duration of pressure was significantly larger in the DM patients with callus than in those without callus. Assuming that an average person takes about 10,000 steps a day, they discussed that the callus skin is exposed to the excessive pressure of 18.600 kg per day!

Third, callus is one of the most important predisposing factors of ulcer formation in DM patients (Edmonds & Foster, 2006). As stated in the Introduction, diabetic patients with sensory neuropathy often overlooked their callus because of absence of the pain. They continue walking on the insensitive feet, and subcutaneous hemorrhage, autolytic seroma and subsequent skin breakdown are easily developed at the callus in DM patients (Apelqvist et al., 2000; Apelqvist et al., 2008; Edmonds & Foster, 2006). Indeed, it was reported that callus formation preceded ulceration in 82.4 % of diabetic foot ulcer patients (Sage et al., 2001). Murray et al. (Murray et al., 1996) also reported a relative risk of 11.0 for an ulcer developing under an area of callus in DM patients with neuropathy.

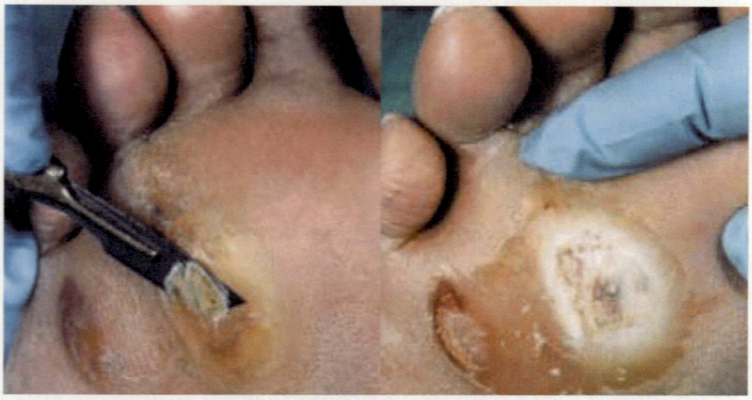

Fig. 4. Callus removal by sharp debridement. Whitish, macerated, moist tissue is found under surface of callus, indicating imminent ulceration. Reproduced from British Medical Journal, Diabetic foot ulcers, Edmonds, M. E. & Foster, A. V. Vol. 332, p.407-410, 2006. with permission from BMJ Publishing Group Ltd.

It is noteworthy that foot ulceration derived from the callus may be quite rare in healthy population, although callus is commonly seen in non-diabetic subjects. This may be due to insensitivity to inflammatory pain in the neuropathic patients, and also due to difficulty of noticing inflammatory edema and erythema associated with ulcer progression, because the plantar skin has thicker layer of the stratum corneum. Even if the surface of the callus is seemingly dry in DM patients, macerated, moist tissue can occasionally be found underneath the callus when the surface is debrided, indicating that the foot is close to ulceration (Fig.4)(Edmonds & Foster, 2006). Then, how can we detect such latent inflammation in the callus before ulcer formation is completed? Is the latent inflammation in the callus absent in healthy population?

3.2 Our strategy of screening for latent inflammation in the callus: Thermography and ultrasonography

In order to solve these problems, we decided to use thermography and ultrasonography in the next study (Nishide et al., 2009). Because the DM patients have a difficulty in noticing inflammation in their calluses by themselves, and because inflammatory calluses may be difficult to detect by the physical inspection and examination, "latent inflammation" was operationally defined in this study when both of the two following findings were observed in order to reduce the possibility of the false positive case: skin temperature elevation by thermography, and identification of low echoic lesion by ultrasonography (Nishide et al., 2009).

In this study, we compared 30 DM neuropathy patients having plantar calluses (the DM group) with 30 non-diabetic callus patients of matched age and sex (the non-DM group) (Nishide et al., 2009). The DM group was recruited from the patients at the Diabetic Foot Outpatient Clinic at the University of Tokyo Hospital between November 2006 and October 2007. The non-DM group was the volunteers selected by the snowball sample method. Diagnosis of associated neuropathy was required as an inclusion criterion for the DM group. It was defined by the criteria by Japanese Diabetic Neuropathy Association, or by detection of sensory loss using 5.07 (10g) monofilament touch test in at least one of the three plantar regions (Pham et al., 2000). All the patients and volunteers were inspected and examined by a dermatologist and two experienced and certified Wound, Ostomy and Continence Nurses (WOCNs.) The subjects with visible inflammation, pain around the calluses, preformed foot ulcers, autoimmune diseases or other acute inflammatory diseases were exluded from the study.

IR thermographic measurement of the skin temperature was performed as described in the previous chapter, with 15 minutes equilibration (Nagase et al., 2011; Nishide et al., 2009). In this study, we focused on temperature of the callus and the surrounding skin. The callus temperature was defined as an average temperature value of the 4 mm x 4 mm square, the center of which was on the highest temperature point. The temperature of the surrounding skin was defined as an average of the 4 mm x 4 mm square in an adjacent area unaffected by the temperature change of the callus. Previous studies suggested different criteria of temperature elevation in inflammatory skin: 2.2°C for prevention of diabetic foot disorder (Armstrong et al., 2007; Lavery et al., 2007), and 1.2°C for inflammatory leg ulcers (Sayre et al., 2007). We selected 1.2°C as a criterion of temperature elevation since our focus of this study was early screening and prevention.

We also used ultrasonography (LOGIQ Book XP, GE Medical Systems, UK. 10 MHz, B-mode) for detecting edematous and fluid-filled changes of the latent inflammatory callus (Nishide et al., 2009). Identification of low echoic lesion was defined in this study when lowered ultrasonographic signal was clearly observed in either the dermal, subdermal or muscle layers. Ultrasonography has been increasingly used as a diagnostic and assessment tool in the field of skin care. 20 MHz ultrasonography is more popular among dermatologic specialists because of higher image resolution of the more superficial skin layer such as the epidermis and the dermis (Schmid-Wendtner & Burgdorf, 2005). However, 20 MHz ultrasonography can only produce images 20 mm below the skin surface (Yabunaka et al., 2009). We selected 10MHz ultrasonography in this study for focusing on the subcutaneous or muscle layers which may be more prone to be damaged by external forces (Nishide et al., 2009). Our group routinely uses 10 MHz ultrasonography for obtaining sufficient visualization of the pressure-related deep tissue injury (Aoi et al., 2009; Nagase et al., 2007; Yabunaka et al., 2009), providing considerable justification for our choice in this study.

3.3 Inflammation was detected in 10% of the diabetic foot callus

In this study, 63 and 94 calluses were observed in the 30 DM group participants and in the 30 non-DM group participants, respectively (Nishide et al., 2009). 40 (63.5%) and 23 (36.5%) calluses were located in the toes and metatarsal areas in the DM group, respectively. 50 (53.2%) and 44 (46.8%) calluses were located in the toes and metatarsal areas in the non-DM group, respectively. There were no significant differences in the number per person, location and size of the calluses between the two groups.

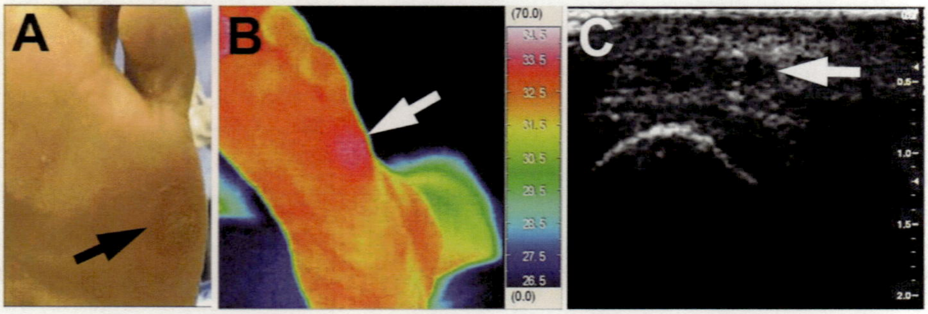

Fig. 5. An example of latent inflammation identified by thermography and ultrasonography. (A) Photograph. An arrow indicates the callus. (B) Thermography. An arrow indicates elevated temperature. (C) Ultrasonography. An arrow indicates low echoic lesion in the subcutaneous layer. Reprinted from Diabetes Research and Clinical Practice, Vol. 85 No.3. Nishide, K. et al. Ultrasonographic and thermographic screening for latent inflammation in diabetic foot callus. p.304-309, 2009. with permission from Elsevier.

Both thermographic and ultrasonographic data were available in 50 calluses in the DM group and 65 calluses in the non-DM group. These calluses were assessed for latent inflammation. Notably, no inflammatory findings were observed by thermography and ultrasonography in the non-DM group. Whereas, five (10%) calluses in the DM group were regarded as positive inflammation. Skin temperature increase could be clearly detected by thermography (Nishide et al., 2009) (Figs. 5A, B). Low echoic lesion was also sufficiently identified using ultrasonography (Fig. 5C).

More detailed explanations of the five inflammatory calluses are given below.

Case 1: The callus was located at the base of the first metatarsus. Temperature elevation was 2.3 °C. Low echoic lesion was noted in the muscle layer.

Case 2 (Fig.5): The callus was located at the base of the fifth metatarsus. Temperature elevation was 1.6 °C. Low echoic lesion was noted in the subcutaneous fatty layer.

Case 3: The callus was located at the lateral side of the great toe. Temperature elevation was 2.8 °C. Low echoic lesions were noted in the epidermis, dermis and muscle layers.

Case 4: The callus was located at the tip of the fourth toe. Temperature elevation was 1.6 °C. Low echoic lesion was noted in the muscle layer.

Case 5: The callus was located at the lateral side of the fifth toe. Temperature elevation was 1.9 °C. Low echoic lesion was noted in the subcutaneous fatty layer.

3.4 Discussion and future perspectives

This study was the first paper demonstrating significant versatility of thermography and ultrasonography as screening tools for latent asymptomatic inflammation underneath the foot callus in DM patients. As stated above, inflammatory change in the callus has been considered as a high risk factor for later ulcer development. In this study, 10% of the calluses in the DM group had the inflammatory findings, whereas none in the non-DM group.

In this study, it is noteworthy that thermography and ultrasonography were able to detect latent inflammatory changes in the callus, which could not be identified even by physical examination by the wound care specialists including a dermatologist and two certified WOCNs. This fact indicates that the inflammation underneath the seemingly dry callus can be easily overlooked by physicians and medical staffs not specialized in wound and foot care and by patients themselves. We consider that 10% of inflammatory rate in our DM group is awfully high. Although callus is a very common phenomenon often seen in healthy people, we should not underestimate clinical relevance of callus as a predisposing status of ulcer formation in DM population.

As stated earlier, thermometry has been proposed as a promising way of identifying "at risk" foot, as shown in the randomized controlled trials by Armstrong et al. (Armstrong et al., 2007) and Lavery et al. (Lavery et al., 2004; Lavery et al., 2007). We again consider that thermography has several great advantages for identifying latent inflammation in the foot callus, compared with their pinpoint thermometric measurements in the bilateral plantar landmark points. First, their methods may overlook the inflammatory site not located in the anatomical landmark points. Second, temperature differences of bilateral landmark points are estimated in their methods. However, calluses are often developed in the same location of both feet, which makes the bilateral comparison difficult. Third, thermography enables clear visualization of morphological temperature distribution as stated in the previous chapter, and this advantage may also be of importance for finding the inflammation of the callus "at a glance."

We could identify subcutaneous inflammatory changes underneath the calluses by 10 MHz ultrasonography. Ultrasonography is a non-invasive, inexpensive and portable technique, and thus it has been gradually used in the broad area of medicine. For the assessment of the skin, a 20 MHz probe is more widely used for the search and imaging of lymph nodes, chronic ulcers and subcutaneous tumors in a variety of clinical settings (Schmid-Wendtner & Burgdorf, 2005; Yabunaka et al., 2009). However, we focused on the subcutaneous tissue damage using a 10 MHz probe in this study, because it is known that the deep tissue damages precede skin breakdown when the callus is developed into the full thickness skin ulcer (Apelqvist et al., 2000; Apelqvist et al., 2008; Edmonds & Foster, 2006). Indeed, our current study using ultrasonography revealed that three of the five inflammatory calluses had tissue damage downward to the muscle layer. This fact clearly indicates that the calluses in the diabetic foot may not be just a thickening of the horny layer. We also consider that the thermography should be used for the initial screening of inflammation, and that ultrasonography may be useful for determining severity of tissue damage after thermographic assessment. It is also of note that latent inflammatory findings by combination of thermography and ultrasonography were detected only in the DM group, without any observational symptoms and pains. Our data strongly suggests that "asymptomatic inflammation" in the callus may be a specific feature in the DM population.

There were several limitations in this study. Because this study was cross-sectional, we could not follow up patients with latent inflammation until subsequent ulceration develop. Our study provides no evidence to suggest that the calluses with latent inflammation eventually ulcerated. Future prospective observation is needed to confirm whether our findings of "latent inflammation" really result in diabetic foot ulcers. It should also be kept in mind that we used the strict criteria of latent inflammation by two methods, that is, both elevated temperature and low echoic lesion. Although this method can reduce the probability of the false positive, which ensures the patients with latent inflammatory callus were truly at risk, there would be more than 10 % of the cases if we used more sensitive method. (Please remember that there were four feet with hot spots identified by only thermography in the normal controls, and that some of them were associated with the callus in the previous chapter.) It will be necessary in future to determine the most suitable cut-off point.

In summary, although there were such limitations in this study, we believe that thermographic and ultrasonographic screening for latent inflammation will effectively prevent callus-derived foot ulceration in DM patients in future.

4. Concluding remarks

Through the two abovementioned studies, we successfully showed that the non-invasive imaging modalities such as thermography and ultrasonography are very promising tools for evaluating blood circulation and inflammatory status and for preventing ulcer formation in the diabetic foot. The latter study (Nishide et al., 2009) was completed and published before the thermographic classification in the former study (Nagase et al., 2011) was established. One of the reasons why the work by Nishide et al. (Nishide et al., 2009) was successful without the classification was, probably, that we focused on the thermographic findings of the callus, a clinically visible skin disorder. For the broader application of thermography to a variety of clinical spectrum of diabetic foot in future, the knowledge about the normal thermographic findings should be essential as a reference. In this sense, we believe that future clinical importance of thermographic and ultrasonographic evaluation of the diabetic foot will be based on our classification described above.

We consider that there may be some difficulties in interpreting atypical temperature increase in thermography. Temperature increase can be caused by not only latent inflammation, but also A-V shunting and increased plantar pressure as seen in the atypical diabetic foot with increased loading of the hallux and fifth toe described in section 2.6. For discriminating these causes, we consider that careful inspection of the foot and parallel use of ultrasonography will be helpful. Further research will provide us with a key to solve this problem.

Management of diabetic foot requires intimate contact between medical staffs and patients. Behavioral factors, such as patients' poor compliance with self foot care, also contribute to the deterioration of diabetic foot. We previously reported that prevalence of onycomychosis, another important predisposing factor of diabetic foot ulcers, was significantly associated with not washing of feet every day (Takehara et al., 2011). Temperature measurement by patients themselves at home will also become an important part of self care in future. The preventive strategies of self monitoring of the foot temperature using a handheld IR thermometer or recent LC thermography have a reasonable advantage in this regard

(Armstrong et al., 2007; Frykberg et al., 2009; Lavery et al., 2004; Lavery et al., 2007). On the contrary, IR thermography and ultrasonography have been previously performed mainly by medical doctors, radiologists and related technologists, because they require considerable expertise in their handling and data analyses. In order to popularize our strategy described above using IR thermography and ultrasonography in a community based manner, specific education of handling these modalities should be needed for staffs engaged in community health (such as nurse practitioners in United States). How is it possible?

Our research group is composed of multidisciplinary scientists. The first author of this chapter (Nagase) is a plastic surgeon. Our laboratory also includes research nurses (including WOCNs), molecular biologists and engineering specialists. As our research described above has been progressed, the nursing staffs in our group have increasingly showed a great improvement in their technique of using thermography and ultrasonography. Now we routinely use these modalities without any difficulties. Our experience may support the idea that these modalities will be well handled by community based medical staffs in future under the appropriate educational system. As these technologies are non-invasive and "patient-friendly" without any pain and discomfort, they are really promising as future nursing tools. In this regard, our researches described above can be regarded as a pioneering attempt integrating medical technologies and nursing care, based on the intimate discussion and collaboration among our multidisciplinary research members.

5. References

Abouaesha, F., van Schie, C. H., Griffths, G. D., Young, R. J., & Boulton, A. J. (2001). Plantar tissue thickness is related to peak plantar pressure in the high-risk diabetic foot. *Diabetes Care*, Vol.24, No.7, (July 2001), pp. 1270-1274, ISSN 0149-5992

Adachi, B. (1928). *Das Arteriensystem der Japaner. Band II*, Maruzen, Kyoto, Japan.

Aoi, N., Yoshimura, K., Kadono, T., Nakagami, G., Iizuka, S., Higashino, T., Araki, J., Koshima, I., & Sanada, H. (2009). Ultrasound assessment of deep tissue injury in pressure ulcers: possible prediction of pressure ulcer progression. *Plastic and Reconstructive Surgery*, Vol.124, No.2, (August 2009), pp. 540-550, ISSN 1529-4242

Apelqvist, J., Bakker, K., van Houtum, W. H., Nabuurs-Franssen, M. H., & Schaper, N. C. (2000). International consensus and practical guidelines on the management and the prevention of the diabetic foot. International Working Group on the Diabetic Foot. *Diabetes/Metabolism Research and Reviews*, Vol.16 Suppl 1, (September-October 2000), pp. S84-92, ISSN 1520-7552

Apelqvist, J., Bakker, K., van Houtum, W. H., & Schaper, N. C. (2008). Practical guidelines on the management and prevention of the diabetic foot: based upon the International Consensus on the Diabetic Foot (2007) Prepared by the International Working Group on the Diabetic Foot. *Diabetes/Metabolism Research and Reviews,*, Vol.24 Suppl 1, (May-June 2008), pp. S181-187, ISSN 1520-7552

Armstrong, D. G., Holtz-Neiderer, K., Wendel, C., Mohler, M. J., Kimbriel, H. R., & Lavery, L. A. (2007). Skin temperature monitoring reduces the risk for diabetic foot ulceration in high-risk patients. *The American Journal of Medicine*, Vol.120, No.12, (December 2007), pp. 1042-1046, ISSN 0002-9343

Attinger, C., Cooper, P., & Blume, P. (1997). Vascular anatomy of the foot and ankle. *Operative Techniques in Plastic and Reconstructive Surgery*, Vol.4, No.4, (November 1997), pp. 183-198, ISSN 1071-0949

Attinger, C. E., Evans, K. K., Bulan, E., Blume, P., & Cooper, P. (2006). Angiosomes of the foot and ankle and clinical implications for limb salvage: reconstruction, incisions, and revascularization. *Plastic and Reconstructive Surgery*, Vol.117, No.7 Suppl, (June 2006), pp. 261S-293S, ISSN 0007-1226

Benbow, S. J., Chan, A. W., Bowsher, D. R., Williams, G., & Macfarlane, I. A. (1994). The prediction of diabetic neuropathic plantar foot ulceration by liquid-crystal contact thermography. *Diabetes Care*, Vol.17, No.8, (August 1994), pp. 835-839, ISSN 0149-5992

Bharara, M., Cobb, J. E., & Claremont, D. J. (2006). Thermography and thermometry in the assessment of diabetic neuropathic foot: a case for furthering the role of thermal techniques. *The International Journal of Lower Extremity Wounds*, Vol.5, No.4, (December 2006), pp. 250-260, ISSN 1534-7346

Bharara, M., Schoess, J., Nouvong, A., & Armstrong, D. G. (2010). Wound inflammatory index: a "proof of concept" study to assess wound healing trajectory. *Journal of Diabetes Science and Technology*, Vol.4, No.4, (July 2010), pp. 773-779, ISSN 1932-2968

Bharara, M., Viswanathan, V., & Cobb, J. E. (2008a). Cold immersion recovery responses in the diabetic foot with neuropathy. *International Wound Journal*, Vol.5, No.4, (October 2008), pp. 562-569, ISSN 1742-481X

Bharara, M., Viswanathan, V., & Cobb, J. E. (2008b). Warm immersion recovery test in assessment of diabetic neuropathy--a proof of concept study. *International Wound Journal*, Vol.5, No.4, (October 2008), pp. 570-576, ISSN 1742-481X

Brem, H., Sheehan, P., Rosenberg, H. J., Schneider, J. S., & Boulton, A. J. (2006). Evidence-based protocol for diabetic foot ulcers. *Plastic and Reconstructive Surgery*, Vol.117, No.7 Suppl, (June 2006), pp. 193S-209S, ISSN 0007-1226

Bus, S. A. (2008). Foot structure and footwear prescription in diabetes mellitus. *Diabetes/Metabolism Research and Reviews*, Vol.24 Suppl 1, (May-June 2008), pp. S90-95, ISSN 1520-7552

Chan, A. W., MacFarlane, I. A., & Bowsher, D. R. (1991). Contact thermography of painful diabetic neuropathic foot. *Diabetes Care*, Vol.14, No.10, (October 1991), pp. 918-922, ISSN 0149-5992

Edmonds, M. E., & Foster, A. V. (2006). Diabetic foot ulcers. *British Medical Journal*, Vol.332, No.7538, (February 2006), pp. 407-410, ISSN 1468-5833

Flynn, M. D., & Tooke, J. E. (1995). Diabetic neuropathy and the microcirculation. *Diabetic Medicine*, Vol.12, No.4, (April 1995), pp. 298-301, ISSN 0742-3071

Frykberg, R. G., Tallis, A., & Tierney, E. (2009). Diabetic foot self examination with the TempstatTM as an integral component of a comprehensive prevension program. *The Journal of Diabetic Foot Complications*, Vol.1, No.1, (2009), pp. 13-18

Harii, K., Omori, K., & Omori, S. (1974). Hair transplantation with free scalp flaps. *Plastic and Reconstructive Surgery*, Vol.53, No.4, (April 1974), pp. 410-413, ISSN 0032-1052

Kang, P. B., Hoffman, S. N., Krimitsos, E., & Rutkove, S. B. (2003). Ambulatory foot temperature measurement: a new technique in polyneuropathy evaluation. *Muscle & Nerve*, Vol.27, No.6, (June 2003), pp. 737-742, ISSN 0148-639X

Lavery, L. A., Armstrong, D. G., Vela, S. A., Quebedeaux, T. L., & Fleischli, J. G. (1998). Practical criteria for screening patients at high risk for diabetic foot ulceration. *Archives of Internal Medicine*, Vol.158, No.2, (January 1998), pp. 157-162, ISSN 0003-9926

Lavery, L. A., Higgins, K. R., Lanctot, D. R., Constantinides, G. P., Zamorano, R. G., Armstrong, D. G., Athanasiou, K. A., & Agrawal, C. M. (2004). Home monitoring of foot skin temperatures to prevent ulceration. *Diabetes Care*, Vol.27, No.11, (November 2004), pp. 2642-2647, ISSN 0149-5992

Lavery, L. A., Higgins, K. R., Lanctot, D. R., Constantinides, G. P., Zamorano, R. G., Athanasiou, K. A., Armstrong, D. G., & Agrawal, C. M. (2007). Preventing diabetic foot ulcer recurrence in high-risk patients: use of temperature monitoring as a self-assessment tool. *Diabetes Care*, Vol.30, No.1, (January 2007), pp. 14-20, ISSN 0149-5992

Lavery, L. A., Peters, E. J., Williams, J. R., Murdoch, D. P., Hudson, A., & Lavery, D. C. (2008). Reevaluating the way we classify the diabetic foot: restructuring the diabetic foot risk classification system of the International Working Group on the Diabetic Foot. *Diabetes Care*, Vol.31, No.1, (January 2008), pp. 154-156, ISSN 0149-5992

Murray, H. J., Young, M. J., Hollis, S., & Boulton, A. J. (1996). The association between callus formation, high pressures and neuropathy in diabetic foot ulceration. *Diabetic Medicine*, Vol.13, No.11, (November 1996), pp. 979-982, ISSN 0742-3071

Nagase, T., Koshima, I., Maekawa, T., Kaneko, J., Sugawara, Y., Makuuchi, M., Koyanagi, H., Nakagami, G., & Sanada, H. (2007). Ultrasonographic evaluation of an unusual peri-anal induration: a possible case of deep tissue injury. *Journal of Wound Care*, Vol.16, No.8, (September 2007), pp. 365-367, ISSN 0969-0700

Nagase, T., Sanada, H., Takehara, K., Oe, M., Iizaka, S., Ohashi, Y., Oba, M., Kadowaki, T., & Nakagami, G. (2011). Variations of plantar thermographic patterns in normal controls and non-ulcer diabetic patients: Novel classification using angiosome concept. *Journal of Plastic, Reconstructive & Aesthet Surg*, Vol.64, No.7, (July 2011), pp. 860-866, ISSN 1748-6815

Nagase, T., Sekiguchi, J., & Ohmori, K. (1996). Finger replantation in a 12-month-old child: a long-term follow-up. *British Journal of Plastic Surgery*, Vol.49, No.8, (December 1996), pp. 555-558, ISSN 0007-1226

Nakagami, G., Sanada, H., Iizaka, S., Kadono, T., Higashino, T., Koyanagi, H., & Haga, N. (2010). Predicting delayed pressure ulcer healing using thermography: a prospective cohort study. *Journal of Wound Care*, Vol.19, No.11, (November 2010), pp. 465-470, ISSN 0969-0700

Nishide, K., Nagase, T., Oba, M., Oe, M., Ohashi, Y., Iizaka, S., Nakagami, G., Kadowaki, T., & Sanada, H. (2009). Ultrasonographic and thermographic screening for latent inflammation in diabetic foot callus. *Diabetes Research and Clinical Practice*, Vol.85, No.3, (September 2009), pp. 304-309, ISSN 0168-8227

Pataky, Z., Golay, A., Faravel, L., Da Silva, J., Makoundou, V., Peter-Riesch, B., & Assal, J. P. (2002). The impact of callosities on the magnitude and duration of plantar pressure in patients with diabetes mellitus. A callus may cause 18,600 kilograms of excess plantar pressure per day. *Diabetes & Metabolism*, Vol.28, No.5, (November 2002), pp. 356-361, ISSN 1262-3636

Pavicic, T., & Korting, H. C. (2006). Xerosis and callus formation as a key to the diabetic foot syndrome: dermatologic view of the problem and its management. *Journal der Deutschen Dermatologischen Gesellschaft*, Vol.4, No.11, (November 2006), pp. 935-941, ISSN 1610-0389

Peters, E. J., & Lavery, L. A. (2001). Effectiveness of the diabetic foot risk classification system of the International Working Group on the Diabetic Foot. *Diabetes Care*, Vol.24, No.8, (August 2001), pp. 1442-1447, ISSN 0149-5992

Pham, H., Armstrong, D. G., Harvey, C., Harkless, L. B., Giurini, J. M., & Veves, A. (2000). Screening techniques to identify people at high risk for diabetic foot ulceration: a prospective multicenter trial. *Diabetes Care*, Vol.23, No.5, (May 2000), pp. 606-611, ISSN 0149-5992

Roback, K., Johansson, M., & Starkhammar, A. (2009). Feasibility of a thermographic method for early detection of foot disorders in diabetes. *Diabetes Technology & Therapeutics*, Vol.11, No.10, (Oct 2009), pp. 663-667, ISSN 1520-9156

Rutkove, S. B., Chapman, K. M., Acosta, J. A., & Larrabee, J. E. (2005). Foot temperature in diabetic polyneuropathy: innocent bystander or unrecognized accomplice? *Diabetic Medicine*, Vol.22, No.3, (March 2005), pp. 231-238, ISSN 0742-3071

Sage, R. A., Webster, J. K., & Fisher, S. G. (2001). Outpatient care and morbidity reduction in diabetic foot ulcers associated with chronic pressure callus. *Journal of American Podiatric Medical Association*, Vol.91, No.6, (June 2001), pp. 275-279, ISSN 8750-7315

Sayre, E. K., Kelechi, T. J., & Neal, D. (2007). Sudden increase in skin temperature predicts venous ulcers: a case study. *Journal of Vascular Nursing*, Vol.25, No.3, (September 2007), pp. 46-50, ISSN 1062-0303

Schmid-Wendtner, M. H., & Burgdorf, W. (2005). Ultrasound scanning in dermatology. *Archives of Dermatology*, Vol.141, No.2, (February 2005), pp. 217-224, ISSN 0003-987X

Stess, R. M., Sisney, P. C., Moss, K. M., Graf, P. M., Louie, K. S., Gooding, G. A., & Grunfeld, C. (1986). Use of liquid crystal thermography in the evaluation of the diabetic foot. *Diabetes Care*, Vol.9, No.3, (May-June 1986), pp. 267-272, ISSN 0149-5992

Sun, P. C., Jao, S. H., & Cheng, C. K. (2005). Assessing foot temperature using infrared thermography. *Foot & Ankle International*, Vol.26, No.10, (October 2005), pp. 847-853, ISSN 1071-1007

Sun, P. C., Lin, H. D., Jao, S. H., Chan, R. C., Kao, M. J., & Cheng, C. K. (2008). Thermoregulatory sudomotor dysfunction and diabetic neuropathy develop in parallel in at-risk feet. *Diabetic Medicine*, Vol.25, No.4, (April 2008), pp. 413-418, ISSN 0742-3071

Sun, P. C., Lin, H. D., Jao, S. H., Ku, Y. C., Chan, R. C., & Cheng, C. K. (2006). Relationship of skin temperature to sympathetic dysfunction in diabetic at-risk feet. *Diabetes Research and Clinical Practice*, Vol.73, No.1, (July 2006), pp. 41-46, ISSN 0168-8227

Takehara, K., Oe, M., Tsunemi, Y., Nagase, T., Ohashi, Y., Iizaka, S., Ueki, K., Tsukamoto, K., Kadowaki, T., & Sanada, H. (2011). Factors associated with presence and severity of toenail onychomycosis in patients with diabetes: A cross-sectional study. *International Journal of Nursing Studies*, Vol.48, No.9, (September 2011), pp. 1101-1108, ISSN 0020-7489

Taylor, G. I., & Palmer, J. H. (1987). The vascular territories (angiosomes) of the body: experimental study and clinical applications. *British Journal of Plastic Surgery*, Vol.40, No.2, (March 1987), pp. 113-141, ISSN 0007-1226

The International Working Group on the Diabetic Foot (1999). *International Consensus on the Diabetic Foot*, The International Working Group on the Diabetic Foot, ISBN 90-9012716-x, Maastricht, Netherlands.

Wang, H., Wade, D. R. J., & Kam, J. (2004). IR imaging of blood circulation of patients with vascular disease. *Proceeding of Thermosense XXVI*, ISBN 9780819453280, Bellingham, WA, USA, April, 2004.

Yabunaka, K., Iizaka, S., Nakagami, G., Aoi, N., Kadono, T., Koyanagi, H., Uno, M., Ohue, M., Sanada, S., & Sanada, H. (2009). Can ultrasonographic evaluation of subcutaneous fat predict pressure ulceration? *Journal of Wound Care*, Vol.18, No.5, (May 2009), pp. 192-196 ISSN 0969-0700

Yamada, T., Gloviczki, P., Bower, T. C., Naessens, J. M., & Carmichael, S. W. (1993). Variations of the arterial anatomy of the foot. *American Journal of Surgery*, Vol.166, No.2, (August 1993), pp. 130-135, ISSN 0002-9610

4

Wound Fluid Diagnostics in Diabetic Foot Ulcers

Markus Löffler[1,2], Michael Schmohl[3],
Nicole Schneiderhan-Marra[3] and Stefan Beckert[2]
[1]*Department of Immunology, University of Tuebingen,*
[2]*Department of General, Visceral and Transplant Surgery, University of Tuebingen,*
[3]*NMI-Natural and Medical sciences Institute at the University of Tuebingen, Reutlingen, Germany*

1. Introduction

Wound fluid seems -at least theoretically- easily accessible and might open a new window to the local wound microenvironment that cannot be evaluated by the analysis of serum or plasma markers. Recently, this strategy has been supported by a first time wound fluid proteome analysis comparing acute and chronic wounds (Eming et al. 2010). Interestingly, there seem to be essential differences with respect to wound fluid protein composition when comparing acute and chronic wounds. The wound fluid proteome of healing tissue is characterised by proteins involved in tissue growth and protection from inflammatory activity, whereas non-healing wounds are characterised by a chronic inflammatory environment primarily consisting of leukocyte proteases and inflammatory mediators (Eming et al. 2010). This is particularly striking since the non-healing state in diabetic foot ulcers has previously been linked to persistent inflammatory activity (Acosta et al. 2008). Thus, the wound fluid of chronic wounds seems to be characterised by an altered wound micro-milieu and may, therefore, provide deeper insights into the causes of delayed wound healing.

Tissue repair can be clearly characterised as an ubiquitous process and a wound is more precisely described as a transitional tissue rather than a static tissue. Physiological wound healing can be recognised as continuous change, which might be seen as a dynamic and interactive process resulting in remodelling and tissue restitution. This nature of transitional tissues comes down to the difficulty of obtaining appropriate sample materials. Nevertheless, the classical phases of healing are useful as a broad roadmap of the course of healing, since more precise models and clear landmarks are not available. The historical view on wound healing categorises the healing process in separate phases: starting with acute injury > I. coagulation > II. an early inflammatory phase > III. a late inflammatory phase > IV. a proliferative phase, and > V. remodelling, which ends with tissue restitution (Velnar, Bailey, and Smrkolj 2009).

Changes in wound fluid markers, cytokines or cell populations are more suitable for describing the local wound microenvironment than are alterations of systemic markers. The nature of systemic serum-based markers is likely the sum of different effects all over the body. Of course distinct and rather exceptional markers obtained from blood -such as PSA (prostate specific antigen) (Balk, Ko, and Bubley 2003) or troponin- have been proven to be tissue specific (Apple 1999) and can therefore reveal insights into local processes. However, most of the markers found in the bloodstream instead result from systemic alterations rather than from local changes. Wound healing takes place simultaneously at a variety of locations in the body. Therefore, the impact of serum markers on the assessment of the wound microenvironment is questionable so long as there is no systemic affection by septicaemia. In addition, many systemic inflammatory markers are altered in response to a variety of immune mediators which in turn are triggered by inflammatory events somewhere in the body. In this context, the secretion of CRP by the liver upon stimulation by circulatory cytokines such as IL-6 (Pepys and Hirschfield 2003) can be exemplified. In line with this concept, several studies evaluating CRP as a valuable marker of infection in diabetic foot ulcers were judged to be unable to underline its sole effectiveness (Dinh, Snyder, and Veves 2010).

Since most systemic markers do not exhibit clear tissue specificity, it might be of special interest to gain insights into the local wound microenvironment by assessing biochemical markers in wound fluid, which in turn might give us a clue about the local processes reflecting the current status of wound healing.

In the diabetic foot in particular -which is characterised by delayed healing- local biomarkers facilitating the evaluation of the wound may be of great clinical value. Being able to determine the probability of healing and the risk of infection by assessing markers in wound fluid might have a great impact on clinical practice.

2. Wound fluid

Wound fluid is an interesting object of investigation because its composition is influenced by the state of the wound and the phase of healing (Mani 1999; Trengove, Langton, and Stacey 1996). Wound fluid generally consists of an inhomogeneous mixture of different endogenous and exogenous sources. It is constituted by a provisional matrix of exudates or transudates that originate from the blood, which in turn has already been altered by multiple independent pathologic and physiological factors (such as cardiac failure or hydration status as well as vasoconstriction or diabetes). In addition, wound fluid composition is further modified by factors which are secreted by local cells in the wound or by cells that migrate into the wound, as well as by supplementary factors derived from microbial contamination. Since the wound cellular population is constantly changing during the physiological course of healing, wound fluid should exhibit altered characteristics over time (especially regarding its proteome).

Ideally, wound fluid should be collected non-invasively and with little effort, resulting in a better patient as well as greater physician acceptance. This is in contrast to tissue biopsies or techniques -which are defined as the gold standard in animal models- such as subcutaneously implanted wire mesh cylinders (Hunt Schilling Cylinders), which are inadequate for monitoring wound healing in humans (Hunt et al. 1967; Schilling, Joel, and

Shurley 1959). Thus, non-invasive techniques hold a relevant advantage for the future, allowing the assessment of longitudinal profiles and changes in wound fluid composition.

2.1 Sampling techniques

2.1.1 Sampling of chronic wound fluids

Covering wounds with occlusive dressings and harvesting the accumulated exudate underneath is probably the most common technique for obtaining wound fluid in chronic wounds. Various modifications of this technique have been described with respect to used materials, patient preparation and time scales, as well as with respect to wound bed preparation (Trengove et al. 1999; Trengove, Bielefeldt-Ohmann, and Stacey 2000; Yager et al. 1996; Wysocki and Grinnell 1990; James et al. 2000; Wallace and Stacey 1998; Chen et al. 1997; Wysocki et al. 1999; Gohel et al. 2008). Even very comprehensive protocols aiming for standardisation have been proposed, including the prior fasting of patients for eight hours as well as grading their hydration status by drinking one litre of water while hanging down the leg (Trengove, Langton, and Stacey 1996). However, this is not suitable for daily clinical routines. In addition, there is also major variability with respect to the time frames defined for exudate accumulation, ranging from about one hour (Trengove et al. 1999) to five days (Ono et al. 1994). Therefore, the technique of wound fluid collection may indeed impact upon subsequent analytic results.

For chronic wounds in particular, techniques for harvesting even small amounts of wound fluid directly from the wound surface have been described. For this purpose, blunt-end glass micro-capillaries have been used to collect fluid directly from the wound surface (Weckroth et al. 1996). In venous leg ulcers, even the manual expression of wound fluid from absorptive dressings has been proposed (Hoffman, Starkey, and Coad 1998).

Another method for obtaining wound fluid is to cover the wound surface with different types of dressings from which it is then mechanically extracted. In the past, this particular technique has frequently been modified. Protocols describing the extraction of fluids directly from dressings have been reported multiple times (Fivenson et al. 1997; Seah et al. 2005). For example, wound exudate trapped in a foam dressing has been obtained by squeezing the dressing material through a syringe (Seah et al. 2005).

Another option is placing a sterile mesh onto the wound which absorbs the wound fluid into a sterilised pre-weighed whatman paper, which was described as allowing the recovery of 50-200µl of sample material. Subsequently, wound fluid was extracted from the filters by washouts employing a suitable buffer (Moor, Vachon, and Gould 2009). Similarly, glass microfibre circle filters were inserted into wound centres in order to saturate for 2 hours with wound exudate. Wound fluid was then extracted by phosphate buffered saline (Schmidtchen 2000).

A further technique described for the acquisition of wound fluid is a modification of the methodology used by the Schirmer´s test, which was originally invented to measure tear secretion in an ophthalmologic setting (Schirmer 1903, cited by Kallarackal et al. 2002). This attempt consists of absorbent paper strips which are placed on the wound surface thereby soaking with fluid for 5 minutes. Subsequently, the sample material is recovered by stirring the paper strips in a buffer for 2 hours (Muller et al. 2008).

Also, hydrophilic dextranomer beads layered on wounds have been used. In preliminary experiments with defined amounts of proteins, a recovery of 88-98% was described when extracting the beads with equal volumes of phosphate buffered saline for 12 hours (Cooper et al. 1994).

One potential drawback to these approaches is the issue of sample dilution, thus altering the analyte containing matrix as well as leaving the precise amount of fluid enclosed and remaining in the dressing material undetermined. Furthermore, huge inter-patient variability in cytokine concentrations -possibly due to technical problems during wound fluid aspiration from under occlusive Tegaderm® dressings- was observed in one study (Gohel et al. 2008).

To overcome the obstacles of methodological limitations in sample material and sampling difficulties, a technique using washouts of wound areas by the application of 5ml of sterile saline to wounds and subsequent collection of the fluid again by needle aspiration has been proposed (Ambrosch et al. 2008). However, a relevant dilution of the sample may again occur and so exert undetermined effects on the original fluid matrix.

Microdialysis has also been proposed for collecting wound fluid. However, this is an invasive technique and it is not undisputed since the insertion of foreign material may affect the wound microenvironment and induce confounding effects on the expression of signalling molecules (Stenken et al. 2010; Mellergard et al. 2008). Nevertheless, this technique is well established for sampling the fluid of the interstitial space and the samples obtained are usually of high quality (Simonsen et al. 1998; Clough and Noble 2003).

A possible major issue in all these techniques -covering wounds with foreign material to a minor or major extent- is the fact that the collection materials may influence the biochemical or immunological properties of the wound (Schmidtchen 2000; Hoffman, Noble, and Eagle 1999) or else interfere with the analytes that are to be measured.

Given these findings, we have considered implementing a novel way of obtaining wound fluid which might overcome some of the shortcomings of the earlier proposed techniques. Being convinced that wound fluid is a complex substrate (displaying the recent condition of the wound healing process), the sample material should be rapidly harvested within a short processing time so as to remain unaltered. The new protocol should be neither time-consuming nor cause much logistical effort, and thereby be suitable for daily clinical routines.

The issue of limited sample volumes is diminishing in importance since novel analytic techniques and devices still provide good and reproducible measurements, even when using very little amounts of fluid (see section 4). However, the issue of acquiring suitable and high-quality material in a reproducible, standardised manner is increasingly relevant and has been sought for years (Yager, Kulina, and Gilman 2007).

Therefore, we performed wound swabs without pressure using micro-flocked swabs (Minitip Flocked Swabs; nylon flocked swabs with moulded breakpoint, MicroRheologics, Brescia, Italy) that adsorb the wound exudate through capillary action, coating nylon fibres without entrapment. In our setting, wound fluid was collected from diabetic foot ulcers by swabbing -after sharp debridement and haemostasis- using the Levine technique (Wound infection in clinical practice. An international consensus 2008). Subsequently, the wound fluid was recovered by immediate centrifugation of swab tips at 10 000 rpm for 3 minutes at room temperature, using eppendorf cups equipped with a filter to hold the swab tip in place (Oxy Fill centrifugal filters without RoTrac capillary pore membrane, Carl Roth GmbH, Karlsruhe, Germany). The resulting cell free supernatant could then be used for subsequent analysis (Löffler et al. 2011).

2.1.2 Sampling of acute wound fluids

Techniques for harvesting acute wound fluid usually differ considerably from the methods described above for chronic wounds. This can be attributed to the different availability of wound exudates in the acute setting, as well as the different time frame until tissue restitution is reached. In several studies, wound fluid was obtained from suction drains, which have been inserted intra-operatively (Yager et al. 1996; Trengove et al. 1999; Baker and Leaper 2000). The collection of blister fluid is another opportunity for acquiring sample material (Oono et al. 1997; Ortega, Ganz, and Milner 2000).

Negative pressure therapy (Vacuum Assisted Closure, V.A.C.) permits additional access to wound fluid (Duckworth et al. 2004), which is also a suitable technique in diabetic foot ulcers (Noble-Bell and Forbes 2008). However, in this setting the disparity between methods seems quite obvious, so long as rather passive methods are compared to negative pressure therapy (Yager, Kulina, and Gilman 2007). Wound fluid obtained by V.A.C. therapy is characterised by an increased protein concentration. In a study of Dealey et al., the attempt to establish a suitable and valid technique for comparison failed due to technical reasons, causing the cessation of a second study arm (Dealey, Cameron, and Arrowsmith 2006).

Nevertheless, when interpreting the results with some caution, comparisons of the values from acute and chronic wound fluid can be worthwhile and can give important hints as to the differences between non-healing and healing wounds. Furthermore, the opportunity of analysing wound fluid over time will surely facilitate the discovery of relevant healing factors.

3. Sample requirements and challenges dependent on the choice of analytes

Besides all the obstacles that have been experienced in harvesting wound fluid and the interconnected high logistical effort to some extent also with respect to patient preparation, it is reasonable to assume that the sampling technique itself is likely to influence subsequent analysis.

So far, there is no gold standard to which a new sampling technique could be referenced to, nor any overview of the different methods that could elucidate the advantages and disadvantages of each particular technique. This lack of knowledge, along with the inherent variations in wound fluid composition -particularly in chronic wounds- complicates the picture and renders wound fluid a fairly complex analytic material. The missing standardisation in sampling wound fluid is likely to result in wound fluid being seen as an *undefined soup,* as termed decades ago by Trengove et al. (Trengove, Langton, and Stacey 1996). However, wound fluid might also be recognised as part of the problem in recalcitrant non-healing wounds and it might reflect the wound healing physiology better than any other sample material (Widgerow 2011).

Consequently, there are several inherent challenges in assaying chronic wound fluid. Very early comparisons between acute and chronic wound fluids showed a relevant difference in protease levels (Tarnuzzer and Schultz 1996) that has been confirmed by various authors subsequently (Chen et al. 1997; Moor, Vachon, and Gould 2009; Schmidtchen 2000). The issue of a proteolytic microenvironment in chronic wounds may be an important factor contributing to the non-healing phenotype, as growth factors and matrix components are subject to degradation (Widgerow 2011). This is not only true for growth factors and cytokines, but may also apply to receptors and signalling targets, which may thereby result in considerable loss of function. Therefore, merely quantifying analytes probably rather overestimates their protein bioactivity rather than reflecting the actual situation in the wound.

The composition and texture of wound fluid is influenced by the amount of exudate produced over a defined period of time as well as by its evaporation and absorption. Similarly, general factors such as leg positioning and the hydration status of the patient significantly alter the quality of wound fluid (Trengove, Langton, and Stacey 1996). Years ago, it had already been shown that the wound fluid of healing chronic leg ulcers showed relevant differences in global components -such as albumin and total protein content- when compared to the wound fluid of non-healing ulcers (James et al. 2000). Albumin reflects the plasma compartment of wound exudate and is, therefore, influenced by vascular leakage or acute vascular injury as well as by intravascular pressure.

When measuring protein biomarkers in wound fluid, the technical approach for how to obtain sample material must not be underestimated. It is still under discussion, whether values should be normalised to volume measures or total protein content for instance. Obtaining meaningful results is especially problematic when protease activity is high. Therefore, it is highly relevant to harvest immediate and unaltered sample material which is likely to reflect the original matrix of the wound microenvironment. In any cases, when intending to assess the amounts of peptide growth factors or other proteins in wound fluid, it should be recommended to determine the proteolytic activity of the environment in order to complete the picture. In this context, inert metabolites such as lactate might be considered advantageous since many of the limitations that apply to proteins do not apply here (Löffler et al. 2011).

There has been rapid progress in analytic techniques and devices, which allow for the accurate and sensitive determination of wound fluid composition. On the other hand, the techniques and methods used to obtain wound fluid need to catch up with this pace and should be thoroughly re-evaluated with regard to the requirements that have to be met for producing sound and meaningful results.

4. Protein arrays for the analysis of minute sample amounts

The analysis of cytokines and matrix metalloproteinases in complex biological fluids requires sensitive, accurate and reliable methods. This is usually accomplished using classical solid phase sandwich immunoassays, such as ELISA (de Jager and Rijkers 2006). However these methods are characterised by high sample consumption and the single analysis of only one mediator per experiment. Due to the frequently found low exudate levels in chronic wounds along with the inherent complexity of wound fluid, appropriate technologies are needed to accurately and reliably determine multiple parameters with minimal sample consumption. In this context, protein microarrays are important tools for the simultaneous detection and quantification of multiple parameters in complex biological mixtures, such as plasma (Cassatella et al. 1997) or tissue lysates (Beidler et al. 2008). This technology has been shown to exhibit high sensitivity and optimal signal to noise ratios even in the case of low target concentrations (Ekins 1989, 1998).

There are two different types of microarray systems -planar and bead based arrays can be employed for multiplexed immunoassays. Whereas planar microarrays can be generated with hundreds and thousands of different capture spots, which are distinguished by their corresponding xy-coordinates, bead-based systems (e.g. Luminex) represent an interesting and flexible alternative, especially when the number of parameters to be determined in parallel is rather low. All bead-based array systems employ colour or size coded microspheres as solid support for the capture molecules. Beads are identified in a flow cytometer and the amount of captured target molecules is quantified on each individual bead using an appropriate reporter system. Sensitivity, reliability and accuracy are similar to those observed with standard ELISA procedures. Using bead-based technology, thousands of samples can be screened within a short time. Throughput neither seems to be a problem anymore, nor does sample volume (Stoll 2004; Templin et al. 2004).

Inflammatory processes such as wound healing involve a complex network of immunoregulatory molecules such as chemokines, cytokines, proteases and their respective counter-regulatory mediators (Hahm, Glaser, and Elster 2011). The analysis of a complete set of mediators can therefore be considered to be of more value than the single analysis of only one single analyte (Gardy et al. 2009; de Jager et al. 2003). Although protein microarray technology has been successfully applied for the analysis of multiple analytes in complex biological mixtures -such as plasma, serum, urine and cerebrospinal fluid- publications using protein arrays for the analysis of wound status are rare (Hsu et al. 2008; Weigelt et al. 2009; Craig-Schapiro et al. 2011; Swain et al. 2011). For instance, Grimstad et al. measured the concentration of 27 different cytokines in wound fluid derived from acute wounds using a bead-based system (Grimstad et al. 2011). Beidler et al. applied this technology to measure the concentrations of matrix metalloproteinases and cytokines in wound tissue lysate (Beidler et al. 2008, 2009). In combination with appropriate wound sampling procedures, the complex protein-composition of wound exudate together with limitations in the anticipated sample volume renders protein array technology -be it planar or bead-based- as an interesting tool for the analysis of wound-associated biomarkers (see section 6.1). Due to the inherent heterogeneity of wound exudate samples from chronic leg ulcers, the normalisation of the data needs to be discussed. In this context, the levels of albumin and total protein in wound fluid might represent an interesting reference value.

5. Infection in the diabetic foot

Foot pathologies are among the most frequent causes of hospitalisation in diabetic patients (Tecilazich, Dinh, and Veves 2011), with infection being the most dangerous complication. However, local processes triggered by microbial activity in the wound microenvironment have not gathered much interest until now. Apart from the classical means of diagnosing infection by clinical examination and microbiological swabbing, analysing wound fluid might provide additional important information. Furthermore, it is crucial to understand that microbiological sampling should be considered as a tool for proving the clinical suspicion of infection rather than as a diagnostic instrument itself (Richard, Sotto, and Lavigne 2011).

Diagnosing infection in diabetic foot ulcers is challenging. This is especially true when the clinical assessment is not conclusive. The clinical signs for the diagnosis of infection may even be diminished by comorbidities -such as peripheral arterial disease, impaired leukocyte function and neuropathy- thereby reducing local signs of inflammation (Edmonds 2005; Williams, Hilton, and Harding 2004). However, since infection is a major cause of diabetes-related morbidity and mortality (Prompers et al. 2008) and as it paves the way towards limb amputation (Armstrong and Lipsky 2004), novel diagnostic tools that support prompt decision-making are urgently needed.

Currently there is ample room for the misclassification and delayed treatment of infection in the diabetic foot, and many issues in diagnosing diabetic foot infections are left unsolved (Jeffcoate et al. 2008). Furthermore, infection can show rapid onset and progression in diabetic foot ulcers.

In daily clinical practise, systemic markers of infection are the most established way of supporting the clinical suspicion of infection at present. The classical markers in this context include leukocyte count and C-reactive protein (CRP) as well as the erythrocyte sedimentation rate. Additionally, systemic markers specific to bacterial infection -such as procalcitonin, a peptide precursor of calcitonin, orosomucoid and haptoglobin- have been evaluated in serum of diabetic foot ulcers patients for the determination of infection (Jeandrot et al. 2008). Consecutively, a variety of immune mediators -including acute phase proteins, cytokines and chemokines- were examined in the plasma of patients with diabetic foot syndrome. These markers included CRP and fibrinogen as well as IL-6, IL-8, IL-18, macrophage inflammatory protein 1α (MIP1α), interferon γ-inducible protein-10 (IP10), macrophage migration inhibitory factor (MIF), macrophage chemoattractant protein 1 (MCP1) and RANTES (Weigelt et al. 2009). Both of the studies just cited were able to connect the occurrence of certain systemic inflammatory markers with the presence of infection in the diabetic foot.

In the first of these studies, serum CRP and procalcitonin were found to be significantly elevated during infection. CRP was discovered to be of a higher performance than procalcitonin, probably triggered by TNFα, IL-6 and IL-1 derived from the site of inflammation (Jeandrot et al. 2008). Still, the diagnosis of infection was principally determined by clinical assessment and the treatment was chosen accordingly.

Although various studies have been investigating CRP as a possible marker of infection in diabetic foot ulcers, sufficient support is not available for underlining its sole effectiveness (Dinh, Snyder, and Veves 2010) but it does add relevant supplementary information to the clinical assessment.

In the study conducted by Weigelt et al., besides CRP both IL-6 and fibrinogen -as acute phase reactants- were observed to be associated with the severity of foot ulcerations (88% type 2 diabetics) but not with the grade of infection. The overall findings in this fairly large study population can be interpreted to underline a specific alteration of the immune status of in diabetic patients, opposed to a rather general immune activation (IL-6 ↑, CRP ↑, fibrinogen ↑, MIP1α ↑, MIF↑, IP-10↑, RANTES↓, MCP-1 →, IL-8→ upon infection) (Weigelt et al. 2009). This is a further important hint towards suspecting determined alterations in the immune response in diabetes, which may prove relevant to the future detection and assessment of diabetic foot ulcers. Anyhow, it should be noted that even low levels of most of the cytokines in circulation would reach toxic levels relatively fast, whereas -in principle- at their site of action in the local environment their levels can rise manifold higher.

When analysing serological markers and cytokine patterns in wounds together with wound microbiology, local IL-6 concentrations are rather likely to support the clinical suspicion of infection than serological markers can. The analysis of local IL-6 and TNFα was shown to be able to discriminate between monomicrobial and polymicrobial infections in contrast to serum CRP and liposaccharide binding protein (LBP). Furthermore, local IL-6 was reported to reflect higher bacterial loads and infection, especially with pseudomonas (Ambrosch et al. 2008). The determination of CRP as well as LBP as serological parameters, together with the semi-quantitative analysis of bacterial load and microbial identification, was performed. In this setting, the assessment of wounds was shifted to a first primary appraisal of microbiological rather than clinical examination. Although critical levels of bacterial loads in wounds have been proposed (Bowler, Duerden, and Armstrong 2001), the types of pathogen species are equally important. Nevertheless, in neuropathic diabetic foot ulcers the healing rate was also found to be inversely correlated with high bacterial loads (Xu et al. 2007). Furthermore, in a study by Ambrosch et al., a good correlation between local CRP and TNFα levels in wound washouts and tissue punch biopsies could be shown (Ambrosch et al. 2008).

In addition to the controversial findings on CRP, the upstream marker IL-6 seems to become even more meaningful in the local context. Overall, local alterations are likely to precede systemic changes. On the basis of this rationale, we advocate the investigation of the local microenvironment and possibly the correlation of these findings with circulatory markers. We are convinced that this local approach is more suitable for discovering useful markers for the assessment of infection in diabetic foot ulcer patients than the opposite approach of searching for alterations in the complicated circulatory proteome.

Of course, this local approach is not always suitable as -for instance- in the acute Charcot foot, which is a widely unresolved problem in diabetic foot care. Notably in this context, it would be of great interest to find circulatory markers disclosing the disease state and having possible therapeutic implications on hand. Initial attempts have already been made in this direction (Mabilleau et al. 2011).

6. Wound fluid - a window reflecting the wound microenvironment?

The question of whether wound fluid could serve as a valuable *window into the wound environment* has already been asked -years ago- by Dorne R. Yager et al. (Yager, Kulina, and Gilman 2007). Therefore, it is not a novel aspect but it is indeed an exciting option for having a closer look into the wound microenvironment. Recently, it has even been proposed that the corrosive nature of the chronic wound environment and the continuous breakdown of the extracellular matrix mediated by proteases may link wound fluid directly to the phenotype of chronic non-healing wounds (Widgerow 2011). If this were the case, the science of assessing wound fluid should be an important stepping stone in obtaining access to the problem of chronic non-healing wounds. Wound fluid -which has been investigated in a variety of studies- has added much to our understanding of wound healing. Nevertheless, to date there are neither techniques nor markers that have found their way into clinical practise.

6.1 Biomarkers

A biomarker can be defined as a substance that is used as an indicator of normal biological processes, pathologic conditions and therapeutic interventions (Hahm, Glaser, and Elster 2011). They are widely attributed as playing a key role in the diagnosis, prognosis and clinical management of a broad range of disease states (Mueller, Muller, and Perruchoud 2008). Prominent examples are prostate specific antigen (PSA) (Makarov et al. 2009), or Her-2. However, due to complex disease pathologies and aetiological heterogeneity, it turns out that standalone markers are rather unlikely to be specific or else applicable on a wide-scale and a whole set of candidate markers are considered to be more promising e.g. as demonstrated by Domenici et al. (Domenici et al. 2010). According to Yager et al. there are as yet no accepted biomarkers, which allow the evaluation of the wound status and this critically hampers the improvement of appropriate treatments and effective therapies. Among the most promising candidate biomarkers are matrix metalloproteinases, cytokines and chemokines (Yager, Kulina, and Gilman 2007).

6.2 Proteases and their inhibitors

Chronic ulcers are characterised by a highly proteolytic microenvironment. Therefore, the four major biochemical classes of proteases (serine proteases, metalloproteinases, cysteine proteases and aspartic proteases) have generated great interest in the context of wound healing. In particular, matrix metalloproteinases (MMPs) and their tissue inhibitors (TIMPs) are critically involved in wound healing. Using protein array technology, Beidler et al. (Beidler et al. 2008) demonstrated that MMPs are differentially expressed in ulcerative and healthy tissue lysates. They demonstrated that MMP-8 and -9 in particular are strongly increased in ulcer tissue and decreased after the onset of the healing process. Yager et al.showed that MMP-2 and MMP-9 are elevated in chronic wound fluid compared with fluid from acute surgical wounds (Yager et al. 1996). Ladwig et al. (Ladwig et al. 2002) and Liu et al. (Liu et al. 2009) reported an increased ratio of MMP-9 to TIMP-1 in chronic non-healing wound fluid compared with healing wounds. Together with the finding that the MMP2:TIMP-2 ratio is elevated in non-healing compared with healing leg ulcers (Mwaura et al. 2006), this suggests that a disturbed homeostasis between MMPs and TIMPs might be correlated with the non-healing status. Also, in chronic non-healing diabetic foot ulcers, MMPs and their inhibitors (TIMPs) have received much interest. In a study by Lobmann et al., higher concentrations of the MMPs -2, -8 and -9, in conjunction with lower concentrations of TIMP-2, were determined in tissue biopsies when comparing diabetic wounds to healthy controls (Lobmann et al. 2002). The study by Liu et al. extended these findings of elevated MMP-9 in diabetic foot ulcers to healing rates. Elevated MMP-9 -in these ulcers- was suggested to be linked to inflammatory processes and poor healing. Furthermore, in conjunction with low TIMP-1 and TGFβ, high MMP-9 was proposed as being indicative of poor wound healing (Liu et al. 2009). These findings are coincident with other previous findings - for instance, in pressure ulcers where diminished healing rates have been described in a high MMP-9/low TIMP-1 environment (Ladwig et al. 2002) and with a slightly different setting regarding the MMP-9:TIMP-2 ratio in diabetic foot ulcers (Lobmann et al. 2006). The interconnection of elevated MMP-9/MMP-8 levels and poor healing has further been described in neuropathic diabetic foot ulcers, but furthermore here an association between high levels of MMP-1 and TIMP-1 and better healing rates has been shown (Muller et al. 2008). Recently, Widgerow proposed a theory focusing on neutrophil-derived proteases -especially elevated MMP-9 in chronic wound fluid- as being involved in a vicious circle and stating that the corrosive nature of wound fluid was not only actively involved in matrix breakdown but also causative for non-healing a state probably further aggravated by bacterial factors (Widgerow 2011). According to this view, continued inflammation and leukocyte infiltration is triggered in chronic non-healing wounds, thereby perpetuating tissue destruction (Rayment, Upton, and Shooter 2008; cited by Widgerow 2011). Together with an imbalance towards a proteolytic microenvironment and in conjunction with bacterial colonisation causing the continuous breakdown of extracellular matrix and growth factors, this milieu keeps wounds in a prolonged destructive state and so averts healing (Rayment, Upton, and Shooter 2008).

In conclusion, we can see various overlapping motifs concerning an imbalance of MMPs and their inhibitory factors (TIMPs) in different types of wounds, which is also true for diabetic foot ulcers. MMPs seem to constitute some of the key players in this microenvironment and are probably linked to inflammatory activity and bacterial load, as well as the critical degradation of growth factors and extracellular matrix components. Nevertheless, as there are various MMPs involved in healing, such as MMP-1 to MMP-10, MMP-12 and MMP-13 and several of their inhibitors (Armstrong and Jude 2002; Gill and Parks 2008); they are also important for physiological wound healing, although in a timely and ordinary fashion. As MMPs also have physiological roles and intimate links with inflammatory processes, an overview investigation of their roles with regard to inflammatory activity and wound healing rates would be desirable for coming to novel conclusions notably in non-healing wounds. For this endeavour, wound fluid might constitute a nearly ideal sample material.

6.3 Cytokines and growth factors

Besides MMPs, cytokines and chemokines are frequently discussed as potential indicators for the status of wound healing. In general, there is an ample variety of factors which can be found in the wound microenvironment and that play a role in wound healing. Nevertheless, the cytokines found in the local microenvironment are usually produced by local cells (Holzheimer and Steinmetz 2000) and may, therefore, provide us with interesting information on the local environment. The issue of mediators being found in wounds is already complex in physiological terms, and confounding factors -such as the chronic wound environment and exogenous factors from bacterial colonisation and the endogenous reactions to this scenario- make it even more complicated. Besides this, it is a fact that the pathogenesis of wound healing on the molecular level is poorly understood and may be diverse according to various different wound entities. Nevertheless, we will attempt a concise digression on the topic without the intent to give a comprehensive impression of chemokines, cytokines and growth factors in wound fluids.

To our knowledge, there are no broad analyses available of these mediators in conjunction with clinical endpoints from chronic ulcers. Therefore, it may be prudent to begin with a glance at acute wound healing.

In a study by Grimstad et al. (already mentioned above) an attempt to characterise acute wound fluid from surgical drains at the first postoperative day after mastectomy was undertaken. This aspect therefore best describes the initial phase of the acute inflammatory response, which is particularly interesting in this relatively broad investigation assessing the levels of 27 different cytokines, chemokines and growth factors (Grimstad et al. 2011). Information as to this amount is generally scarce and will therefore be looked at in more detail here. In this context, the cytokines IL-6 and IL-8 -such as TNFα and IFNγ- were found in high abundance in acute wound fluid. In contrast with this pro-inflammatory pattern, the IL-1 receptor antagonist (IL-1RA) was also detected in high concentrations here. Interestingly, at this context the amounts of IL-1β detected and the anti-inflammatory cytokine IL-10 were found to be relatively low.

This pattern just as observed in wound fluid at the onset of inflammation suggests a distinct but contained local inflammatory environment. The picture witnessed in this phase of wound healing can be interpreted -in our view- as an inflammatory response with strong inhibitory and restorative stimuli. This might be the case, as IL-8 constitutes a chemotactic factor for neutrophil recruitment (Baggiolini and Clark-Lewis 1992) as well as a factor promoting epidermal cell proliferation (Tuschil et al. 1992); moreover, IL-6 plays an ambivalent role with pro- as well as anti-inflammatory properties, such as inhibiting TNFα and repressing IL-1β as well as inducing IL-1RA and IL-10 (Tilg et al. 1994). The low levels of the key pro-inflammatory marker IL-1β, which is -for instance- associated with inflammasome activity and the control of infection (Schroder and Tschopp 2010) is also notable in this early postoperative setting.

With regard to chronic non-healing wounds, a connection with persistent inflammatory activity is a guiding principle, which is observed in various entities of impaired healing (Acosta et al. 2008; Pukstad et al. 2010). In a longitudinal study in chronic venous leg ulcers, decreases in IL-1α and IL-1β were observed in healing ulcers, whereas increases in IL-8 and MIP-1α were associated with non-healing. This was observed in conjunction with decreased levels of toll-like receptor (TLR) activities in healing ulcers (Pukstad et al. 2010). The persistent activation of innate immune responses, in dividing the healing and non-healing entities of wounds by TLR activation and distinct cytokine patterns (IL-1α ↑, IL1-β↑, IL-8↓ and MIP-1α↓), may even be interpreted in favour of a constant bacterial challenge in non-healers with relevant effects on the wound microenvironment.

The elevated expression of IL-1β and excessive TNFα in non-healing wounds (Wallace and Stacey 1998) may, therefore, be linked to the distinct properties observed in this microenvironment. This may be the case, as high TNFα has been described not only as inducing IL-1β and its own synthesis but also their synergistic effects resulting in the suppression of extracellular matrix synthesis, whereas MMP synthesis is induced and TIMP synthesis is inhibited (Mast and Schultz 1996), thus contributing to persistent inflammatory activity and tissue destruction in diabetes (Nwomeh, Yager, and Cohen 1998; Naguib et al. 2004). This link may, therefore, constitute a part of the vicious circle that we know of, linking alterations observed in the microenvironment of non-healing wounds to persistent inflammatory activity.

For instance, levels of TNFα have been found to be elevated in non-healing compared to healing leg ulcers (Wallace and Stacey 1998). Trengove et al. found elevated levels of the pro-inflammatory cytokines IL-1, IL-6 and TNFα in non-healing compared with healing ulcers and that these mediators decreased over the course of healing (Trengove, Bielefeldt-Ohmann, and Stacey 2000). Beidler and co-workers measured 22 mediators in healthy and ulcerative tissue lysates and found that IL-1α, IL-1β, IL-4, IL-6, IL-8, IL-10, IL-12p40, G-CSF, GM-CSF, MCP-1, IFNγ, TNFα, MIP-1α, MIP-1β and TGFβ1 were expressed at significantly higher levels in ulcer tissue compared with healthy controls. Moreover, they found the analytes IL-1α, IL-1β, IFNγ, IL-12p40, GM-CSF and IL-1RA to be differentially expressed in rapid versus delayed healing ulcers (Beidler et al. 2009).

In summary, there are promising candidates that might be used as indicators of the healing status of chronic and acute wounds. However, additional efforts are needed to further validate the existing candidates and to discover new potential biomarkers. In this context, the use of entire biomarker panels instead of standalone molecules should be taken into account.

Especially in diabetes, it is established that a local over-secretion of pro-inflammatory cytokines (notably TNFα, IL-6 and IL-1) is observed, impacting the wound healing microenvironment and opposing healing (Acosta et al. 2008). These factors have been multiply observed in the context of failure to heal and are linked with other processes observed in the wound environment, such as elevated proteolysis and the degradation of growth factors and their receptors.

When it comes to growth factors, it is conceivable that beneath the mere abundance of these factors in wound fluid the aspect of bioactivity is of primary relevance. This may be best demonstrated by the reactions that have been described for ages, when comparing the diverse effects of wound fluids on cells in culture. The most important aspect of this may be the positive effect evoked by acute wound fluid on cellular proliferation. When acute wound fluid is added to cells in culture, increased proliferation of vascular endothelial cells, fibroblasts and endothelial cells was observed (Greenburg and Hunt 1978; Katz et al. 1991). Furthermore, the deposition of extracellular matrix and migration of cells are enhanced by acute wound fluid supplemented to cell cultures. In opposition to this, chronic wound fluid has been observed numerous times as inhibiting proliferation *in vitro* (Trengove, Bielefeldt-Ohmann, and Stacey 2000; Bucalo, Eaglstein, and Falanga 1993; Phillips et al. 1998), thus hampering tissue restoration. Of course, the converse argument that the lack of proliferative stimulus in chronic wound fluid may be attributed to a mere lack of growth factors is invalid. To underline this thesis, Trengove et al. were not able to detect significant changes within the levels of platelet-derived growth factor (PDGF), epidermal growth factor (EGF), basic fibroblast growth factor (bFGF) or transforming growth factor beta (TGFβ) from healing and non-healing ulcers. However, in mitogenic assays in fibroblasts, wound fluid from healing ulcers was able to provoke a significantly enhanced proliferative response (Trengove, Bielefeldt-Ohmann, and Stacey 2000). Furthermore, additional growth factors have been implicated as playing an important role in wound healing, such as insulin-like growth factor (IGF) (Wagner et al. 2003) or keratinocyte growth factor (KGF) (Gibbs et al. 2000).

In a study by He et al., it was demonstrated that the addition of platelet derived growth factor (PDGF) to chronic wound fluid was able to synergistically enhance proliferation in fibroblasts, whereas chronic wound fluid alone also enhanced fibroblast proliferation at lower levels (He et al. 1999). Nevertheless, the original matrix in this study was not preserved and the results suggest that essential factors can be found in wound fluid enhancing proliferation that can be stimulated by the addition of growth factors from external sources, whereas the original fluid matrix is suited to suppressing proliferative effects. To sum up the findings, a mere lack of growth factors does not seem to be responsible for impaired wound healing. In fact, other factors that characterise the wound environment seem to be of relevance in impairing local proliferation. For instance, it has been shown that high glucose levels are suited to inhibit fibroblast proliferation and to induce resistance to growth factors (Hehenberger and Hansson 1997). Furthermore, in fibroblasts from chronic diabetic wounds, lactate levels above 7 mM have been shown to abrogate cell proliferation as a specific effect of elevated L-lactate levels (Hehenberger et al. 1998). Another aspect that may be of relevance within this context is the enhanced degradation of growth factors by proteases which is observed in chronic wound fluid when compared with its acute counterpart (Trengove et al. 1999).

Eventually, cellular factors (such as reaching the end of their replicative life span, which was suggested for fibroblasts in chronic ulcers that had not healed for 3 years, and were non-responding to PDGF while exhibiting a normal expression of their respective receptors compared to their normal counterparts) are another possibility that may explain the lack of proliferation (Agren et al. 1999) together with the demand for antecedent therapeutic intervention. Interestingly, this condition of environmentally-driven cellular aging has been shown not to be correlated with telomere shortening but to be induced by other factors; possibly decreased resistance to oxidative stress (Wall et al. 2008), including the possibility of reversing this induced phenotype. Nevertheless, fibroblast dysfunction in late non-healing ulcers seems to constitute an important factor propagating this condition that cannot be overcome anymore by mere basic growth factor supplementation.

6.4 Role of lactate

Tissue lactate accumulates during the physiological course of healing to concentrations of ~ 10-12 mM as opposed to 1–3 mM normally found in blood and most uninjured, resting tissues (Ghani et al. 2004). Even though it has been shown that these high lactate concentrations persist irrespective of tissue oxygenation (Ghani et al. 2004), the concept of lactate as *a dead end product* in hypoxia has survived for many years still. Nowadays, it is widely accepted that tissue lactate is mainly derived from aerobic glycolysis.

Lactate is understood to have many fundamental metabolic and signalling functions (Gladden 2004). Thus, lactate enhances wound healing by the stimulation of extracellular matrix synthesis (Hussain, Ghani, and Hunt 1989; Green and Goldberg 1964) and angiogenesis (Beckert et al. 2006; Hunt et al. 2007). However, at higher concentrations these positive effects seem to deteriorate. In fibroblast experiments, a threshold for cell proliferation could be determined (Hehenberger et al. 1998). Cellular proliferation was enhanced so long as lactate levels were lower than this particular threshold but inhibited when raised above.

In chronic wounds, tissue lactate concentrations reach far higher levels compared with acute wounds. Inflammatory cells that are ubiquitously present in chronic wounds cover their energy demand mainly through aerobic glycolysis and they generate lactate as a by-product and in huge amounts. Next, lactate leaves the cytosol to the extracellular space by monocarboxylic transferases (MCT) (Gladden 2004).

Almost every chronic wound is more or less subject to bacterial contamination. Even though bacterial contamination does not necessarily lead to immediate subsequent infection, wound healing is impaired when the bacterial load reaches a certain level. In addition, many bacterial strains that have been detected in chronic wounds -and in the diabetic foot in particular- cover their energy demand by fermentation, thus producing additional lactate.

Lactate levels in wound fluid of diabetic foot ulcers (DFU)

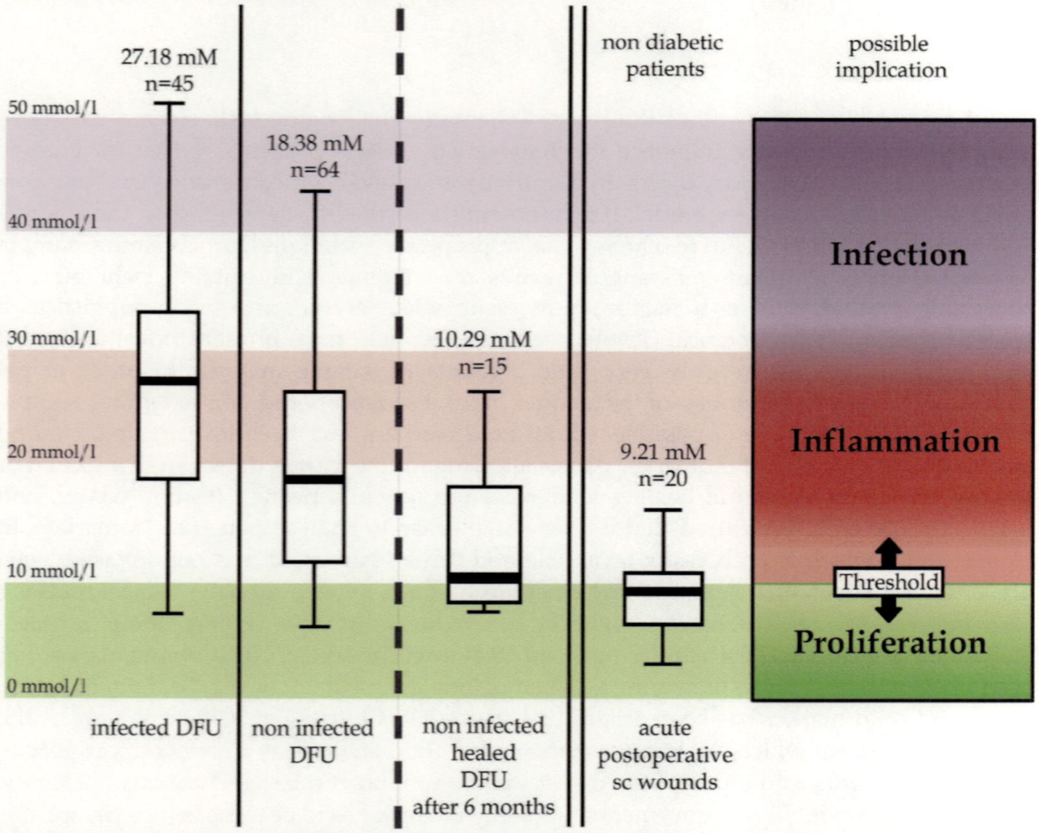

Fig. 1. Lactate levels in diabetic foot ulcers (DFU) with clinical signs of soft-infection are shown on the left side of the continuous line as opposed to non-infected DFU on the right. In addition, lactate concentrations of DFU that healed within a follow-up period of 6 months are given to the right of the dotted line. Further right, wound fluid lactate concentrations in surgical wounds are shown. Wound fluid lactate concentrations are given as box plots (median, minimum - maximum as well as the 25th and 75th percentiles). The respective median lactate concentrations are given above the corresponding box plots. The possible clinical implications of lactate are presented in coloured boxes (modified according to Löffler et al. 2011).

In diabetic foot ulcers, a correlation between elevated wound fluid lactate levels and the clinical signs of soft-tissue infection could be demonstrated. Wounds with clinical signs of soft-tissue infection showed significantly higher wound fluid lactate concentrations as opposed to those without soft-tissue infection. Out of the wound sub-population, without clinical signs of soft-tissue infection, wounds that healed within a 6 months follow-up period were characterised by wound fluid lactate concentrations comparable with those found in acute healing wounds (Löffler et al. 2011). In summary, elevated lactate levels seem to be attributed both to inflammatory and bacterial activity. Nevertheless, lactate is likely to favour healing unless its concentration exceeds a certain threshold. On the other hand, lactate in wound fluid might be a diagnostic marker both for impaired healing and soft-tissue-infection (Figure 1).

7. Conclusions

Sampling and analysing wound fluid is an inherently challenging task, since a variety of local and systemic factors influence its composition. This is particularly true for chronic wounds and for diabetic foot ulcers. In addition, there is no clear consensus yet about how to obtain adequate sample material. It is important nevertheless, depending on the analysis intended to be undertaken to choose the appropriate technique for obtaining sample material. Hence, to obtain meaningful results an adequate and suitable technique for harvesting wound fluid is a major pre-requisite when considering using sophisticated analytic methods. The technical developments in this field have brought novel analytical opportunities that require only very little amounts of sample material in order to get meaningful results. A variety of techniques have been proposed for obtaining sample materials and a multitude of possible wound fluid markers have been investigated. Finding meaningful biomarkers or biomarker panels allowing for the instant detection of infection or the determination of wound healing tendencies are urgently needed (Hahm, Glaser, and Elster 2011). We are convinced that it does make sense to analyse potential biomarkers in wound fluid, which is both easily accessible and can be harvested in a non-invasive way. The obstacle to overcome here is to implement techniques suitable for daily clinical routines, allowing for fast and reliable diagnostic procedures. In this setting, there are less confounding factors to deal with as opposed to systemic markers. No systemic marker has been proven to be capable of serving as a standalone diagnostic tool yet. To date, however, no wound fluid marker has been established that might fill this gap neither. We are at the beginning of an era which might appreciate wound fluid analysis as a novel opportunity to get deeper insights into a complicated and widely unknown micro-environment. There is still substantial room for improvement and plenty of work has to be done before we are able to understand the elementary mechanisms of non-healing.

8. Perspective

Valuable markers for clinical wound assessment are urgently needed. Wound fluid biomarkers are probably the best option for reaching this aim. For this purpose, wound fluid components -such as proteases and their inhibitors as well as cytokines and growth factors and other elements associated with the local inflammatory response- are worthwhile investigating. The wound fluid degradation products of the extracellular matrix represent another interesting aspect in assessing the pathophysiology of non-healing wounds

(Moseley et al. 2004). This is by virtue of the fact that the course of chronic wound healing may be directly reflected in matrix turnover due to a highly proteolytic and pro-oxidative environment. In addition, markers of oxidative stress and simple metabolites such as lactate may also give us important information on the state of wound healing. However, there is still ample room for the discovery of both valuable and inert wound fluid biomarkers. It can be anticipated that novel technical opportunities along with reproducible sampling methods will bring forward new biomarkers, which may aid in future wound assessment. The need is there, especially in the diabetic foot, and hopefully meaningful studies will soon be under way to bridge this gap, thereby substantiating the valour of wound fluid diagnostics.

9. Acknowledgment

This work was supported by a fortune grant (1780-0-0 and 1780-0-1) of Tuebingen University (ML).

10. References

Acosta, J. B., D. G. del Barco, D. C. Vera, W. Savigne, P. Lopez-Saura, G. Guillen Nieto, and G. S. Schultz. 2008. The pro-inflammatory environment in recalcitrant diabetic foot wounds. *Int Wound J* 5 (4):530-9.

Agren, M. S., H. H. Steenfos, S. Dabelsteen, J. B. Hansen, and E. Dabelsteen. 1999. Proliferation and mitogenic response to PDGF-BB of fibroblasts isolated from chronic venous leg ulcers is ulcer-age dependent. *J Invest Dermatol* 112 (4):463-9.

Ambrosch, A., R. Lobmann, A. Pott, and J. Preissler. 2008. Interleukin-6 concentrations in wound fluids rather than serological markers are useful in assessing bacterial triggers of ulcer inflammation. *Int Wound J* 5 (1):99-106.

Apple, F. S. 1999. Tissue specificity of cardiac troponin I, cardiac troponin T and creatine kinase-MB. *Clin Chim Acta* 284 (2):151-9.

Armstrong, D. G., and E. B. Jude. 2002. The role of matrix metalloproteinases in wound healing. *J Am Podiatr Med Assoc* 92 (1):12-8.

Armstrong, D. G., and B. A. Lipsky. 2004. Diabetic foot infections: stepwise medical and surgical management. *Int Wound J* 1 (2):123-32.

Baggiolini, M., and I. Clark-Lewis. 1992. Interleukin-8, a chemotactic and inflammatory cytokine. *FEBS Lett* 307 (1):97-101.

Baker, E. A., and D. J. Leaper. 2000. Proteinases, their inhibitors, and cytokine profiles in acute wound fluid. *Wound Repair Regen* 8 (5):392-8.

Balk, S. P., Y. J. Ko, and G. J. Bubley. 2003. Biology of prostate-specific antigen. *J Clin Oncol* 21 (2):383-91.

Beckert, S., F. Farrahi, R. S. Aslam, H. Scheuenstuhl, A. Konigsrainer, M. Z. Hussain, and T. K. Hunt. 2006. Lactate stimulates endothelial cell migration. *Wound Repair Regen* 14 (3):321-4.

Beidler, S. K., C. D. Douillet, D. F. Berndt, B. A. Keagy, P. B. Rich, and W. A. Marston. 2008. Multiplexed analysis of matrix metalloproteinases in leg ulcer tissue of patients with chronic venous insufficiency before and after compression therapy. *Wound Repair Regen* 16 (5):642-8.

Beidler, S. K., C. D. Douillet, D. F. Berndt, B. A. Keagy, P. B. Rich, and W. A. Marston. 2009. Inflammatory cytokine levels in chronic venous insufficiency ulcer tissue before and after compression therapy. *J Vasc Surg* 49 (4):1013-20.

Bowler, P. G., B. I. Duerden, and D. G. Armstrong. 2001. Wound microbiology and associated approaches to wound management. *Clin Microbiol Rev* 14 (2):244-69.

Bucalo, B., W. H. Eaglstein, and V. Falanga. 1993. Inhibition of cell proliferation by chronic wound fluid. *Wound Repair Regen* 1 (3):181-6.

Cassatella, M. A., S. Gasperini, F. Calzetti, A. Bertagnin, A. D. Luster, and P. P. McDonald. 1997. Regulated production of the interferon-gamma-inducible protein-10 (IP-10) chemokine by human neutrophils. *Eur J Immunol* 27 (1):111-5.

Chen, S. M., S. I. Ward, O. O. Olutoye, R. F. Diegelmann, and I. Kelman Cohen. 1997. Ability of chronic wound fluids to degrade peptide growth factors is associated with increased levels of elastase activity and diminished levels of proteinase inhibitors. *Wound Repair Regen* 5 (1):23-32.

Clough, G., and M. Noble. 2003. Microdialysis--a model for studying chronic wounds. *Int J Low Extrem Wounds* 2 (4):233-9.

Cooper, D. M., E. Z. Yu, P. Hennessey, F. Ko, and M. C. Robson. 1994. Determination of endogenous cytokines in chronic wounds. *Ann Surg* 219 (6):688-91; discussion 691-2.

Craig-Schapiro, R., M. Kuhn, C. Xiong, E. H. Pickering, J. Liu, T. P. Misko, R. J. Perrin, K. R. Bales, H. Soares, A. M. Fagan, and D. M. Holtzman. 2011. Multiplexed immunoassay panel identifies novel CSF biomarkers for Alzheimer's disease diagnosis and prognosis. *PLoS One* 6 (4):e18850.

de Jager, W., and G. T. Rijkers. 2006. Solid-phase and bead-based cytokine immunoassay: a comparison. *Methods* 38 (4):294-303.

de Jager, W., H. te Velthuis, B. J. Prakken, W. Kuis, and G. T. Rijkers. 2003. Simultaneous detection of 15 human cytokines in a single sample of stimulated peripheral blood mononuclear cells. *Clin Diagn Lab Immunol* 10 (1):133-9.

Dealey, C., J. Cameron, and M. Arrowsmith. 2006. A study comparing two objective methods of quantifying the production of wound exudate. *J Wound Care* 15 (4):149-53.

Dinh, T., G. Snyder, and A. Veves. 2010. Current techniques to detect foot infection in the diabetic patient. *Int J Low Extrem Wounds* 9 (1):24-30.

Domenici, E., D. R. Wille, F. Tozzi, I. Prokopenko, S. Miller, A. McKeown, C. Brittain, D. Rujescu, I. Giegling, C. W. Turck, F. Holsboer, E. T. Bullmore, L. Middleton, E. Merlo-Pich, R. C. Alexander, and P. Muglia. 2010. Plasma protein biomarkers for depression and schizophrenia by multi analyte profiling of case-control collections. *PLoS One* 5 (2):e9166.

Duckworth, W. C., J. Fawcett, S. Reddy, and J. C. Page. 2004. Insulin-degrading activity in wound fluid. *J Clin Endocrinol Metab* 89 (2):847-51.

Edmonds, M. 2005. Infection in the neuroischemic foot. *Int J Low Extrem Wounds* 4 (3):145-53.

Ekins, R. P. 1989. Multi-analyte immunoassay. *J Pharm Biomed Anal* 7 (2):155-68.

Ekins, R. P. 1998. Ligand assays: from electrophoresis to miniaturized microarrays. *Clin Chem* 44 (9):2015-30.

Eming, S. A., M. Koch, A. Krieger, B. Brachvogel, S. Kreft, L. Bruckner-Tuderman, T. Krieg, J. D. Shannon, and J. W. Fox. 2010. Differential proteomic analysis distinguishes tissue repair biomarker signatures in wound exudates obtained from normal healing and chronic wounds. *J Proteome Res* 9 (9):4758-66.

Ertugrul, B. M., O. Savk, B. Ozturk, M. Cobanoglu, S. Oncu, and S. Sakarya. 2009. The diagnosis of diabetic foot osteomyelitis: examination findings and laboratory values. *Med Sci Monit* 15 (6):CR307-12.

Fivenson, D. P., D. T. Faria, B. J. Nickoloff, P. J. Poverini, S. Kunkel, M. Burdick, and R. M. Strieter. 1997. Chemokine and inflammatory cytokine changes during chronic wound healing. *Wound Repair Regen* 5 (4):310-22.

Gardy, J. L., D. J. Lynn, F. S. Brinkman, and R. E. Hancock. 2009. Enabling a systems biology approach to immunology: focus on innate immunity. *Trends Immunol* 30 (6):249-62.

Ghani, Q. P., S. Wagner, H. D. Becker, T. K. Hunt, and M. Z. Hussain. 2004. Regulatory role of lactate in wound repair. *Methods Enzymol* 381:565-75.

Gibbs, S., A. N. Silva Pinto, S. Murli, M. Huber, D. Hohl, and M. Ponec. 2000. Epidermal growth factor and keratinocyte growth factor differentially regulate epidermal migration, growth, and differentiation. *Wound Repair Regen* 8 (3):192-203.

Gill, S. E., and W. C. Parks. 2008. Metalloproteinases and their inhibitors: regulators of wound healing. *Int J Biochem Cell Biol* 40 (6-7):1334-47.

Gladden, L. B. 2004. Lactate metabolism: a new paradigm for the third millennium. *J Physiol* 558 (Pt 1):5-30.

Gohel, M. S., R. A. Windhaber, J. F. Tarlton, M. R. Whyman, and K. R. Poskitt. 2008. The relationship between cytokine concentrations and wound healing in chronic venous ulceration. *J Vasc Surg* 48 (5):1272-7.

Green, H., and B. Goldberg. 1964. Collagen and Cell Protein Synthesis by an Established Mammalian Fibroblast Line. *Nature* 204:347-9.

Greenburg, G. B., and T. K. Hunt. 1978. The proliferative response in vitro of vascular endothelial and smooth muscle cells exposed to wound fluids and macrophages. *J Cell Physiol* 97 (3 Pt 1):353-60.

Grimstad, O., O. Sandanger, L. Ryan, K. Otterdal, J. K. Damaas, B. Pukstad, and T. Espevik. 2011. Cellular sources and inducers of cytokines present in acute wound fluid. *Wound Repair Regen* 19 (3):337-47.

Hahm, G., J. J. Glaser, and E. A. Elster. 2011. Biomarkers to predict wound healing: the future of complex war wound management. *Plast Reconstr Surg* 127 Suppl 1:21S-26S.

He, C., M. A. Hughes, G. W. Cherry, and F. Arnold. 1999. Effects of chronic wound fluid on the bioactivity of platelet-derived growth factor in serum-free medium and its direct effect on fibroblast growth. *Wound Repair Regen* 7 (2):97-105.

Hehenberger, K., and A. Hansson. 1997. High glucose-induced growth factor resistance in human fibroblasts can be reversed by antioxidants and protein kinase C-inhibitors. *Cell Biochem Funct* 15 (3):197-201.

Hehenberger, K., J. D. Heilborn, K. Brismar, and A. Hansson. 1998. Inhibited proliferation of fibroblasts derived from chronic diabetic wounds and normal dermal fibroblasts treated with high glucose is associated with increased formation of l-lactate. *Wound Repair Regen* 6 (2):135-41.

Hoffman, R., J. Noble, and M. Eagle. 1999. The use of proteases as prognostic markers for the healing of venous leg ulcers. *J Wound Care* 8 (6):273-6.

Hoffman, R., S. Starkey, and J. Coad. 1998. Wound fluid from venous leg ulcers degrades plasminogen and reduces plasmin generation by keratinocytes. *J Invest Dermatol* 111 (6):1140-4.

Holzheimer, R. G., and W. Steinmetz. 2000. Local and systemic concentrations of pro- and anti-inflammatory cytokines in human wounds. *Eur J Med Res* 5 (8):347-55.

Hsu, H. Y., S. Wittemann, E. M. Schneider, M. Weiss, and T. O. Joos. 2008. Suspension microarrays for the identification of the response patterns in hyperinflammatory diseases. *Med Eng Phys* 30 (8):976-83.

Hunt, T. K., R. S. Aslam, S. Beckert, S. Wagner, Q. P. Ghani, M. Z. Hussain, S. Roy, and C. K. Sen. 2007. Aerobically derived lactate stimulates revascularization and tissue repair via redox mechanisms. *Antioxid Redox Signal* 9 (8):1115-24.

Hunt, T. K., P. Twomey, B. Zederfeldt, and J. E. Dunphy. 1967. Respiratory gas tensions and pH in healing wounds. *Am J Surg* 114 (2):302-7.

Hussain, M. Z., Q. P. Ghani, and T. K. Hunt. 1989. Inhibition of prolyl hydroxylase by poly(ADP-ribose) and phosphoribosyl-AMP. Possible role of ADP-ribosylation in intracellular prolyl hydroxylase regulation. *J Biol Chem* 264 (14):7850-5.

James, T. J., M. A. Hughes, G. W. Cherry, and R. P. Taylor. 2000. Simple biochemical markers to assess chronic wounds. *Wound Repair Regen* 8 (4):264-9.

Jeandrot, A., J. L. Richard, C. Combescure, N. Jourdan, S. Finge, M. Rodier, P. Corbeau, A. Sotto, and J. P. Lavigne. 2008. Serum procalcitonin and C-reactive protein concentrations to distinguish mildly infected from non-infected diabetic foot ulcers: a pilot study. *Diabetologia* 51 (2):347-52.

Jeffcoate, W. J., B. A. Lipsky, A. R. Berendt, P. R. Cavanagh, S. A. Bus, E. J. Peters, W. H. van Houtum, G. D. Valk, and K. Bakker. 2008. Unresolved issues in the management of ulcers of the foot in diabetes. *Diabet Med* 25 (12):1380-9.

Kallarackal, G. U., E. A. Ansari, N. Amos, J. C. Martin, C. Lane, and J. P. Camilleri. 2002. A comparative study to assess the clinical use of Fluorescein Meniscus Time (FMT) with Tear Break up Time (TBUT) and Schirmer's tests (ST) in the diagnosis of dry eyes. *Eye (Lond)* 16 (5):594-600.

Katz, M. H., A. F. Alvarez, R. S. Kirsner, W. H. Eaglstein, and V. Falanga. 1991. Human wound fluid from acute wounds stimulates fibroblast and endothelial cell growth. *J Am Acad Dermatol* 25 (6 Pt 1):1054-8.

Ladwig, G. P., M. C. Robson, R. Liu, M. A. Kuhn, D. F. Muir, and G. S. Schultz. 2002. Ratios of activated matrix metalloproteinase-9 to tissue inhibitor of matrix metalloproteinase-1 in wound fluids are inversely correlated with healing of pressure ulcers. *Wound Repair Regen* 10 (1):26-37.

Liu, Y., D. Min, T. Bolton, V. Nube, S. M. Twigg, D. K. Yue, and S. V. McLennan. 2009. Increased matrix metalloproteinase-9 predicts poor wound healing in diabetic foot ulcers. *Diabetes Care* 32 (1):117-9.

Lobmann, R., A. Ambrosch, G. Schultz, K. Waldmann, S. Schiweck, and H. Lehnert. 2002. Expression of matrix-metalloproteinases and their inhibitors in the wounds of diabetic and non-diabetic patients. *Diabetologia* 45 (7):1011-6.

Lobmann, R., C. Zemlin, M. Motzkau, K. Reschke, and H. Lehnert. 2006. Expression of matrix metalloproteinases and growth factors in diabetic foot wounds treated with a protease absorbent dressing. *J Diabetes Complications* 20 (5):329-35.

Löffler, M., D. Zieker, J. Weinreich, S. Lob, I. Königsrainer, S. Symons, S. Bühler, A. Königsrainer, H. Northoff, and S. Beckert. 2011. Wound fluid lactate concentration: a helpful marker for diagnosing soft-tissue infection in diabetic foot ulcers? Preliminary findings. *Diabet Med* 28 (2):175-8.

Mabilleau, G., N. Petrova, M. E. Edmonds, and A. Sabokbar. 2011. Number of circulating CD14-positive cells and the serum levels of TNF-alpha are raised in acute charcot foot. *Diabetes Care* 34 (3):e33.

Makarov, D. V., S. Loeb, R. H. Getzenberg, and A. W. Partin. 2009. Biomarkers for prostate cancer. *Annu Rev Med* 60:139-51.

Mani, R. 1999. Science of measurements in wound healing. *Wound Repair Regen* 7 (5):330-4. Mast, B. A., and G. S. Schultz. 1996. Interactions of cytokines, growth factors, and proteases in acute and chronic wounds. *Wound Repair Regen* 4 (4):411-20.

Mellergard, P., O. Aneman, F. Sjogren, P. Pettersson, and J. Hillman. 2008. Changes in extracellular concentrations of some cytokines, chemokines, and neurotrophic factors after insertion of intracerebral microdialysis catheters in neurosurgical patients. *Neurosurgery* 62 (1):151-7; discussion 157-8.

Moor, A. N., D. J. Vachon, and L. J. Gould. 2009. Proteolytic activity in wound fluids and tissues derived from chronic venous leg ulcers. *Wound Repair Regen* 17 (6):832-9.

Moseley, R., J. E. Stewart, P. Stephens, R. J. Waddington, and D. W. Thomas. 2004. Extracellular matrix metabolites as potential biomarkers of disease activity in wound fluid: lessons learned from other inflammatory diseases? *Br J Dermatol* 150 (3):401-13.

Mueller, C., B. Muller, and A. P. Perruchoud. 2008. Biomarkers: past, present, and future. *Swiss Med Wkly* 138 (15-16):225-9.

Muller, M., C. Trocme, B. Lardy, F. Morel, S. Halimi, and P. Y. Benhamou. 2008. Matrix metalloproteinases and diabetic foot ulcers: the ratio of MMP-1 to TIMP-1 is a predictor of wound healing. *Diabet Med* 25 (4):419-26.

Mwaura, B., B. Mahendran, N. Hynes, D. Defreitas, G. Avalos, T. Adegbola, M. Adham, C. E. Connolly, and S. Sultan. 2006. The impact of differential expression of extracellular matrix metalloproteinase inducer, matrix metalloproteinase-2, tissue inhibitor of matrix metalloproteinase-2 and PDGF-AA on the chronicity of venous leg ulcers. *Eur J Vasc Endovasc Surg* 31 (3):306-10.

Naguib, G., H. Al-Mashat, T. Desta, and D. T. Graves. 2004. Diabetes prolongs the inflammatory response to a bacterial stimulus through cytokine dysregulation. *J Invest Dermatol* 123 (1):87-92.

Noble-Bell, G., and A. Forbes. 2008. A systematic review of the effectiveness of negative pressure wound therapy in the management of diabetes foot ulcers. *Int Wound J* 5 (2):233-42.

Nwomeh, B. C., D. R. Yager, and I. K. Cohen. 1998. Physiology of the chronic wound. *Clin Plast Surg* 25 (3):341-56.

Ono, I., H. Gunji, K. Suda, K. Iwatsuki, and F. Kaneko. 1994. Evaluation of cytokines in donor site wound fluids. *Scand J Plast Reconstr Surg Hand Surg* 28 (4):269-73.

Oono, T., Y. Fujiwara, T. Yoshioka, and J. Arata. 1997. Prolidase activity in chronic wound and blister fluids. *J Dermatol* 24 (10):626-9.

Ortega, M. R., T. Ganz, and S. M. Milner. 2000. Human beta defensin is absent in burn blister fluid. *Burns* 26 (8):724-6.

Pepys, M. B., and G. M. Hirschfield. 2003. C-reactive protein: a critical update. *J Clin Invest* 111 (12):1805-12.

Phillips, T. J., H. O. al-Amoudi, M. Leverkus, and H. Y. Park. 1998. Effect of chronic wound fluid on fibroblasts. *J Wound Care* 7 (10):527-32.

Prompers, L., M. Huijberts, N. Schaper, J. Apelqvist, K. Bakker, M. Edmonds, P. Holstein, E. Jude, A. Jirkovska, D. Mauricio, A. Piaggesi, H. Reike, M. Spraul, K. Van Acker, S. Van Baal, F. Van Merode, L. Uccioli, V. Urbancic, and G. Ragnarson Tennvall. 2008. Resource utilisation and costs associated with the treatment of diabetic foot ulcers. Prospective data from the Eurodiale Study. *Diabetologia* 51 (10):1826-34.

Pukstad, B. S., L. Ryan, T. H. Flo, J. Stenvik, R. Moseley, K. Harding, D. W. Thomas, and T. Espevik. 2010. Non-healing is associated with persistent stimulation of the innate immune response in chronic venous leg ulcers. *J Dermatol Sci* 59 (2):115-22.

Rayment, E. A., Z. Upton, and G. K. Shooter. 2008. Increased matrix metalloproteinase-9 (MMP-9) activity observed in chronic wound fluid is related to the clinical severity of the ulcer. *Br J Dermatol* 158 (5):951-61.

Richard, J. L., A. Sotto, and J. P. Lavigne. 2011. New insights in diabetic foot infection. *World J Diabetes* 2 (2):24-32.

Schilling, J. A., W. Joel, and H. M. Shurley. 1959. Wound healing: a comparative study of the histochemical changes in granulation tissue contained in stainless steel wire mesh and polyvinyl sponge cylinders. *Surgery* 46:702-10.

Schirmer, O. 1903. Studien zur Physiologie und Pathologie der Traenenabsonderung und Traenenabfuhr. *Graefes Arch Klin Exp Ophthalmol* 56 (2):197-291.

Schmidtchen, A. 2000. Degradation of antiproteinases, complement and fibronectin in chronic leg ulcers. *Acta Derm Venereol* 80 (3):179-84.

Schroder, K., and J. Tschopp. 2010. The inflammasomes. *Cell* 140 (6):821-32.

Seah, C. C., T. J. Phillips, C. E. Howard, I. P. Panova, C. M. Hayes, A. S. Asandra, and H. Y. Park. 2005. Chronic wound fluid suppresses proliferation of dermal fibroblasts through a Ras-mediated signaling pathway. *J Invest Dermatol* 124 (2):466-74.

Simonsen, L., P. Holstein, K. Larsen, and J. Bulow. 1998. Glucose metabolism in chronic diabetic foot ulcers measured in vivo using microdialysis. *Clin Physiol* 18 (4):355-9.

Stenken, J. A., M. K. Church, C. A. Gill, and G. F. Clough. 2010. How minimally invasive is microdialysis sampling? A cautionary note for cytokine collection in human skin and other clinical studies. *AAPS J* 12 (1):73-8.

Stoll, D. 2004. Microarray technology: an increasing variety of screening tools for proteomic research. *Drug Discovery Today: TARGETS* 3 (1):24-31.

Swain, A., J. Turton, C. L. Scudamore, I. Pereira, N. Viswanathan, R. Smyth, M. Munday, F. McClure, M. Gandhi, S. Sondh, and M. York. 2011. Urinary biomarkers in hexachloro-1:3-butadiene-induced acute kidney injury in the female Hanover Wistar rat; correlation of alpha-glutathione S-transferase, albumin and kidney injury molecule-1 with histopathology and gene expression. *J Appl Toxicol* 31 (4):366-77.

Tarnuzzer, R. W., and G. S. Schultz. 1996. Biochemical analysis of acute and chronic wound environments. *Wound Repair Regen* 4 (3):321-5.

Tecilazich, F., T. Dinh, and A. Veves. 2011. Treating diabetic ulcers. *Expert Opin Pharmacother* 12 (4):593-606.

Templin, M. F., D. Stoll, J. Bachmann, and T. O. Joos. 2004. Protein microarrays and multiplexed sandwich immunoassays: what beats the beads? *Comb Chem High Throughput Screen* 7 (3):223-9.

Tilg, H., E. Trehu, M. B. Atkins, C. A. Dinarello, and J. W. Mier. 1994. Interleukin-6 (IL-6) as an anti-inflammatory cytokine: induction of circulating IL-1 receptor antagonist and soluble tumor necrosis factor receptor p55. *Blood* 83 (1):113-8.

Trengove, N. J., H. Bielefeldt-Ohmann, and M. C. Stacey. 2000. Mitogenic activity and cytokine levels in non-healing and healing chronic leg ulcers. *Wound Repair Regen* 8 (1):13-25.

Trengove, N. J., S. R. Langton, and M. C. Stacey. 1996. Biochemical analysis of wound fluid from nonhealing and healing chronic leg ulcers. *Wound Repair Regen* 4 (2):234-9.

Trengove, N. J., M. C. Stacey, S. MacAuley, N. Bennett, J. Gibson, F. Burslem, G. Murphy, and G. Schultz. 1999. Analysis of the acute and chronic wound environments: the role of proteases and their inhibitors. *Wound Repair Regen* 7 (6):442-52.

Tuschil, A., C. Lam, A. Haslberger, and I. Lindley. 1992. Interleukin-8 stimulates calcium transients and promotes epidermal cell proliferation. *J Invest Dermatol* 99 (3):294-8.

Uzun, G., E. Solmazgul, H. Curuksulu, V. Turhan, N. Ardic, C. Top, S. Yildiz, and M. Cimsit. 2007. Procalcitonin as a diagnostic aid in diabetic foot infections. *Tohoku J Exp Med* 213 (4):305-12.

Velnar, T., T. Bailey, and V. Smrkolj. 2009. The wound healing process: an overview of the cellular and molecular mechanisms. *J Int Med Res* 37 (5):1528-42.

Wagner, S., S. Coerper, J. Fricke, T. K. Hunt, Z. Hussain, M. W. Elmlinger, J. E. Mueller, and H. D. Becker. 2003. Comparison of inflammatory and systemic sources of growth factors in acute and chronic human wounds. *Wound Repair Regen* 11 (4):253-60.

Wall, I. B., R. Moseley, D. M. Baird, D. Kipling, P. Giles, I. Laffafian, P. E. Price, D. W. Thomas, and P. Stephens. 2008. Fibroblast dysfunction is a key factor in the non-healing of chronic venous leg ulcers. *J Invest Dermatol* 128 (10):2526-40.

Wallace, H. J., and M. C. Stacey. 1998. Levels of tumor necrosis factor-alpha (TNF-alpha) and soluble TNF receptors in chronic venous leg ulcers--correlations to healing status. *J Invest Dermatol* 110 (3):292-6.

Weckroth, M., A. Vaheri, J. Lauharanta, T. Sorsa, and Y. T. Konttinen. 1996. Matrix metalloproteinases, gelatinase and collagenase, in chronic leg ulcers. *J Invest Dermatol* 106 (5):1119-24.

Weigelt, C., B. Rose, U. Poschen, D. Ziegler, G. Friese, K. Kempf, W. Koenig, S. Martin, and C. Herder. 2009. Immune mediators in patients with acute diabetic foot syndrome. *Diabetes Care* 32 (8):1491-6.

Widgerow, A. D. 2011. Chronic wound fluid--thinking outside the box. *Wound Repair Regen* 19 (3):287-91.

Williams, D. T., J. R. Hilton, and K. G. Harding. 2004. Diagnosing foot infection in diabetes. *Clin Infect Dis* 39 Suppl 2:S83-6.

Wound infection in clinical practice. An international consensus. 2008. *Int Wound J* 5 Suppl 3:iii-11.

Wysocki, A. B., and F. Grinnell. 1990. Fibronectin profiles in normal and chronic wound fluid. *Lab Invest* 63 (6):825-31.

Wysocki, A. B., A. O. Kusakabe, S. Chang, and T. L. Tuan. 1999. Temporal expression of urokinase plasminogen activator, plasminogen activator inhibitor and gelatinase-B in chronic wound fluid switches from a chronic to acute wound profile with progression to healing. *Wound Repair Regen* 7 (3):154-65.

Xu, L., S. V. McLennan, L. Lo, A. Natfaji, T. Bolton, Y. Liu, S. M. Twigg, and D. K. Yue. 2007. Bacterial load predicts healing rate in neuropathic diabetic foot ulcers. *Diabetes Care* 30 (2):378-80.

Yager, D. R., R. A. Kulina, and L. A. Gilman. 2007. Wound fluids: a window into the wound environment? *Int J Low Extrem Wounds* 6 (4):262-72.

Yager, D. R., L. Y. Zhang, H. X. Liang, R. F. Diegelmann, and I. K. Cohen. 1996. Wound fluids from human pressure ulcers contain elevated matrix metalloproteinase levels and activity compared to surgical wound fluids. *J Invest Dermatol* 107 (5):743-8.

5

Wound Measurement in Diabetic Foot Ulceration

Julia Shaw and Patrick M. Bell
Regional Centre for Endocrinology and Diabetes, Royal Victoria Hospital, Belfast United Kingdom

1. Introduction

In this chapter the authors aim to provide a brief introduction to wound assessment in the diabetic foot and discuss the role of wound measurement within that assessment process. A literature review describing wound measurement in diabetic foot wounds was conducted and a review of wound measurement tools and techniques reported. The results of a wound measurement study using a particular technique and the importance of wound measurement in clinical practice is discussed. Conclusions are drawn and a way forward is suggested.

The prevalence of diabetes worldwide was estimated to be 2.8% in 2000 rising to 4.4% in 2030. The total number of people with diabetes is projected to rise from 171 million in 2000 to 366 million in 2030 (Wilde et al, 2004). As diabetes is the most frequent cause of non-traumatic amputation in the developed world, it is likely that there will be a significant impact on patients' health, their carers and health care systems. Progress has been made in recent years to manage risk factors associated with diabetic foot ulceration and to manage infection, ischaemia and glycaemic control. Multidisciplinary assessment, treatment and education programmes have been developed to prevent damage to insensitive feet. Healing rates and outcomes related to diabetic foot ulceration have been studied by many investigators and various wound measurement techniques have been employed in the quest to quantify outcomes. Outcomes in terms of ulcer healing have been based on ulcer area, ulcer duration and ulcer grade (from the superficial abrasion to the ulcer presenting with exposed bone in the wound base, necrosis, infection and/ or osteomyelitis). Initial wound measurement and regular monitoring is a useful tool in the assessment of treatment effectiveness (Vowden and Vowden, 2005, Gethin, 2006).

2. Wound assessment and the role of wound measurement

Wound assessment is complex and multi-faceted. It includes wound appearance, wound aetiology, prediction and monitoring of healing rates, identification of factors delaying healing and wound documentation. Wound measurement is an important component of this and has the potential to provide baseline measurements and accurately determine the percentage reduction/increase in wound area over time.

In any study involving wound measurement there are key concepts to be considered:

1. Accuracy. This is the ability of the measuring tool to measure the true size of an object.
2. Validity. The ability of the measuring tool to measure what it is intended to measure.
3. Repeatability/test-retest reliability. The ability of the measuring tool to repeat an accurate measurement on more than one occasion with consistency.
4. Reliability and Inter-rater reliability. The consistency of results obtained using the device when used by one or more than one operator.
5. Usability. Do users find the tool convenient, effective and easy to use? (Fette, 2006).

For a measurement tool to be successful it must satisfy these criteria and demonstrate reliability in its application. Failure to do so will result in inappropriate data. In the case of wound measurement systems the most common means of assessing the reliability of a system are test-retest reliability and inter-rater reliability (Gilman, 1990).

Ideally the outcome of any treatment regimen in the management of diabetic foot wounds is complete wound closure. It has been suggested that the ability to measure a percentage area reduction may be important in differentiating between healing and non-healing wounds, and that it is also important for the evaluation of the efficacy of different treatment regimens ((Kantor and Margolis, 2000; Flanagan, 2003; Sheehan et al, 2003; Gethin, 2006; Papazoglou et al, 2010). In wound management, three types of outcome are important: therapeutic efficacy, value for money and patient satisfaction (Gallagher, 2003). Oyibo et al (2001) in a study of diabetic foot ulcers (n=194) investigated the effect of ulcer size and site, patients' age, sex and type/duration of diabetes on the eventual outcome. They found that ulcer area correlated well with healing time, but age, sex, type and duration of diabetes did not affect outcome. They concluded that ulcer area could be a useful predictor of ulcer outcome. This is supported by the work of several authors who concluded that percentage change in ulcer area at 4 weeks was a robust predictor of healing in diabetic foot wounds (Flanagan, 2003; Sheehan et al, 2003; Gethin, 2006; Papazoglou et al, 2010).

3. Wound measurement tools and techniques

A broad search of the literature was conducted to identify search terms and filters that could be used to yield studies specific to wound measurement tools and techniques in wound healing overall and more specifically in diabetic foot wounds. The electronic databases used to identify papers relevant to this review were Pubmed, Medline, and Cinahl (1989-2011). Secondary hand searching was also carried out using relevant journal articles and reference lists, books, and conference proceedings. Papers were included if they reported on trials describing and comparing wound measurement methods and tools. Papers were excluded if they were not written in English.

Quantifying the size of the wound is an important component of wound assessment and has the potential to provide baseline measurements and accurately determine the percentage reduction/increase in wound area over time (Flanagan, 2003; Margolis et al, 2003). There are many methods of wound measurement and each possesses advantages and disadvantages. The ideal tool has been described by Polit & Hungler (1995) as

"one that gives rise to results that are relevant, accurate, unbiased, sensitive, uni-dimensional and efficient".

Wound measurement techniques can be categorised as contact or non-contact in their application. Contact techniques include acetate tracing of the wound, the use of depth gauges, and volume measurement using casts or saline. Non-contact techniques involve the use of structured light and lasers, photography, video image analysis, magnetic resonance imaging and stereophotogrammetry (Williams, 1997). These tools and techniques are described, discussed and compared in detail.

3.1 Simple wound measurement

Simple wound measurement methods include those techniques that use either a length and width measurement or a wound tracing to calculate surface wound area. To determine wound surface area there are two important issues: the identification of the wound margin (typically using a wound tracing or alternatively a digital image) and the calculation of wound area.

It is essential that the wound margin is clearly identified prior to measurement regardless of the measurement tool used. The appearance of the wound may be affected by various factors all of which may influence accurate measurement:

1. Haemorrhage following debridement.
2. The presence of infection and undermining of the wound edges.
3. The presence of excess wound exudate and evidence of maceration of the surrounding skin.

The wound edge may be described clinically as the area where normal skin converts to tissue which is red, yellow or black in colour. Normal skin may be macerated and white in appearance, or there may be lilac coloured tissue (new epithelial tissue) at the leading edge of the wound.

Identification of the wound edge may be difficult and is largely determined by the subjective assessment of the observer who performs the measurement (Plassmann & Jones, 1992; Plassmann et al, 1994; Plassmann, 1995).

Current practice focuses on wound measurement using a simple length and width measurement to calculate surface wound area. This is a crude measurement. Surface wound area is calculated by multiplying the maximum perpendicular length by the maximum width of the wound bed and is typically recorded in cm^2 (Flanagan, 2003). The major flaw in the method is that it is subjective and normally over-estimates wound area by approximately twenty five percent (Majeske, 1992; Dealey, 1994; Goldman and Salcido, 2002; Rodgers et al 2010). This method does not take into account irregularities in the shape of the wound or wound depth. Advantages, however, include ease of use and low cost.

Wound area can also be determined by tracing the outline of the wound (wound circumference) onto a transparent sheet or graph paper divided into 1cm squares. Wound area can then be calculated by manually counting the squares within the "wound". Griffin et al (1993) compared photographic and transparency-based methods for measuring wound area and concluded that both methods provided equally reliable measurements, but that the transparency method was more economical in time and equipment requirements. This is also a subjective measurement and the identification of the actual wound edges can be difficult. The process does not provide information on the 3-dimensional aspect of the wound nor on wound volume and depth. It is also recognised that tracing of the wound edges is where the greatest source of error occurs (Kantor and Margolis, 1998). This is largely dependent on the experience of the clinician (Flanagan, 2003). The main advantage of wound tracing however is that it takes into account body curvature and irregularities of wound circumference.

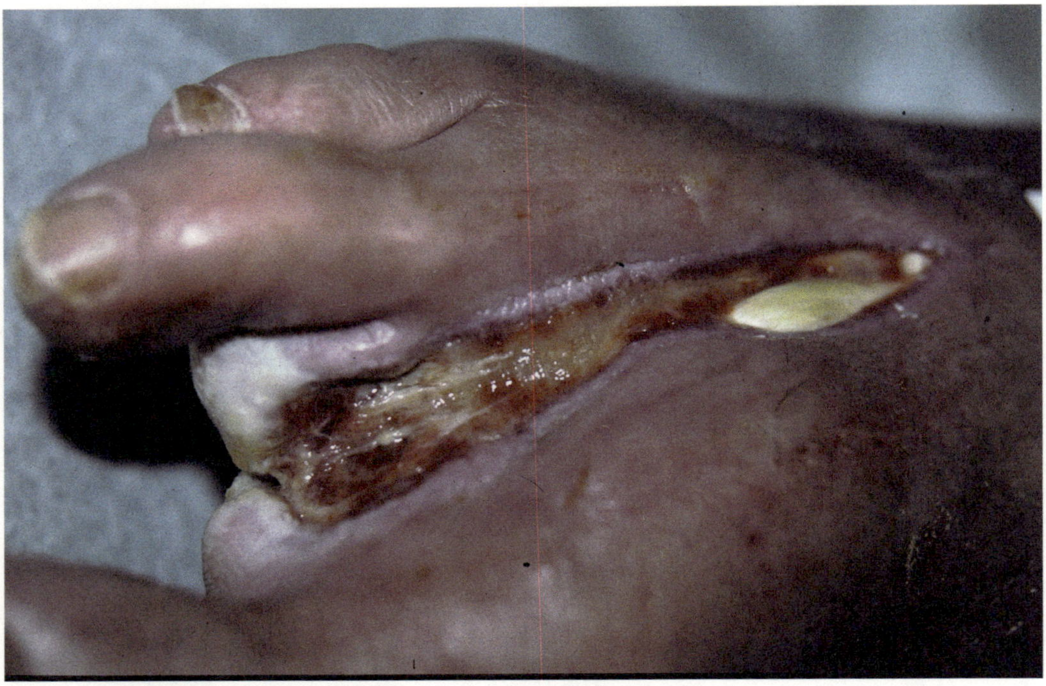

Fig. 1. Photograph illustrating the various types of tissue used to identify the wound edge in a diabetic foot wound

3.2 Mathematical models

It is recognised that simple wound surface area measurements (length x width) are likely to over-estimate the area of the wound by approximately twenty five percent (Goldman and Salcido, 2002). Ruler based schemes tend to be less reliable in wounds >5cm^2 (Oien et al, 2002). Accuracy may be improved by tracing the wound to compensate for body curvature, but this can be difficult to perform in certain areas e.g. the heel. In 1989 Kundin developed the wound gauge to calculate wound area (wound length x width x 0.785) and wound volume (wound area x depth x 0.327). This method appeared to be accurate in the measurement of small wounds but consistently underestimated the size of larger or irregularly shaped wounds (Thomas and Wysocki, 1990).

Oien et al (2002) and Johnson (1995) proposed that various mathematical formulae can be used to improve accuracy in the calculation of wound surface area and volume. They recognised that most foot wounds presented as spherical or elliptical in nature, and that the area of these wounds could be determined using recognised standard mathematical formulae and a wound tracing. This is also likely to produce some over-estimation of ulcer size but less error than the simple area calculation using length and width only (Goldman and Salcido, 2002).

The use of the elliptical method of wound measurement was described by Shaw et al (2007). In a study of measurement of diabetic foot ulcers, wounds were traced, measured with a ruler and the standard formula for the calculation of the area of an ellipse was applied. The surface area was calculated by taking the radius of the longest side of the ellipse (wound), multiplying it by the radius of the shortest side of the ellipse (wound), at 90^0 to the longest side and multiplying that value by π (where $\pi = 3.14$) and r is the radius measurement.

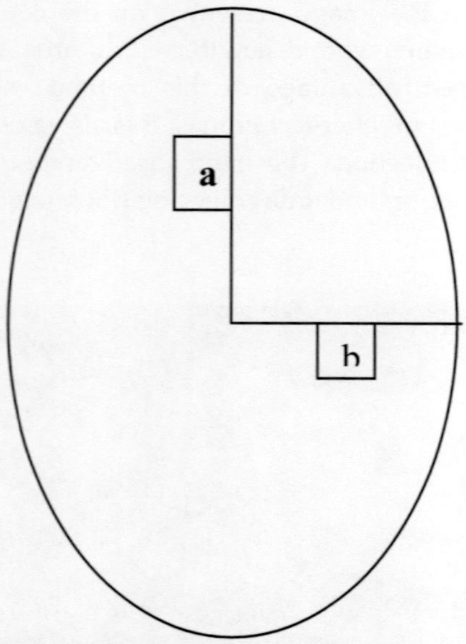

Fig. 2. The area (of the ellipse) is calculated using the formula πab

Johnson (1995) described various mathematical formulae to measure circular, elliptical and irregular wounds. He suggested that if wounds present with an irregular shape, 8 radii can be identified, each taken approximately 45^0 from the next radius and results can be approximated to actual values. The formulae to calculate the surface area is as follows:

$$(r1^2+r2^2.....r8^2)(\pi /8)$$

3.3 Wound planimetry

Wound planimetry is defined as the precise measurement of the area contained within a wound tracing or a digital image (Flanagan, 2003). This measurement can be carried out using a mechanical planimeter or by using an appropriate software package and a digital image. Oien et al (2002) compared four methods of wound measurement in 20 patients with leg and foot ulcers (n=50) of mixed aetiology. Techniques included mechanical planimetry (using a hand held device), digital planimetry, square counting approximations and simple length x width measurements. All methods demonstrated a high degree of agreement for smaller wounds (<10cm^2) but differences occurred as wound size increased. The simple length x width measurement was reported to be the least reliable measure of ulcer size followed by square counting and mechanical planimetry. Digital planimetry was the most reliable of the methods described (Oien et al, 2002).

3.4 Stereophotogrammetry and light techniques

The availability of both contact and non contact methods of wound measurement have already been alluded to. Stereophotogrammetry is a non-contact technique where a stereo camera linked to a computer captures an image of the wound (Plassmann & Jones 1992; Langemo et al, 1998). The image is downloaded to the computer and the wound manually traced with the mouse from the image presented on the computer monitor screen. The software package then calculates wound length, width, area and volume. Langemo et al (1998) reported that the main advantage of this method was that it produced highly reproducible results compared to other techniques. It is also a non-contact technique, and so minimises the risk of cross-infection. The main disadvantage however is that it is time consuming both in terms of set-up and data collection (Plassmann and Jones, 1992).

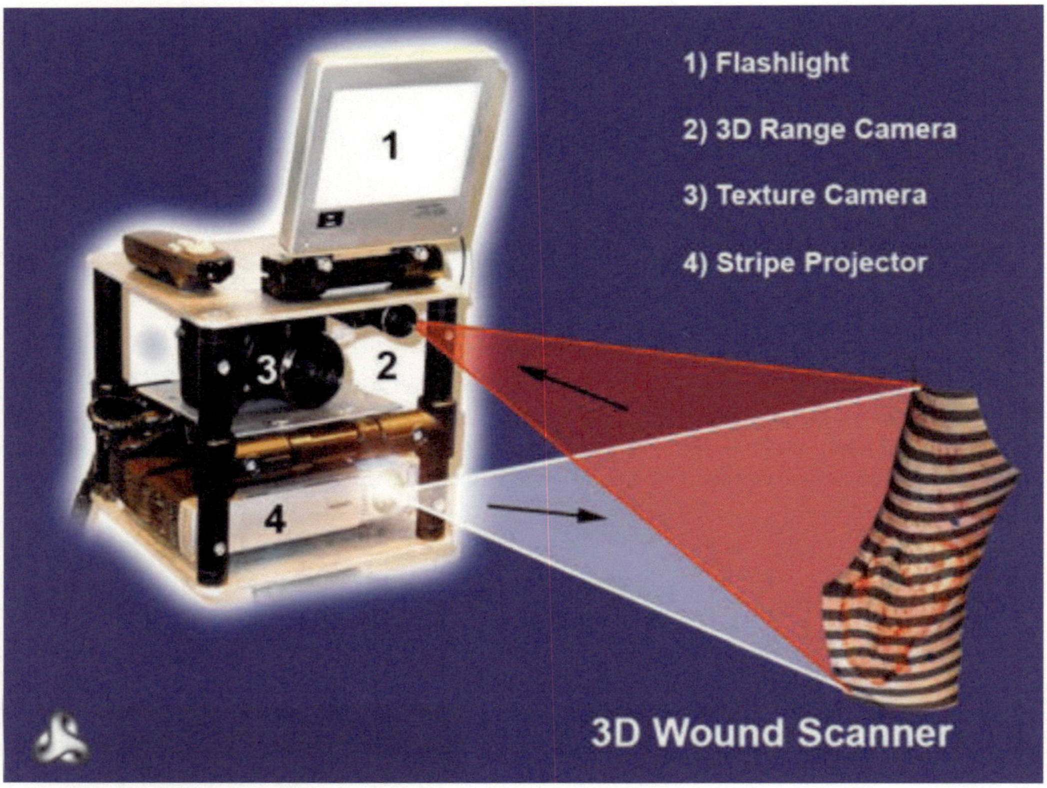

Fig. 3. Illustration of stereophotogrammetry.

A further non-contact method utilising light has been described by Plassmann and Jones,1992; and Melhuish et al, 1994. This structured light triangulation method involves use of a beam of structured light aimed at 45° to the wound. Analysis of the image carried out by computer software provides a 3-dimensional map of the wound allowing accurate measurement of wound area, wound circumference and wound volume. Repeated measurements using this method reported results with a mean error of less than 5% and so it was deemed to be an accurate way of objectively determining the wound boundary and calculating wound area. Melhuish et al (1994) demonstrated a direct correlation between wound circumference and wound area, and wound circumference and wound volume. The authors suggested that it was possible to accurately monitor wound healing by measuring circumference alone, as this measurement was directly linked to both volume and area.

4. Comparison of techniques

None of the methods of wound measurement described is perfect. Clinicians are expected to provide high quality, cost-effective, evidence-based wound care and so the standardisation of wound measurement methods may have important implications for research into the effects of treatments, drugs and disease (Kundin, 1989).

4.1 Simple measurement

Mayrovitz (1997) investigated shape and area measurement in the assessment of diabetic plantar ulcers (n=83). The accuracy of area calculations based on elliptical and rectangular shapes was considered and based on the maximum length and maximum width of the wounds studied. Overall error for both methods was similar with the elliptical model overestimating area (by 10%), and the rectangular method underestimating the area (by 12%) when compared to conventional wound tracing over a sixteen week period. This is in contrast to the results reported by Majeske in 1992, and Goldman and Salcido (2002) who reported that wound area measurement using a simple length and width calculation overestimated wound area by approximately twenty five percent.

4.2 Mathematical models

Gilman (1999) favoured a more complex mathematical model for wound measurement. He argued that in many wound studies there were always wounds of varying sizes and shapes, and so a valid comparison of healing was difficult. He proposed using a mathematical model that described the average distance of advance of the wound margin towards the wound centre over time. This was illustrated in wounds that closed in a uniform and non-uniform way. Bowling et al (2009) reported a strong correlation between elliptical wound measurement and an image processing system in a series of 36 diabetic foot wounds, examined over a 12 week period.

4.3 Wound planimetry

Kantor and Margolis (1998) reported a good correlation between planimetric wound area and wound width, length, width x length, perimeter and area based on the formula for an ellipse. The values for all correlation coefficients were greater than 0.8 for wounds that were less than 40cm^2 in size.

4.4 Stereophotogrammetry and light techniques

In keeping with the work carried out by Mayrovitz (1997), Langemo et al (1998, 2001) compared linear length and width using several methods: a ruler, planimetry, computerised stereophotogrammetry (SPG) length and width and computerised SPG area. They found that the most reliable method was SPG area measurement followed by computerised planimetry. These authors noted that conventional length x width measurement produced the greatest variability in wound area measurement.

The above work was further supported by Lagan et al (2000), who compared the reliability of direct and photographic tracings analysed by planimetry and digital techniques in the measurement of various wound types. The level of repeatability of these methods and the level of variability in wound size was investigated. There was increased variability using planimetry compared to digital techniques and planimetry produced lower readings for wound measurement overall.

Shaw et al (2007) evaluated and compared three wound measurement techniques: the Visitrak system using acetate tracings and planimetry (Smyth and Nephew Healthcare, Hull UK), a digital photography and image processing system (Analyse, Version 6.0; Analyse Direct, Lenexa, KS) and a wound tracing and elliptical measurement method using the standard formula (πab) for the calculation of the area of an ellipse. These methods were used to measure wound surface area for a series of diabetic foot wounds (n=16), of greater than four weeks duration.

Validity within each measurement method was determined using a one-sample t test. Repeatability within each method was investigated by calculating a coefficient of variation (CV) for each wound measurement. An ANOVA was used to complete a calculation of comparability between the methods. A paired t- test was used to examine differences between the elliptical and Visitrak methods.

Validity varied across the three methods but was considered to be acceptable. The Visitrak method measured images <25mm^2 inaccurately and the elliptical method of measurement tended to underestimate size in small wounds. The image processing method was inaccurate for both large and small wounds. Repeatability was acceptable across the three methods. The mean CV for all wounds was calculated as 7.0 for Visitrak, 4.7 for image processing, and 8.5 for the elliptical method. No one method was more repeatable than another. An analysis of comparability between the methods indicated variability particularly between the Visitrak and elliptical methods . The main limitations of the study are that the sample size was small and conclusions can only be drawn for diabetic foot wounds.

5. Implications for clinical practice

Ideally the outcome of any treatment regimen in the management of diabetic foot wounds is complete wound closure. The ability to measure a percentage area reduction may be important in differentiating between healing and non-healing wounds, and for the evaluation of the efficacy of different treatment regimens. Several authors have described the importance of regular wound measurement and reported that a percentage change in wound area over a 4 week period of 30% or more, reliably predicted wound healing (Kantor and Margolis, 2000; Sheehan et al, 2003; Gethin, 2006; Papazoglou et al, 2010).

6. Discussion

Historically wound measurement techniques have focussed on 2-dimensional methods using linear measurement, wound tracings and photography for wound assessment in the clinical setting (Langemo et al, 1998). To date there is still no standardised, universally accepted method with the method chosen largely depending on the level of accuracy required. If a broad indication of wound size is required then a simple technique that is minimally invasive, fast and comfortable for the patient may be adequate. If a more accurate measurement is required (for example in a research study or to enable clinicians to predict wound healing), a more robust method is necessary. Any wound measurement technique has to demonstrate that it is accurate, repeatable and capable of influencing patient care in a positive, cost-effective manner. This can be aided when used in conjunction with a wound measurement protocol (Plassmann and Peters, 2001). Clinicians will inevitably be influenced by the ease of use of a particular tool and efficient use of clinical time.

Simple ruler-based methods provide a crude wound measurement that overestimates wound area by twenty five percent. Complex mathematical models may not be useful for busy clinicians unless incorporated into appropriate software packages that are quick and easy to use. However simple formulae such as those discussed earlier to calculate the area of an ellipse can be used easily in conjunction with wound tracings. The main advantages of this method were that it was quick, easy to use, and non-invasive and that it considered body curvature. Limitations of this method are recognised in that there may be an overestimation of wound area by around 10% (Mayrovitz, 1997). However, diabetic foot wounds are often spherical or elliptical in nature, and Shaw et al (2007) have shown that this is a valid and repeatable method of measurement to use in this group of patients. In contrast in this study, the elliptical method was shown to underestimate wound size compared to tracing and planimetry (Visitrak system) and an image processing system.

Wound planimetry can be carried out within a wound tracing or a digital image. Measurement of wound area is reported to be most accurate in smaller wounds $<10cm^2$. The main advantages of the Visitrak method was that it was quick, easy to use, non-invasive, it considered body curvature and the subjectivity of manually counting squares was removed. The main disadvantage was that it tended to underestimate wound size compared to the elliptical method and was inaccurate in the measurement of wounds $<25mm^2$ (Shaw et al, 2007).

Digital imaging takes considerable time and studies seldom show the total time to capture the image, transfer the image from the camera to the computer, and then calibrate and measure the wound. Computerised methods may be more accurate, but their use is limited due to availability, complicated calibration procedures, cost and clinician time (Plassmann and Jones, 1992; Xiang Liu et al 2006). The advantages of digital imaging are that it facilitates unique calibration at each wound measurement and subjective wound tracing is eliminated. However the accuracy of results does depend on the investigator's ability to take a high quality image in the first instance and the accurate identification of the wound edge from the image. Many additional factors also require management such as lighting, environment and the distance of the camera from the foot. This method clearly has great potential, but depends largely on the clinicians' ability to identify the wound margin accurately, as well as the influence of practical factors in the clinical environment.

7. Conclusions and the way forward

Various methods of wound surface area measurement have been described, and the advantages and disadvantages of each have been discussed. It is essential that an appropriate method is chosen if diabetic foot wounds are to be measured accurately as well as to provide robust results in research wound healing studies.

Historically wound measurement techniques have focussed on 2-dimensional methods using linear measurement, wound tracings and photography for wound assessment in the clinical setting. To date there is still no standardised, universally accepted method used. Digital imaging and computerised methods take considerable time and can be costly and complex mathematical models may not be useful for busy clinicians unless incorporated into appropriate software packages that are quick and easy to use. Computer software that automatically identifies the wound edge thus increasing accuracy and speed of measurement would be a major step forward.

8. References

Bowling FL, King L, Fadavi H, Paterson JA, Preece K, Daniel RW, Matthews DJ, Boulton AJ (2009). An assessment of the accuracy and usability of a novel optical wound measurement system. *Diabetic Medicine,* Jan; 26 (1) pp. 93-96.

Dealey C (1994). *The Care of Wounds.* Blackwell Scientific Publications, Oxford. pp. 76-80.

Fette A (2006). A clinimetric analysis of wound measurement tools. Available from http:// www.worldwide wounds.com/2006/January/Fette Accessed 7/6/2011.

Flanagan M, (2003). Wound Measurement: can it help us to monitor progression to healing? *Journal of Wound Care,* **12**(5), pp. 189-194.

Gallagher S, (2003). Tools of outcome measurement in WOCN practice. *Journal of Wound, Ostomy and Continence Nurses,* **30**, pp. 7-10.

Gethin G, (2006). The importance of continuous wound measuring. *Wounds UK* .2 (2) pp. 60-68.

Gilman TH, (1990). Parameter for measurements of wound closure. *Wounds,* 2(3), pp. 95-101.

Goldman RJ, Salcido R, (2002). More than one way to measure a wound: an overview of tools and techniques. *Advances in Skin and Wound Care,* Sept/Oct, pp. 236-242.Griffin JW, Tolley EA, Tooms RE, Reyes RA, Clifft JK, (1993). A comparison of photographic and transparency-based methods for measuring wound surface area. *Physical Therapy,* 73(2), pp. 117-122.

Johnson JD, (1995). Using ulcer surface area and volume to document wound size. *Journal of the American Podiatric Medical Association,* 85(2), pp. 91-95.

Kantor J, Margolis DJ, (1998). Efficacy and prognostic value of simple wound measurements. *Archives of Dermatology,* 134, pp. 1571-1574.

Kundin JI (1989) A new way to size up a wound. *Am J Nursing.* 89, pp.206-7

Lagan KM, Dusoir AE, McDonagh SM, Baxter D, (2000). Wound Measurement: The comparative reliability of direct versus photographic tracings analysed by planimetry versus digitising techniques. *Archives of Physical Medicine and Rehabilitation,* 81, pp. 1110-1116.

Langemo DK, Melland H, Hanson D, Olson B, Hunter S, Henly SJ, (2001). Comparison of 2 wound volume measurement methods. *Advanced Wound Care,* 14, pp. 190-196.

Liu X, Kim X, Schmidt R, Drerup B, Song J, (2006). Wound measurement by curvature maps: a feasibility study. *Physiological Measurement* 27 pp. 1107-1123.

Majeske C, (1992). Reliability of wound surface area measurements. *Physical Therapy,* 72(2), pp. 138-141.

Margolis DJ, Hoffstad O, Gelfand JM, Berlin JA, (2003). Surrogate end points for the treatment of diabetic neuropathic foot ulcers. *Diabetes Care,* 26(6), pp. 1696-1700.

Mayrovitz HN, (1997). Shape and area measurement considerations in the assessment of diabetic plantar ulcers. *Wounds,* 9(1), pp. 21-28.

Melhuish JM, Plassman P, Harding KG, (1994). Circumference, area and volume of the healing wound. *Journal of Wound Care.* 3(8), pp. 380-384.Öien RF, Hakansson A, Hansen BU, Bjellrup M, 2002. Measuring the size of ulcers by planimetry: a useful method in the clinical setting. *Journal of Wound Care,* 11(5), pp. 165-168.

Oyibo SO, Jude EB, Tarawneh I, Nguyen HC, Armstrong DG, Harkless LB, Boulton AJM, (2001). The effects of ulcer size and site, patient's age, sex and type and duration of diabetes on the outcome of diabetic foot ulcers. *Diabetic Medicine,* 18(2), pp. 133-8.

Papazoglou ES, Zubkov L, Mao X, Neidrauer M, Rannou N, Weingarten MS, (2010). Image Analysis of chronic wounds for determining the surface area. *Wound Repair Regen* Jul-Aug; 18 (4) pp. 349-58.

Plassman P, and Jones BF, (1992). Measuring leg ulcers by colour-coded structured light. *Journal of Wound Care,* 1(3), pp. 35-38.

Plassman P, Melhuish JM, Harding KG, (1994). Methods of measuring wound size: a comparative study. *Wounds,* 40(7), pp. 50-52.

Plassman P, (1995). Measuring wounds. *Journal of Wound Care,* 4(6), pp. 269-272.

Plassman P, Peters JM, (2001). Recording wound care effectiveness. *Journal of Tissue Viability,* **12**(1), pp. 24-28.

Polit DF and Hungler BP, (1995). Nursing *Research, Principles and Methods.* 6th ed Philadelphia: Lipincott. pp. 155-173.

Rodgers LC, Bevilacqua NJ, Armstrong DG, Andros G. (2010). Digital Planimetry results in more accurate wound measurements: a comparison to standard ruler measurements. *J Diabetes Sci Technol.* Jul 1; 4 (4) pp. 799-802.

Shaw J, Hughes CM, Lagan KM, Bell PM, Stevenson MR, (2007). An Evaluation of Three Wound Measurement Techniques in Diabetic Foot Wounds. *Diabetes Care,* 30, pp. 2641-2642.

Sheehan P, Jones P, Caselli A, Giurini J, Veves A (2003). Percentage change in wound area of diabetic foot ulcers over a 4-week period is a robust predictor of complete healing in a 12-week prospective trial. *Diabetes Care* 26 (6) pp. 1879-82.

Thomas AC, Wysocki AB (1990). The healing wound:a comparison of three clinically useful methods of measurement. *Decubitus.* 3 pp. 18-25.

Vowden K, Vowden P, (2005). Moist wound healing for the diabetic foot within the context of TIME. *Wounds UK,* **2** (suppl), pp. 20-23.

Wilde S, Roglig G, Green A, Sicree R, King H, (2004). Global prevalence of diabetes. *Diabetes Care* 27, pp. 1047-1053

Williams C, (1997). Wound-measuring methods. *Nurse Prescriber /Community Nurse,* Sept, pp. 46-48.

6

The Temporary Orthesio-Therapy for Diabetic Foot

Richard Florence
Podiatrist, Peyrehorade, Pédicure – Podologue D.E.
France

1. Introduction

I was taught Temporary Orthesio-therapy by Dr Robert van Lith, a Dutch Podiatrist, who wrote a book called: "Podologie Appliquée"[1].

This therapy technique is used after a very careful examination of the foot, and of the fitting qualities of shoes; an analysis of the involved pathologies and the right use of the tools. It is thus possible to take out the mechanical trauma of the conflicting areas. The knowledge of the foot "biomechanic", together with the knowledge of TOT allows relieving and curing a "keratopathy".

Mechanical stresses are one of the reasons of the foot ulceration appearance; this therapy represents therefore a relevant one for a diabetic patient.

2. Materials and methodology

My purpose is not to deliver a lesson on TOT: it was thoroughly explained in the author's book. As its name says, this technique has to be used just before the permanent orthosis setting up. It is used during the scarring phase.

Doctor Margreet van Putten, Fontys Paramedische Hogeschool manager in Eindhoven, wrote: *"Almost 80% of diabetic ulcers will be cured by offloading the ulcer pressure. Then, you should never take other actions than "unloading the pressure!"(Drôme seminary*[2]).

The list below is not exhaustive but it presents the necessary materials to prepare a temporary orthosis (TO) for the clinical cases described.

2.1 Materials

2.1.1 Adhesive pressure deflection materials

Used products are made by Cuxson Gerrard & Co. Ltd Company, located in England.

---

[1] Van Lith Robert, July 2003, Podologie appliquée, Edition du Lau, ISBN : 2 84750 052 9, Page 67.
[2] Van Putten Margreet, van Lith Marie-Josée, van Lith Robert, The diabetic foot, Montelimar Seminary (Drôme, France), March 2002.

These products are :

- Hapla All Wool Felt ®: pure new wool felt, semi-packed in tight.
- Hapla Gold Felt ®: improved felt with anti-infective agent to protect the foot from fungal and bacterium infection. This product is recommended by Cuxson Gerrard Company to be used on sensitive feet.
- Moleskin ®: thin fleece-lined non stretch cotton
- Hapla Fleecy Web ®: cotton jersey with a fleece-lined cotton surface. Transversally strecht.

2.1.2 Non - adhesive pressure deflection materials

- Plastazote ®: thermoformable polyurethane rubber.
- Walk-line ®: non-rigid thermoformable material.
- Thermoformable Latex foam.

2.1.3 Attachment materials

- Hapla band ® (Cuxson & Gerrard) : thin hypoallergenique bandage.
- Micropore ®: (3 M) micro- porus band-aid with high skin tolerance, air permeable. It doesn't cause contact allergy.
- Chirofix ®: (Cuxson & Gerrard) adhesive bandage with good skin tolerance, micro-porus and transversally strecht.
- Oper fix ®: (Iberhospitex S.A.) strecht tape.

2.1.4 Bandages

- Urgotul S. Ag/S.D. ®: Laboratory URGO
- Mepilex Border ® : Laboratory Mölnlycke Health Care
- Biatain ® : Laboratory Coloplast
- Cellosorb Silver Ag ®: Laboratory URGO
- Actisorb ® : Laboratory Johnson – Johnson Medical ltd

2.2 Methodology

The medical examination is essential to find the first cause of the infection (keropathy, wound or ulceration).

One should observe :

- Deformed foot (hallux or toes)
- Deformed tarsus.

One should look for :

- Neuropathy or arteriopathy presence,
- Static position troubles with hyper hold in toes, metatarsal heads, or fifth metatarsus stiloïd.
- Dynamic troubles,
- Limited joints mobility

The association of all these factors makes the diabetic foot a risky foot.

Pathway to the diabetic foot ulceration[3]:

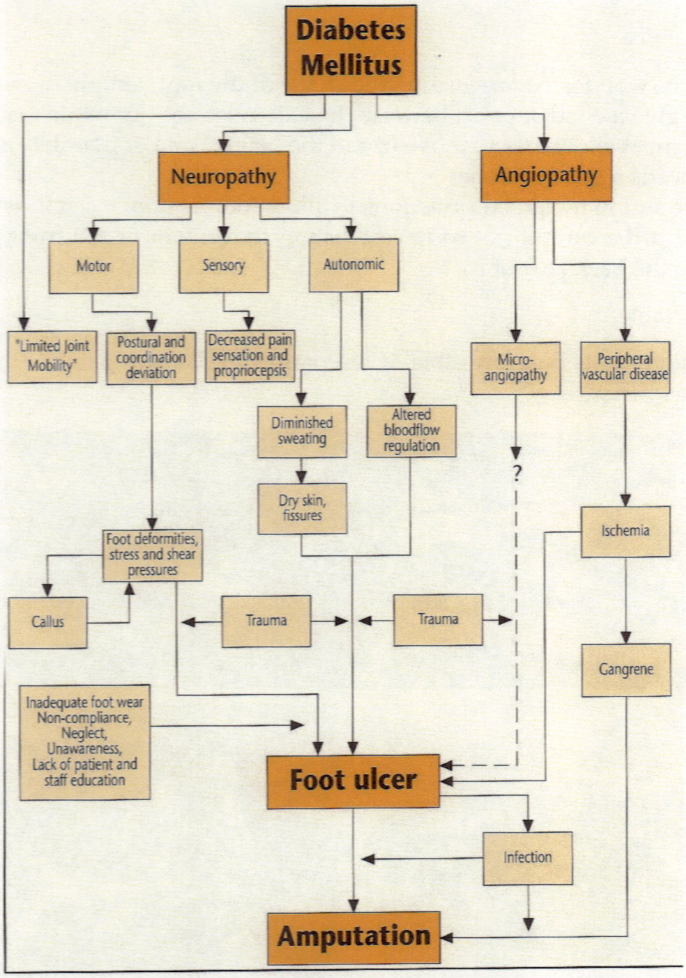

Pathways to diabetic foot ulceration

Fig. 1.

We need to discover what kind of stress is responsible for the pathology (chafing stress, pression or compression, twisting).

Mechanical stresses are responsible for kerathonic pathology. They give skin irritation, accelerate cellular mitosis and enhance hyperkeratosis appearance.

[3] The International Working Group on the Diabetic Foot, may 1999, International Consensus on the Diabetic Foot, Copyright by the International Working Group on the Diabetic Foot, ISBN : 90-9012716-x. (page 29: Pathways to diabetic foot ulceration.)

It is absolutely necessary to know what kind of stress is responsible for the pathology appearance[4]

It is also necessary to analyze the shoes.

Shoes wearing advice :

- Shoes must be well formed regarding the shape of the foot (length and width)
- Shoes must give a good support because the feet must not slip while walking
- Shoe upper must allow toes to move (mind the height) and, if possible, avoid seams
- Shoe back needs a good stiffener
- Sole must be soft in metatarsis junctions to allow foot flexion and it must be hard on the back part of it (be careful not to have twisting movement of the front part of the sole regarding to the back part of it).

It must be confortable.

When compression stress is responsible of the pathology, I use a pair of clips to put out of shape locally the leather.

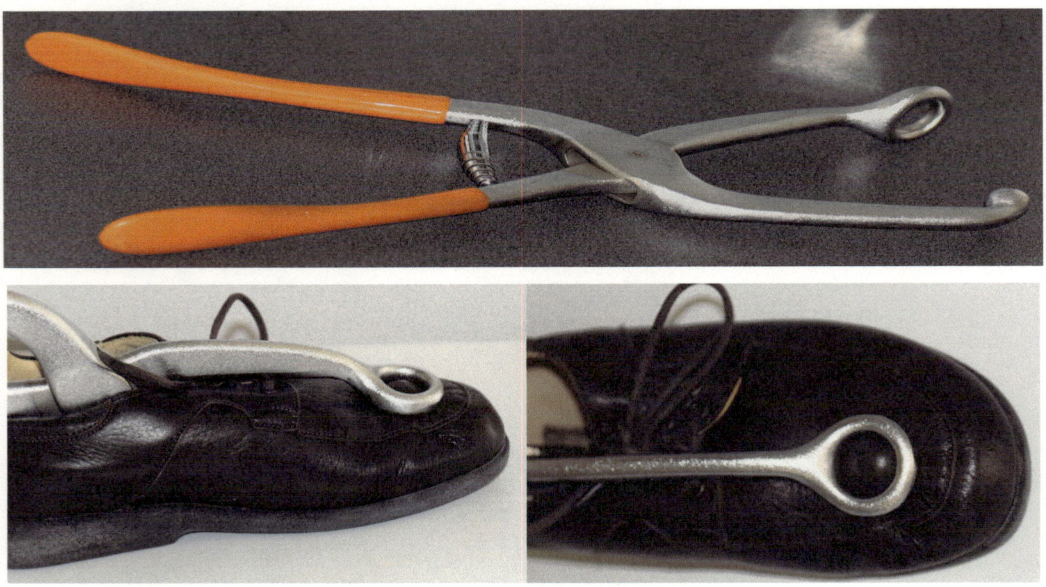

Fig. 2.

Treatment pattern
• Cure the conflictual zone by make the stresses disappear (chafing, pressure and twisting),
• Correct if possible or protect,
• Give a normal function to the articulations again
• If needed, fit with prosthesis to ease step development.
Conclusion: My aim is to enhance the patient autonomy by protecting his or her walking possibilities.

[4] Richard, F., TOT training session notes, Nantes, September, 1998.

In case of a risky foot and when it is hard to find convenient shoes, suitable for the foot out shaping, we need to ask an orthopedist to make made to measure shoes.

After the medical examination, I use to make a prevention assessment, I explain all the different treatment steps (correction, protection, contention with a disease if necessary) and I try to make the patient understand that he or she needs to respect his or her feet.

This treatment is carried out after the instrumental gesture

The used materials allow the therapist to adjust himself to the different clinical cases.

The TO is taped on the skin.

Felt TO is put on to offload the hyper-pressured area in order to eliminate the mechanical stresses of chafing (static and dynamic)

The offloading zone delimitation will be found after the palpation of the zone to be protected, apart from the cellulitis (presence of swelling, erythema and heat indication an inflammatory reaction).

The TO shape is adaptable according to the recovery step.[5]

There is no limit: one has just to be inventive and creative.

Hapla Felt is used in 2 mm size, 5 mm or 7 mm to offload the conflicted area..

One needs to take into account the loading capacity of the product (half of it)

The felt can be doubled, or even triple according to the area which needs to be isolated.

In order to make the TO easy to wear, it is essential to bevel the external sides.

The more important the deformation is, the more material will be needed (felt) to allow a better pressure distribution.

If the inflammation is important, it is absolutely necessary to totally stop walking and so the OT will be bigger.

The basic rules and a good knowledge of the materials allow getting a spectacular result.

Nothing is left to chance because everything can be explained.

The immediate elimination of mechanical stress caused by chafing and pressure allows the patient to put on shoes again without feeling any risk.

In case the patient would suffer neuropathy, the TO would assure scarring.

But this will only be possible provided that everything has been made to constantly offload the injured part during all the scarring time.

As Jean-Louis Richard, Denyse Vannareau et Claire Parer-Richard underlined: offloading the foot is a fundamental measure without which scarring is impossible.[6]

---

[5] Richard, F., Transitory TOT: 28th Podiatry discussions seminary, Paris, 2003.

[6] Richard, J.L. et al. Article : le pied diabétique, Service des maladies de la nutrition et de la diabétologie, CHU de Nîmes, Le Grau du Roi.

Dr Ha Van Georges wrote about this : « the perforating pain cannot be cured if the patient is still walking on it » [7].

The TO will allow the uninterrupted protection of the conflicting zone while the foot is mobilized during the walk.

And this will retain the walking radius, not to say increase it).

Even when confined to bed, the patient's foot is relieved of stress pressures.

That is why I would like to quote again Robert Van Lith's book "Podologie appliquée"[8]

Thanks to the scientific research team, the Cuxson Gerrard & Co. Offers materials with an unique adhesive system.

We are lucky to enjoy an amazing material technological advancement.[9]

	S aureus (NCTC 10788 ATCC 6538)	Ps aeruginosa (NCIMB 8626 ATCC 9027)	C albicans (NCPF 3179 ATCC 10231)
Time	Hapla All Wool Felt Gold		
Inoculum	$4.1x10^6$	$3.6x10^6$	$2.8x10^6$
14 Days	<10	<10	$6.7x10^3$

A greater than 5-Log reduction in S aureus numbers was seen following seven days exposure to the product. A greater than 5-Log reduction in Ps aeruginosa and a 2-Log reduction in C albicans numbers was seen following 14 days exposure to the product.

- Staphylococcus aureus is a gram positive bacteria - common on human skin
- Pseudomonas aeruginosa is a gram negative bacteria
- Candida albicans is a fungus

Results from Independent Laboratory testing Nov 08.
Forty samples of Hapla Gold felt were inoculated with either fungi or bacteria.

Fig. 3.

[7] Dr. Georges Ha Van (Paris), Equilibre N°197 1996 –Qu'est-ce qu'un mal perforant et comment le prévenir ?

[8] Van Lith Robert, July 2003, Podologie appliquée, Edition du Lau, ISBN : 2 84750 052 9 (Pages 70-71 & 108)

[9] Etude éditée par Cuxson et Gerrard montrant le résultat obtenu avec antimicrobial treatment de l'Hapla glod all felt.

3. Results

I would like to highlight this methodology by exposing several clinical cases: domiciliary care, in my podiatric office or in hospital.

I wanted to present different situations because one can notice that ulceration is different regarding to the place and to the limitation of our skills[10].

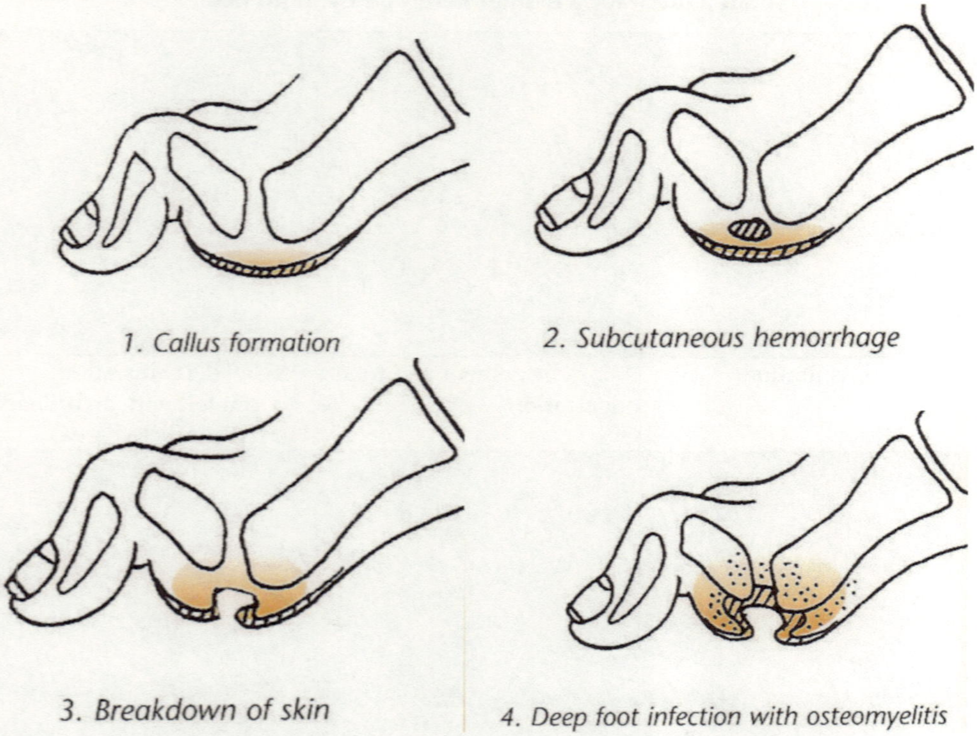

Fig. 4.

The invasive treatment has to be appropriate for the patient's condition.

The follow-up is different when the podiatrist is alone or in a multidisciplinary medical team.

The described cases present treatments on different conflicted areas which helps us to present a wide range of this technique, that is to say:

- Treated patient for a plantar keratopathy , right heel
- Treated patient with plantar keratopathy with a bruise on the metatarsal-phalangeal joint (big toe) reducing and preventing the patient from walking
- TO for an ulceration in order to amputate the fifth toe
- And some impressive cases in hospital.

---

[10] The International Working Group on the Diabetic Foot, may 1999, Practical Guidelines on the Management and the prevention of the Diabetic Foot, Copyright by the International Working Group on the Diabetic Foot, ISBN : 90-9012716-x.) page 2 :Illustration of ulcer due to repetitive stress.)

Here are some results achieved during some consultations:

- Skin scarring is progressive,
- Mechanical stress elimination prevents or postpones the risk of amputation.

3.1 Domiciliary care

3.1.1 CASE A: Treated patient for a plantar keratopathy, right heel

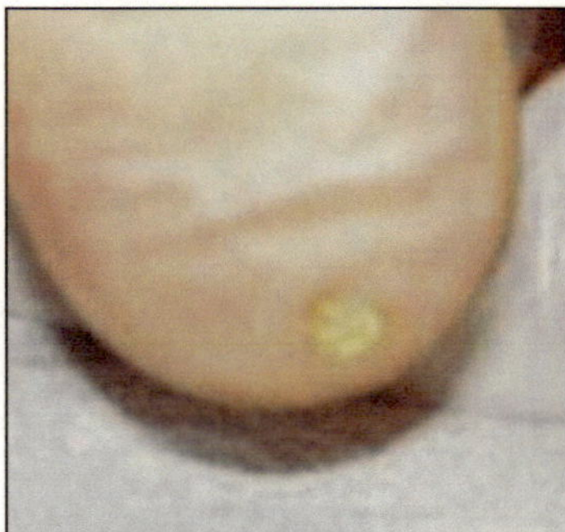	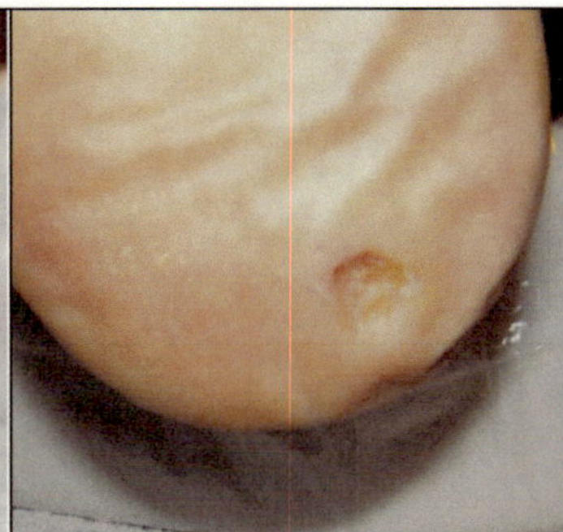	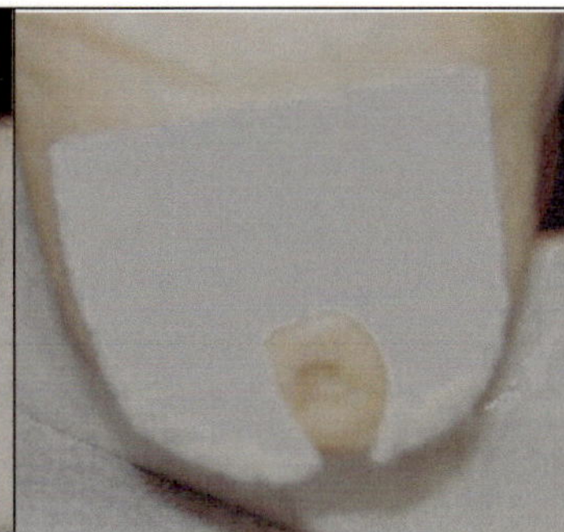
A-1: first consultation	A-2: debridement and total enucleation	A-3: felt TO installing (5 mm felt with an offloading of the conflicted area).
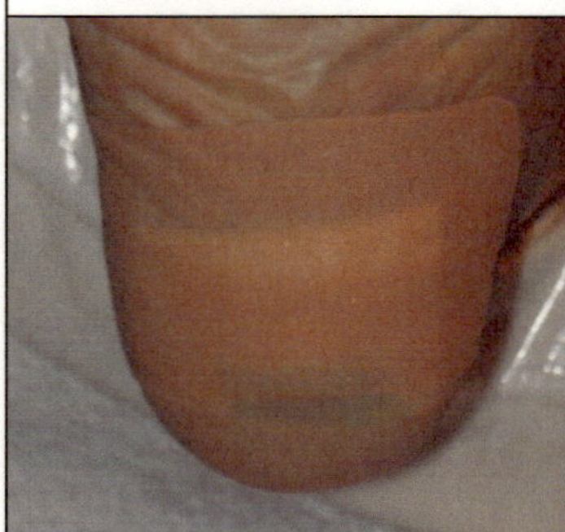	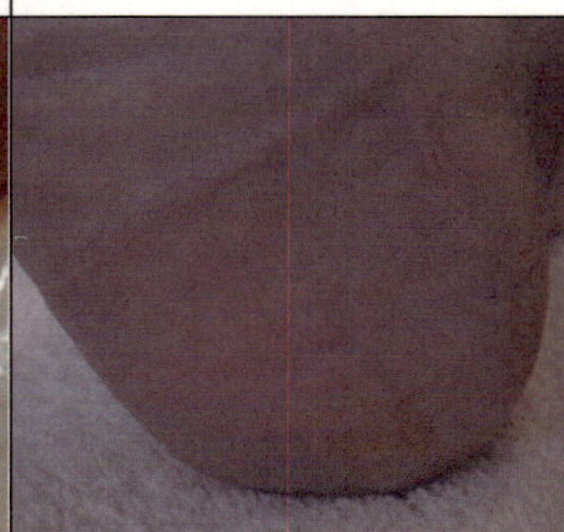	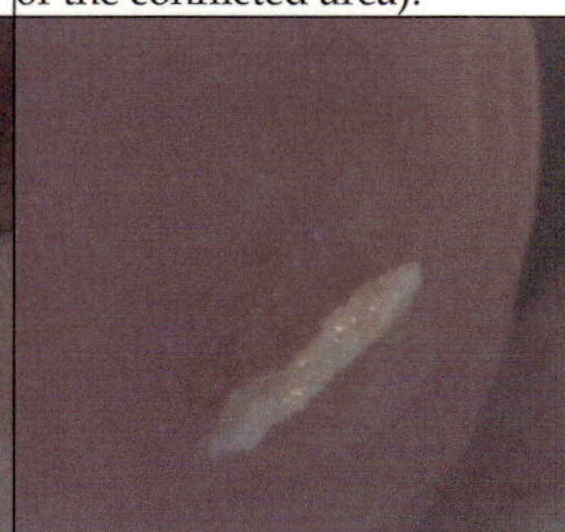
A-4: Bandage installing and fixation with Hapla-band	A-5: after two weeks treatment	A-6 et A-7: two steps enucleation with a set with diamonds cracks burrs
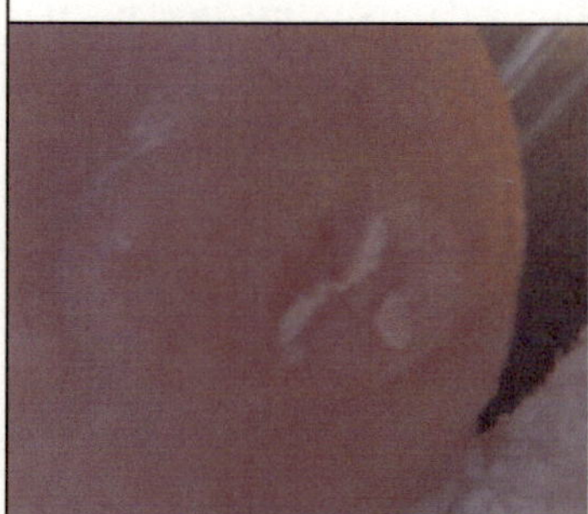	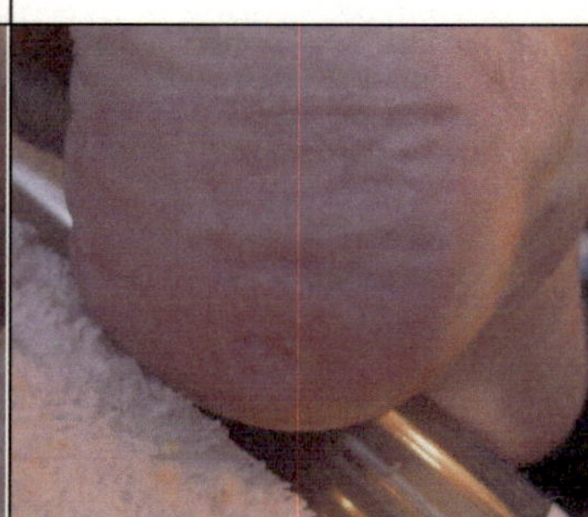	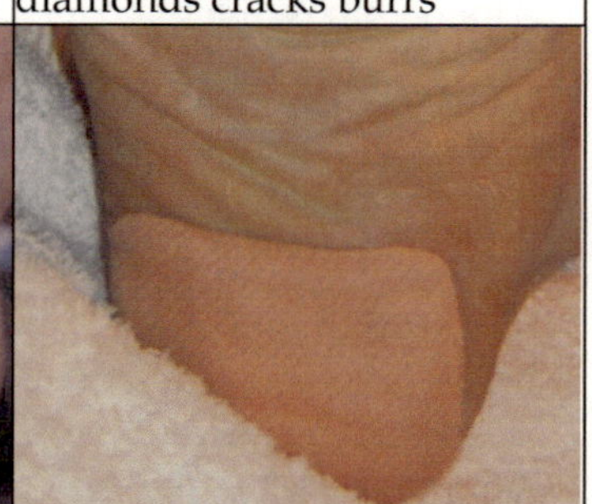
A-6 et A-7: two steps enucleation with a set with diamonds cracks burrs	A-8: End of the instrumental work.	A-9: Moleskine installing. Which covers the back part of the foot.

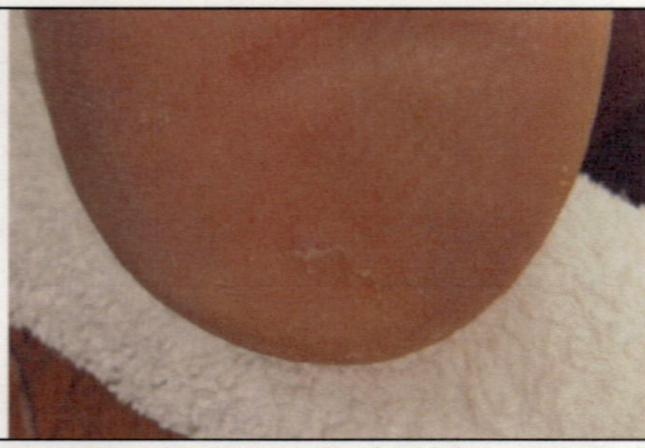

A-10 : After two weeks treatment : skin is totally healthy. Apply Hydra-defense balm or Akildia balm (Asepta-Akiléine laboratory). Which delays the keratin implantation.

Fig. 5.

3.1.2 CASE B: Treated patient with plantar keratopathy with a bruise on the metatarsal-phalangeal joint (big toe) reducing and preventing the patient from walking

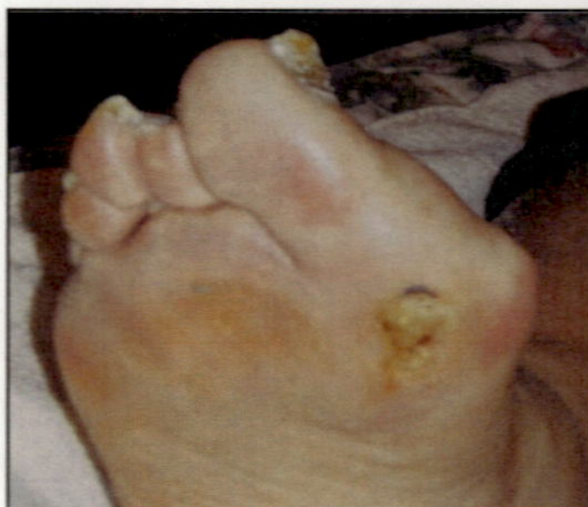

B-1 : First consultation

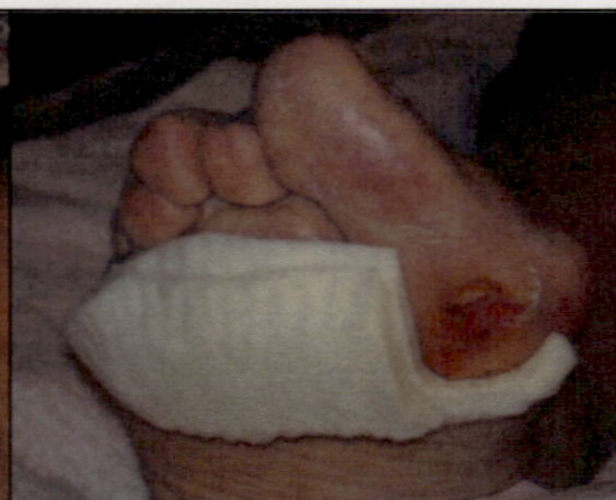

B-2 : TO installing (7 mm felt with two layers)

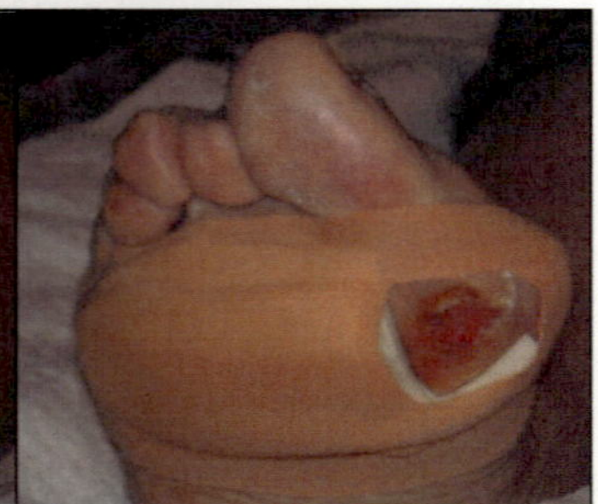

B- 3 : Fixation with Hapla-band with an opening to allow wound access.

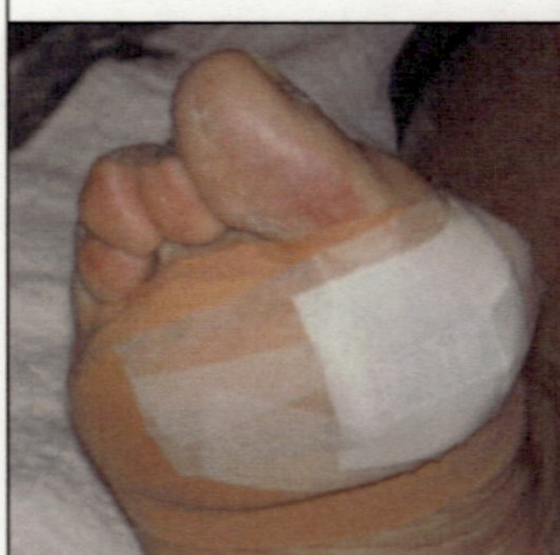

B-4 : Medicinal dressing (Biatain) , which has to be changed every 48 hours by the nurse in charge. After the debridement, new offloading is necessary every one or two weeks by the podiatrist.

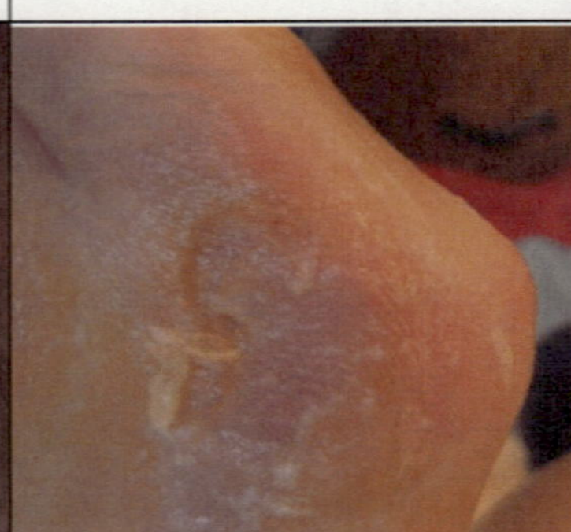

B-5 : Enucleation

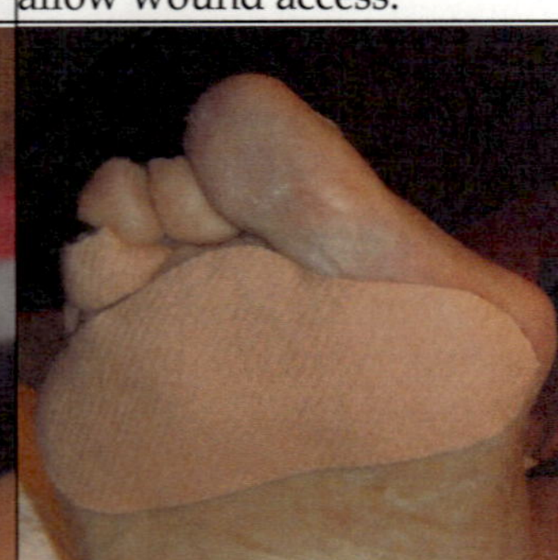

B- 6: TO fitting and Moleskiine fitting.

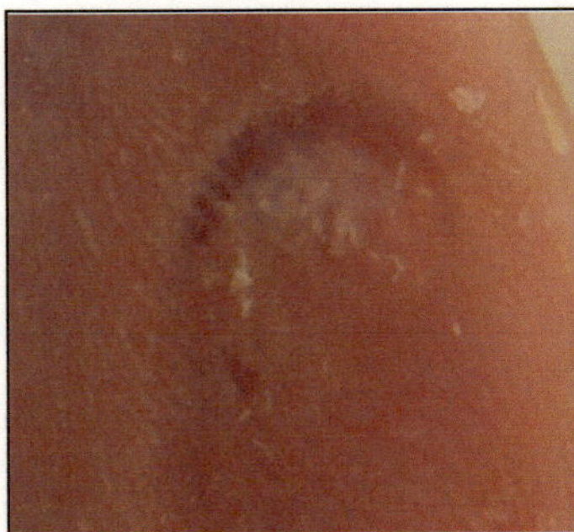	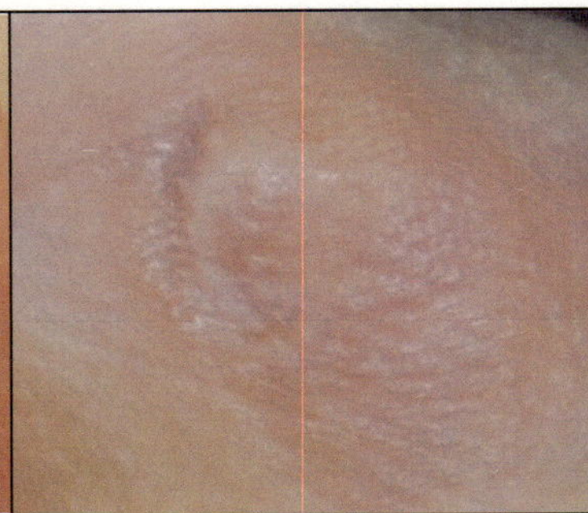	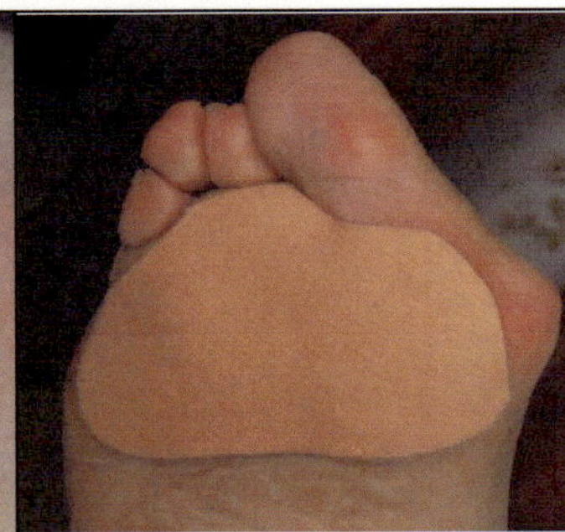
B-7 : After nine weeks, debridement and Moleskine installing.	B-8 : After eleven weeks, debridement	B-9 : Moleskine installing.
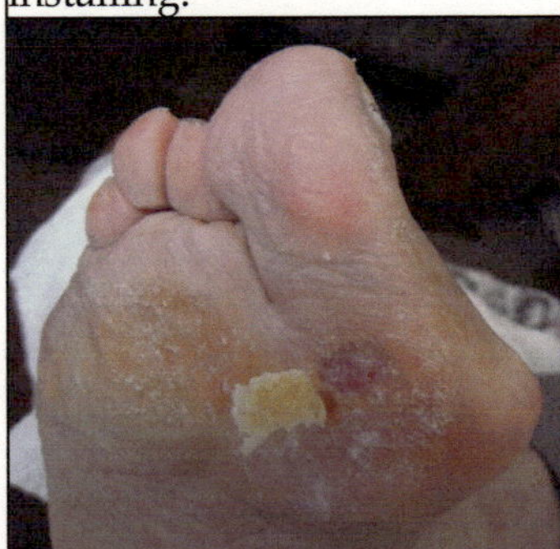	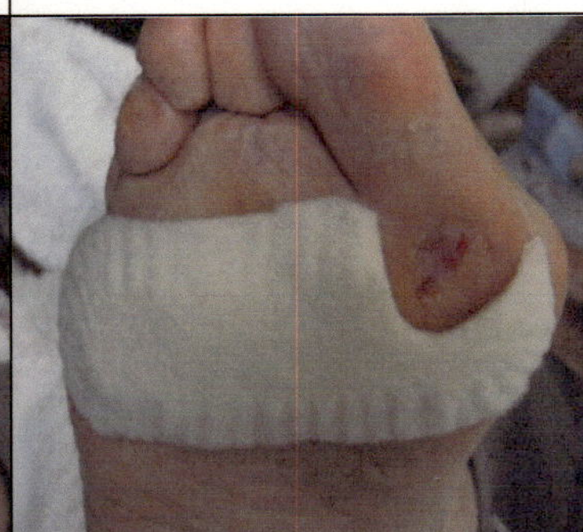	
B-10 : After one month. Without any protection and with an increase of the walking area, skin is wounded.	B-8 : New felt offloading TO fitting. Extra explanation about the importance of this TOT treatment with orthotis device just after the total scarring. Device confection perpetuates the treatment results.	

Fig. 6.

3.2 In my podiatrist office

3.2.1 CASE C: A diabetic patient grade zero, with a fifth metatarsal pain, on the external side

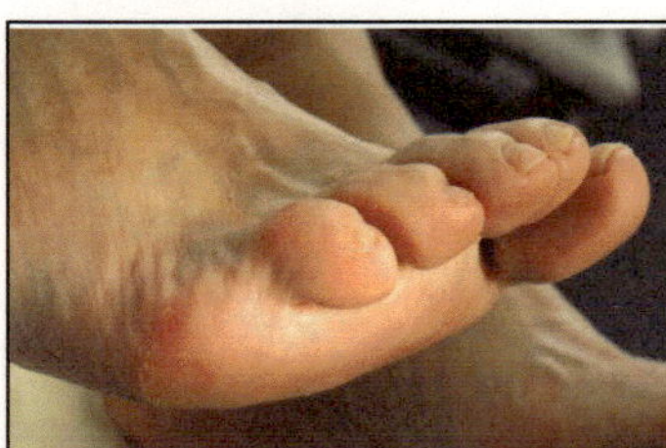	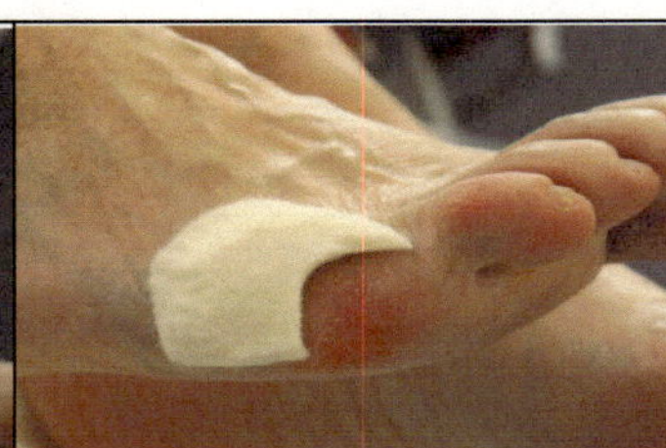	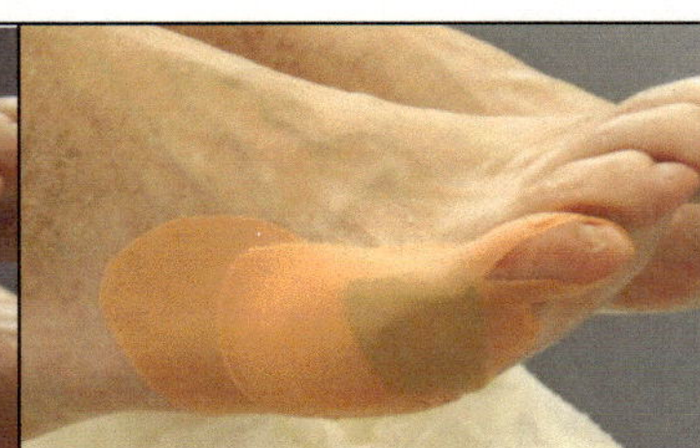
C- 1 : first consultation	C- 2 : TO installing Metatarsis head is totally offloaded (5 mm felt)	C- 3 : OT fixation with Hapla Band

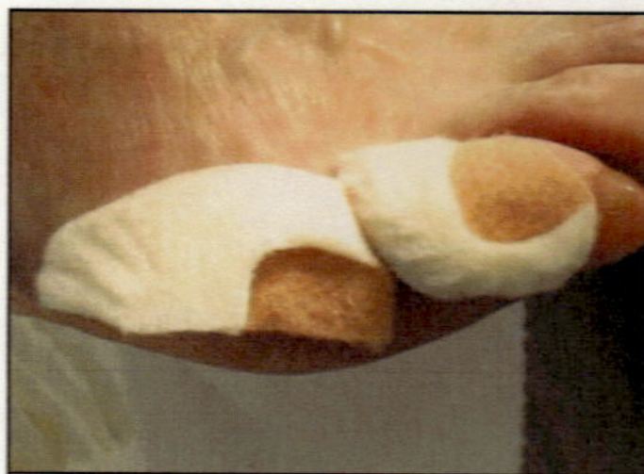	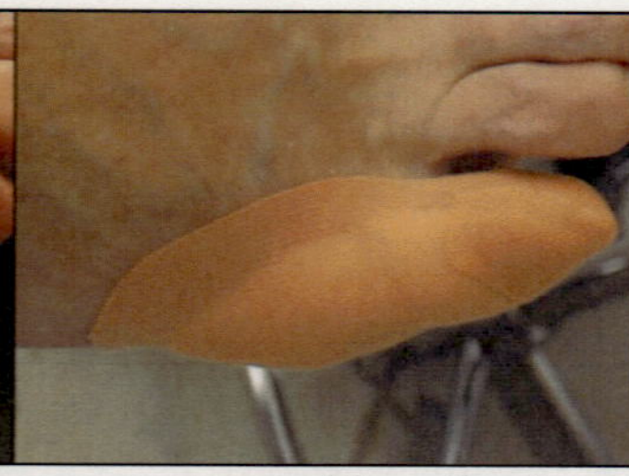	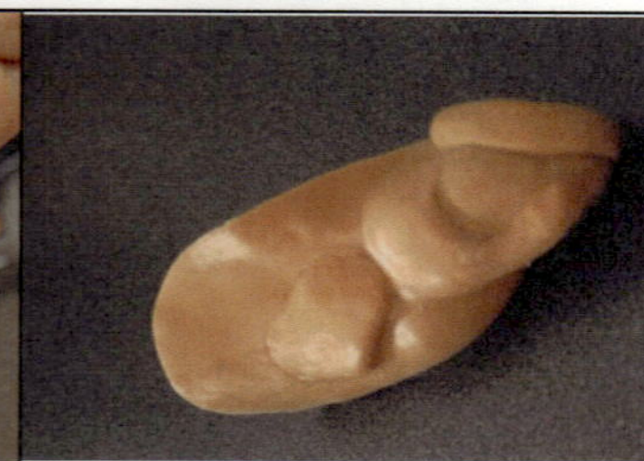
C 4 : after one month. The temporary removable orthosis has been lost. Felt offloading TO installing (offloading M5 and P2/P3 articulation on the fifth toe). Recommendation for a silicone device , equivalent to an TOT but which can be removed.		C 5 : silicone device.

Fig. 7.

3.2.2 CASE D: A diabetic patient grade one (September 2004), she is under oral medication. She presents a bad ulceration on the external side of her third toe, regarding to the distal articulation, due to a too long nail and to the shoes she is wearing (this kind of shoes are to be proscribed for diabetic patients)

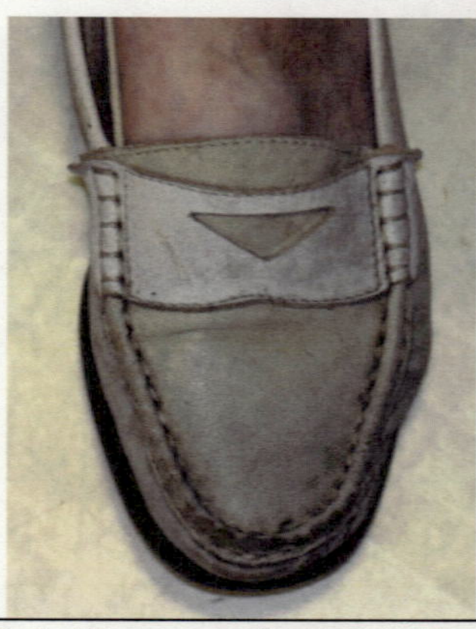	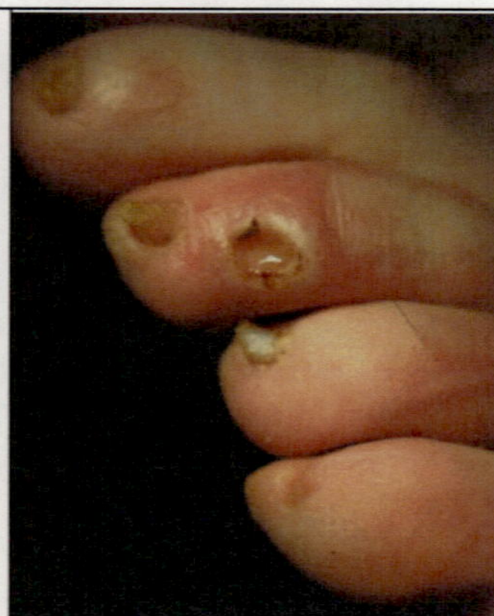	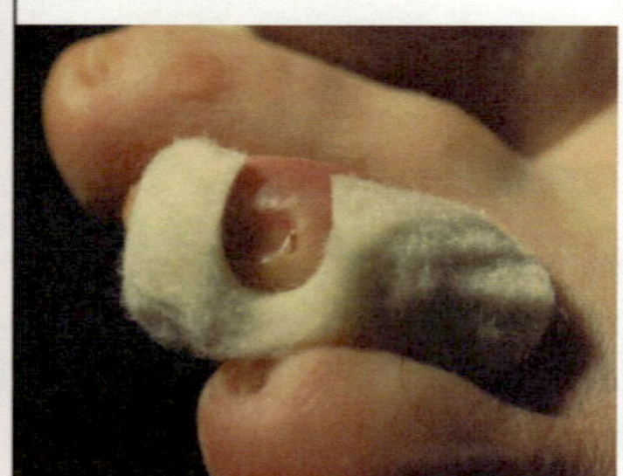
D-1 : First consultation with bad shoes	D-2 : angiopathy ulcer	D-3 : TO installing on September 24th (5 mm felt)
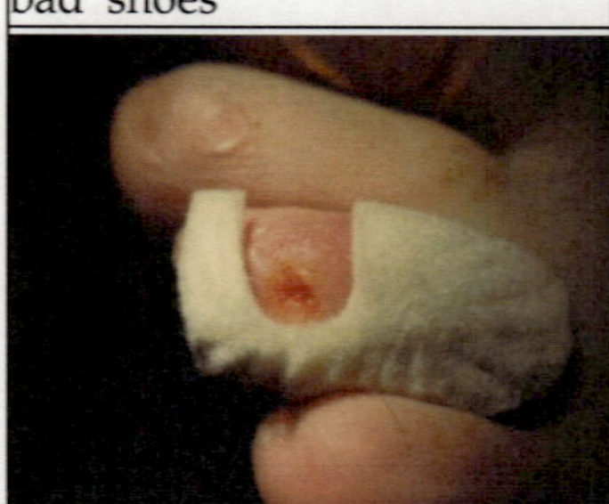	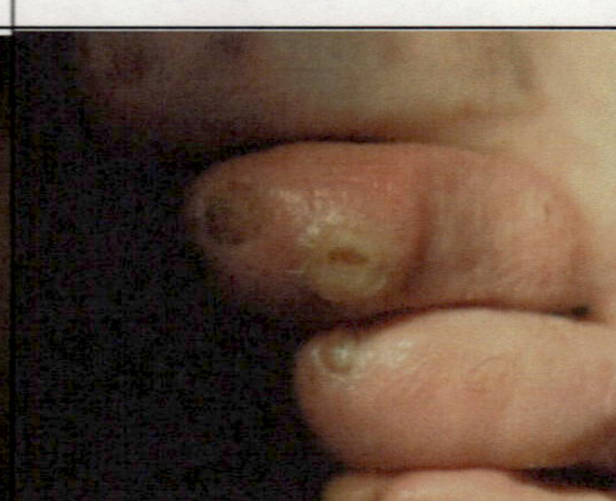	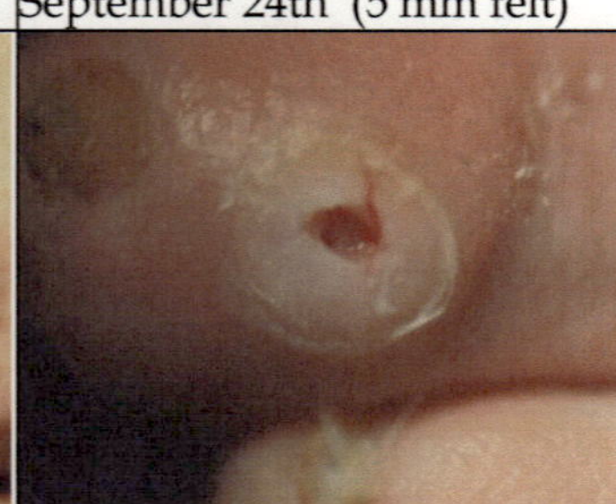
D-4 : TO on September 28th after four days.	D-5 : On October 8th	D-6 : debridement

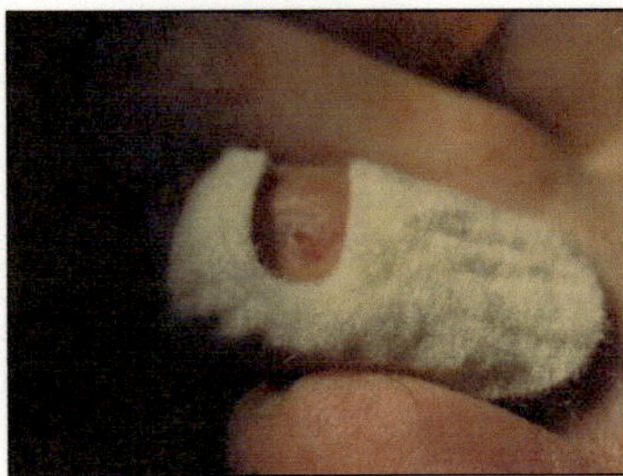	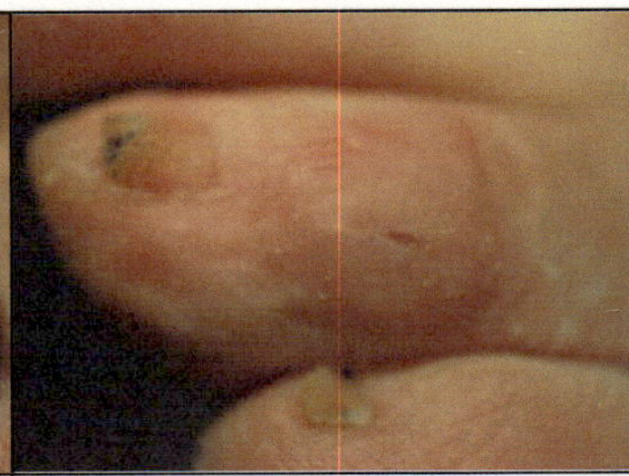	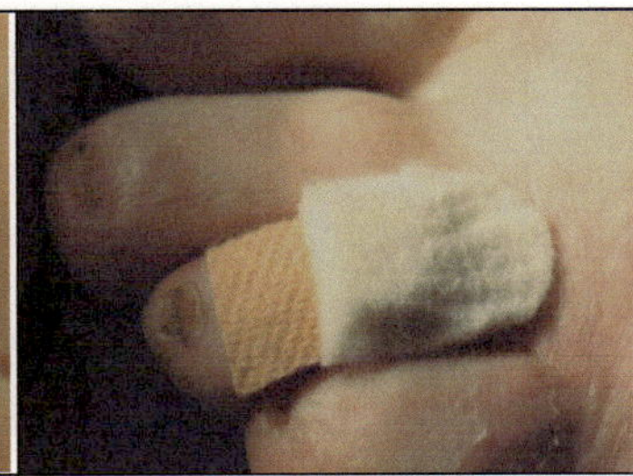
D-7 : TO on October 15th	D-8 : debridement	D-9 : On November 29th, Moleskine fitting to avoid suction with felt TO
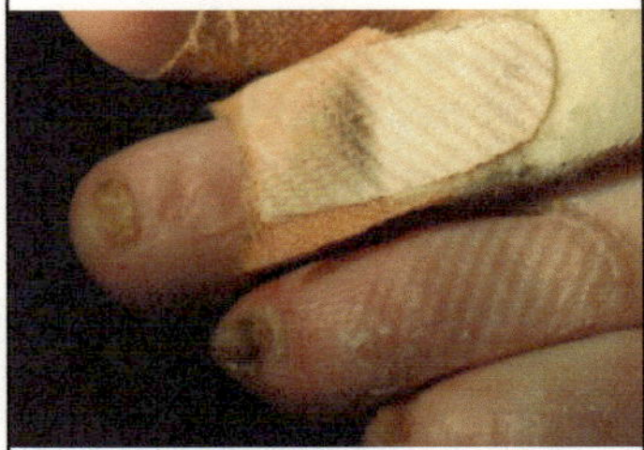	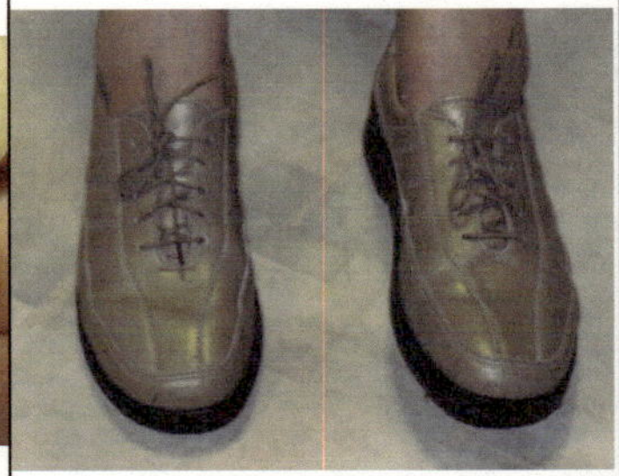	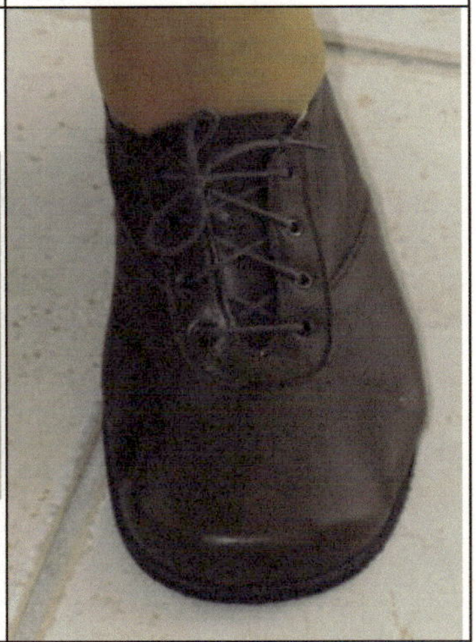
D-10 : TO has been unsticked and returned, then sticked on a neighbor toe to show how the wound has scarred.	D-11 : the patient has bought a new pair of shoes (17/12/2004).	D-12 : orthopaedic shoes in 2011. This patient has now diabete, grade two.

Fig. 8.

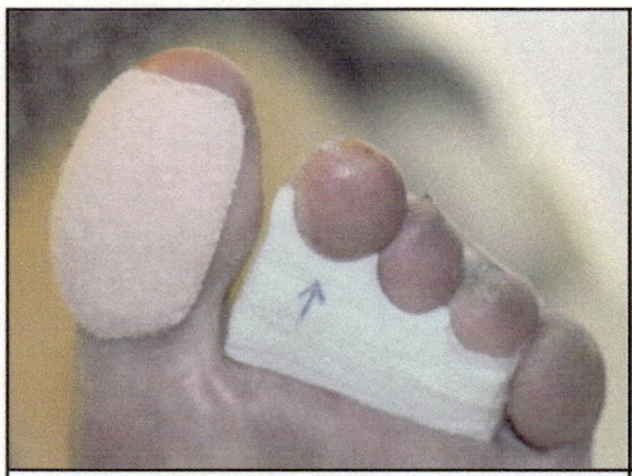	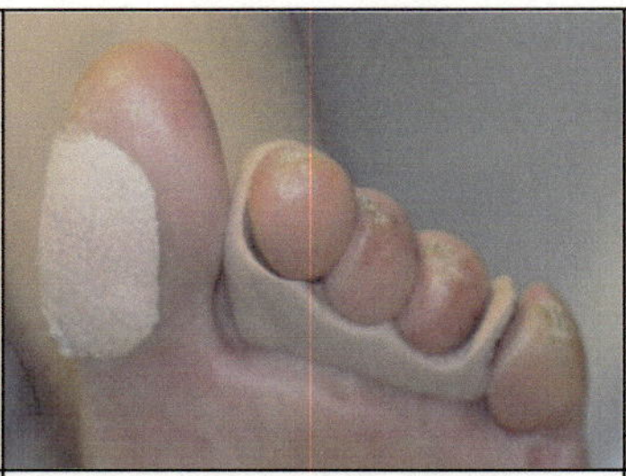	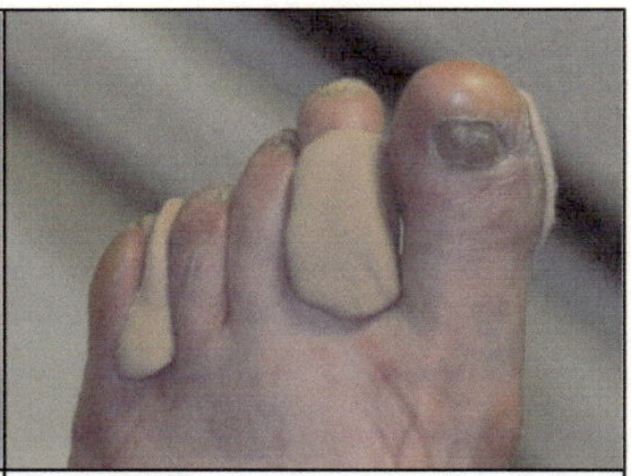
D-13 : Plastazote TO	D-14 : Silicone sub-digital device and Fleecy web under P1/P2 to avoid hyper-keratosis.	D- 15 : Ortho-plastic surgery with second toe protection.

Fig. 9.

This patient's diabete (Diabete Mellitus) comes up to grade 2 in 2009; from then she's insulin-dependent. She has to cope with an angiopathy and suffers a severe neuropathy.

Thanks to a regular medical follow up and to a healthy life, this patient has still got all her toes.

Since 2010, she wears made-to-measure shoes with an appropriate interior shape, seamless. To avoid an ulceration relapse a under- diaphysis protective and corrective orthosis is installed.

With a regular following and a good care of the nails every two months, the patient feet are protected.

3.2.3 CASE E: A patient with a Charcot foot

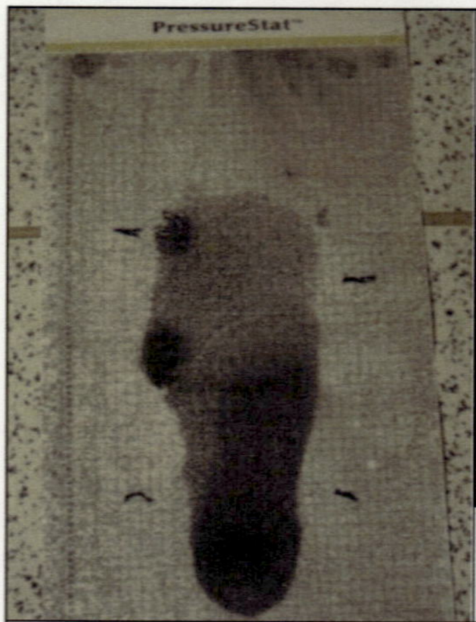	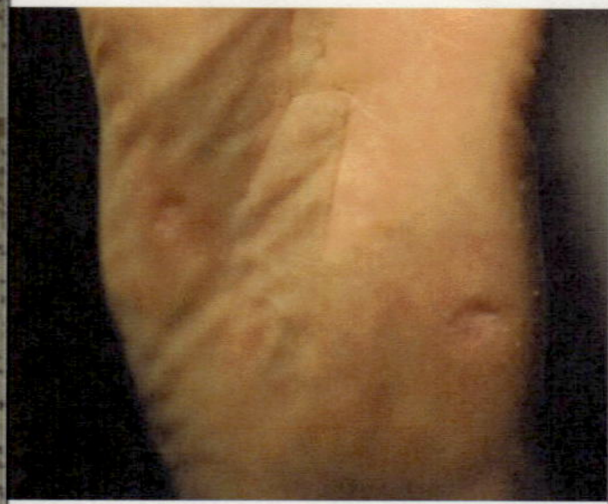	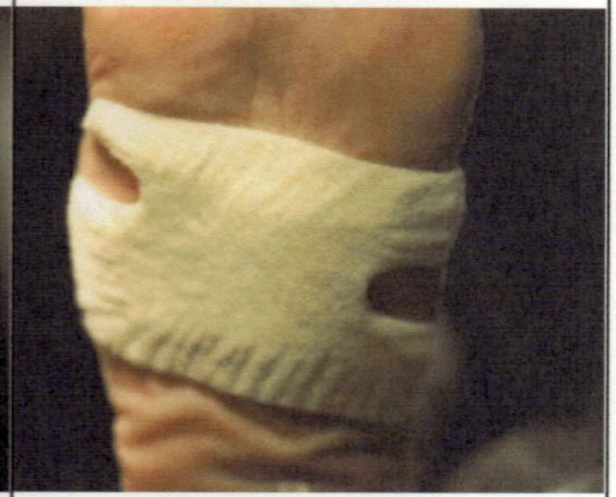
E – 1 : foot print	E-2 : Debridement and enucleation	E-3 : 7 mm TO fitting
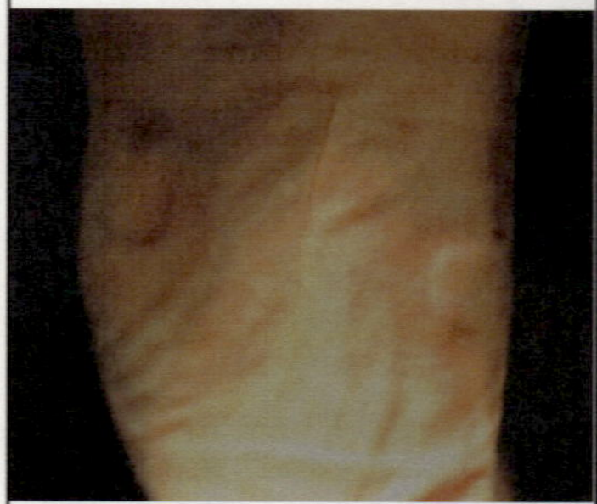	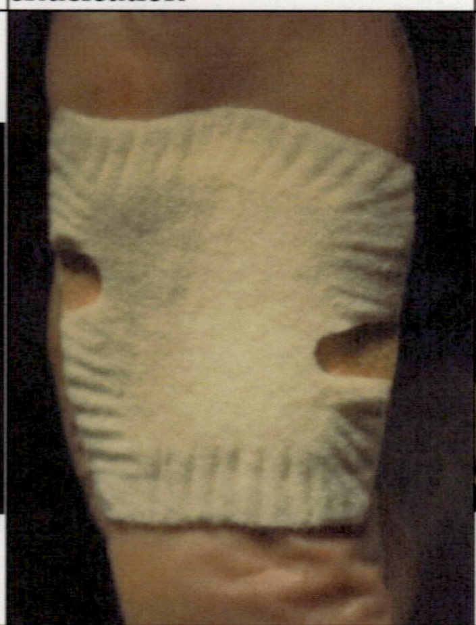	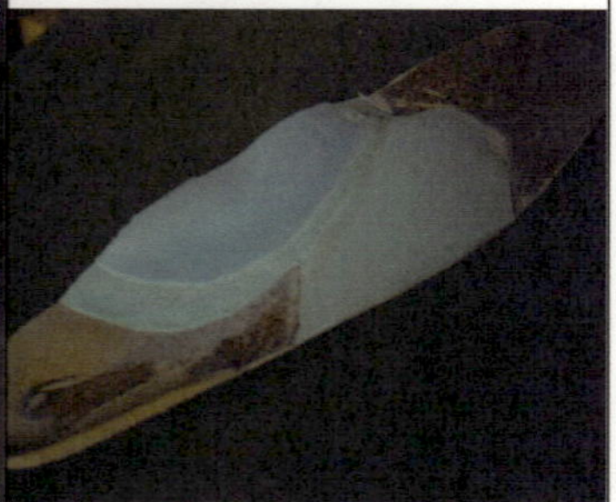
E-4 : after one week.	E-5 : Felt TO installing and Moleskine.	E-6 : Orthotic plantar device

Fig. 10.

3.2.4 CASE F: The patient had her third toe amputated

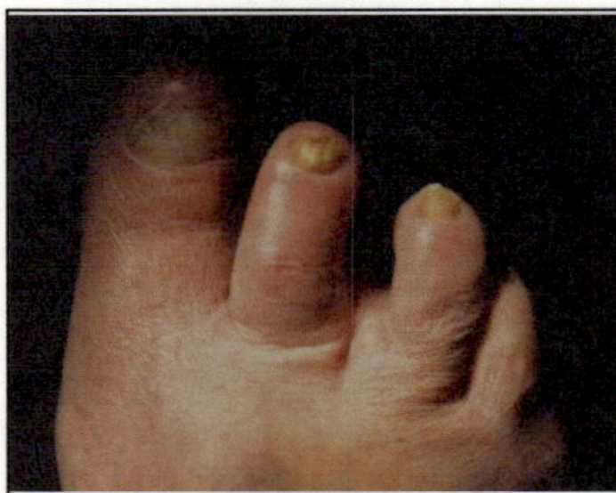	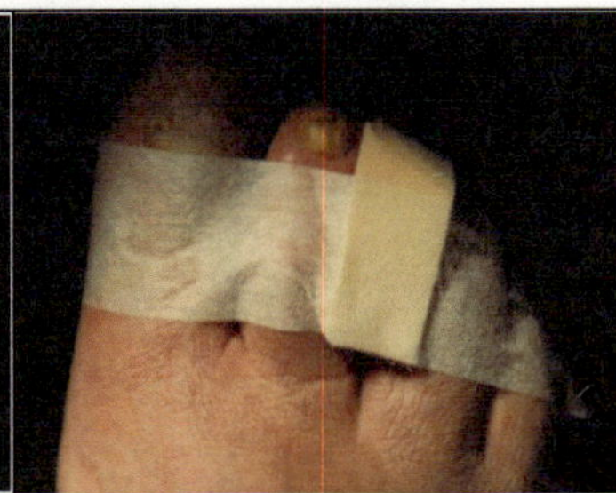	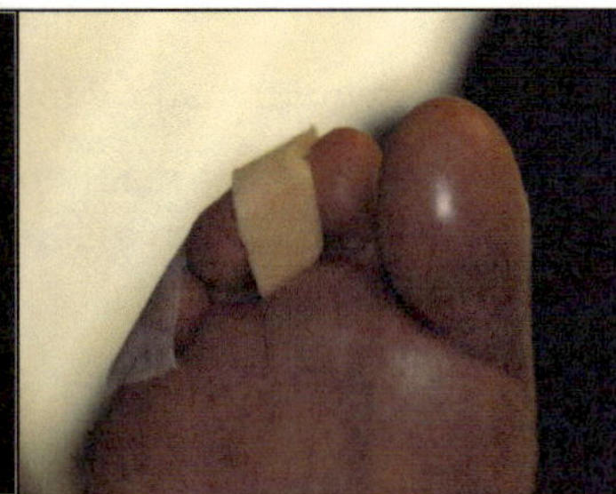
F - 7: First consultation	F-8: Non-rigid Plastazote TO fixed with band-aid	F-9: Plantar view
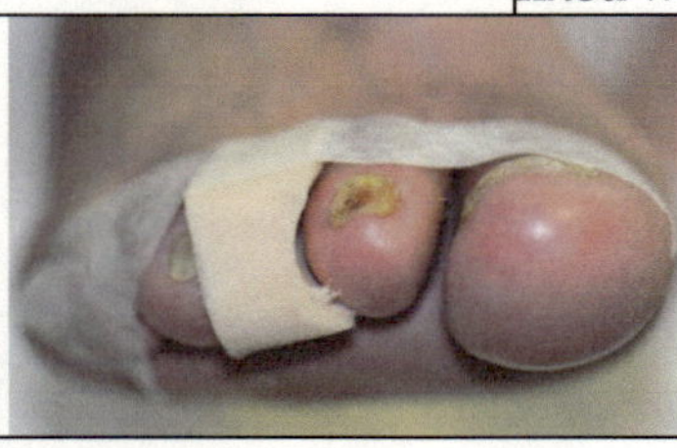	F-10 : front view	

Fig. 11.

3.3 In hospital

Lots of clinical cases are presented in Dr van Lith's book (Podologie appliquée).

The pictures below have been made and interpreted by Mrs. Marie José van Lith. She works in a podiatric office with a multidisciplinary medical team in the Romans hospital's endocrinology department (Drôme, France).

She was kind enough to take part in this article writing.

3.3.1 CASE G: The patient here suffered a diabetic retinopathy which stucked her blind. She also had a kidney insufficiency (she was on dialysis twice a week). She died five within the five years

While she was on hospital, first x-rays show a foot which can't be mobilized therefore no corrective TO is possible, only the protective one can be installed.

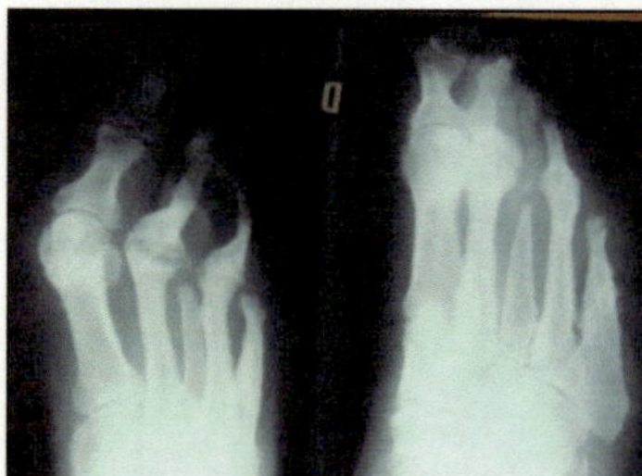	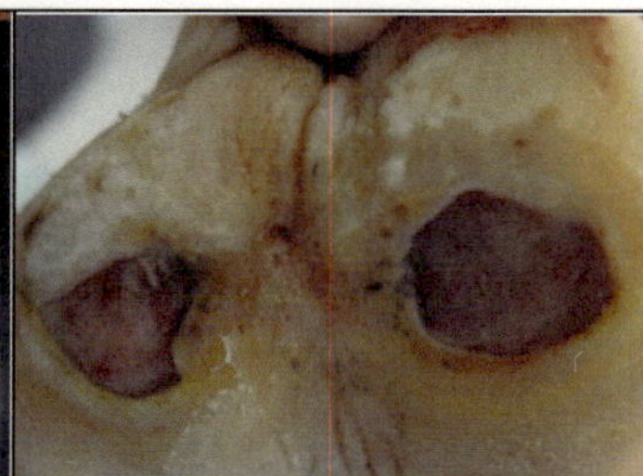	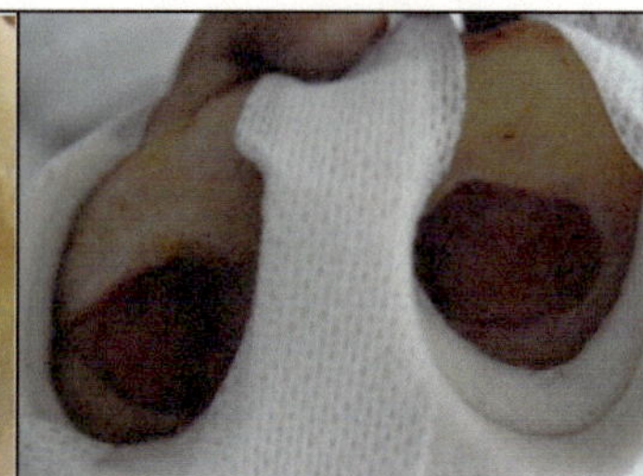
G-1 : The first x-rays	G-2 : On August 29th 2002	G-3 : After debridement of both wounds, felt TO

		installing, sticked with Oper fix bandage but which will be changed only every 8 days.
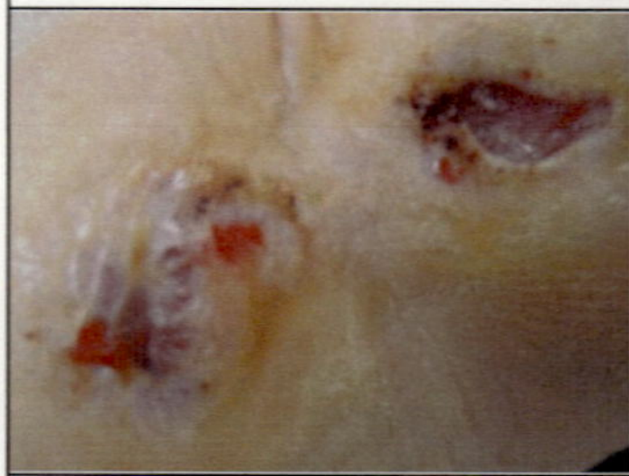	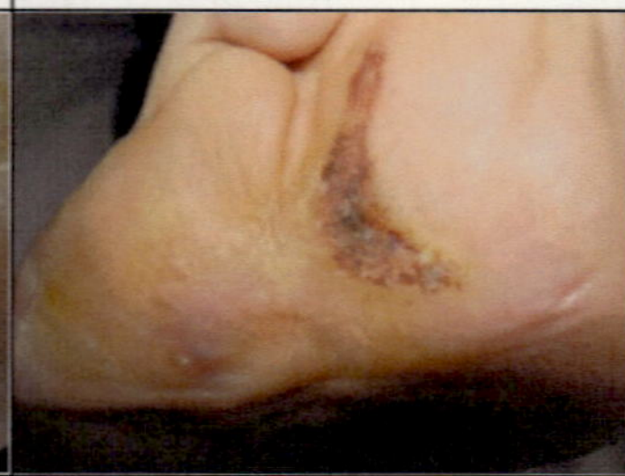	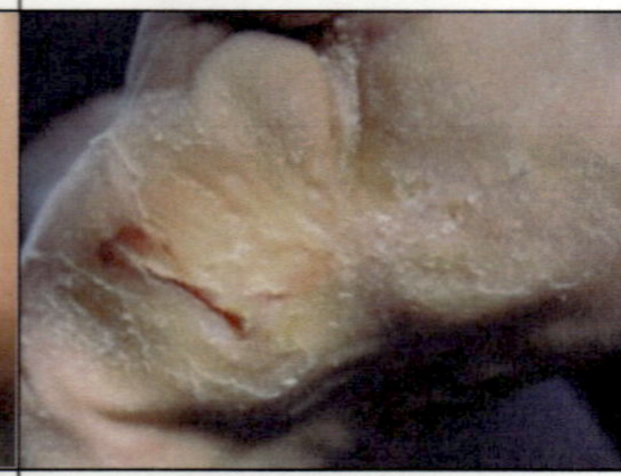
G-4: Wounds were almost totally healed . Some holes made in the TO allows the nurses to dress the wounds every two days (Actisorb Ag+ covered with Cellosorb).	G-5: A new wound appeared.	G-6: On April the 14th , after incision of the hyper-keratosis. Skin started to worsen. The general patient's state is declining.
	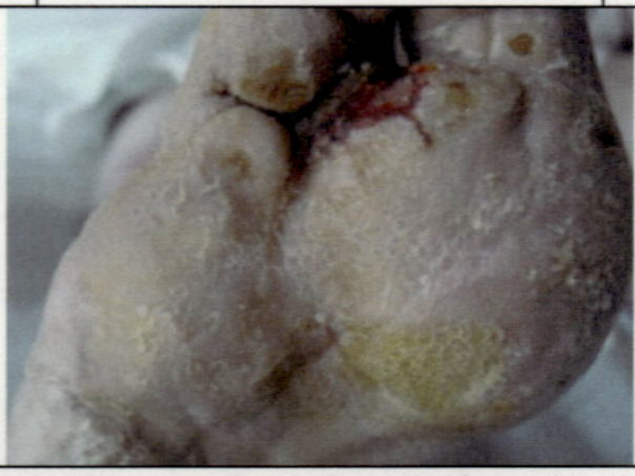	
G-7: This picture has been made three or four days before the death. Hand distal phalanx are bare-skined and the patient is now totally blind. No surgery.		

Fig. 12.

3.3.2 CASE H: The patient suffers a toes deviation. Big toe infraductus and total claw of the second toe. This patient is old, diabetic with a kidney insufficiency. He's only treated by a podiatrist. He has very painful angiopathic wounds

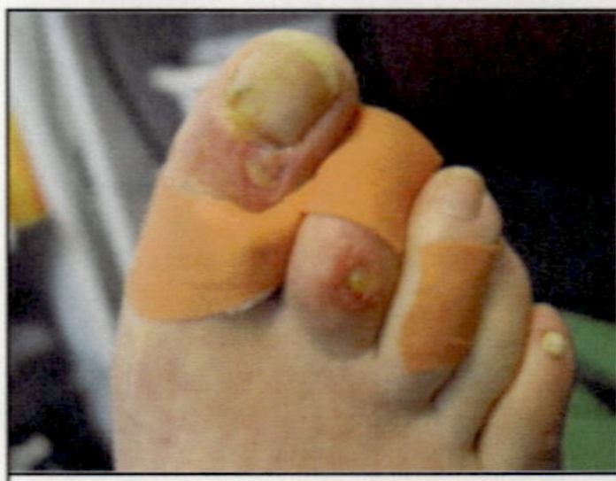	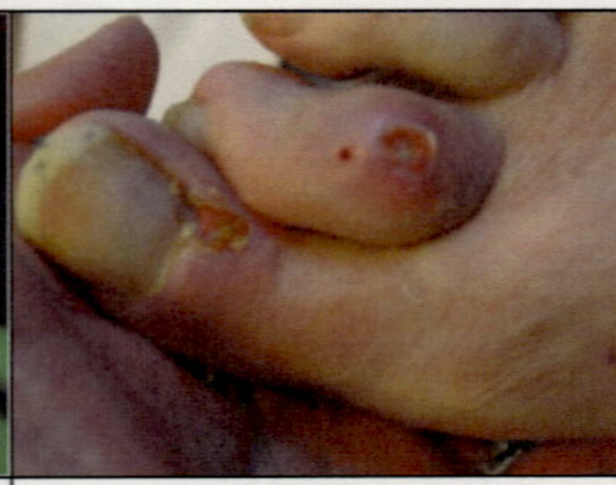	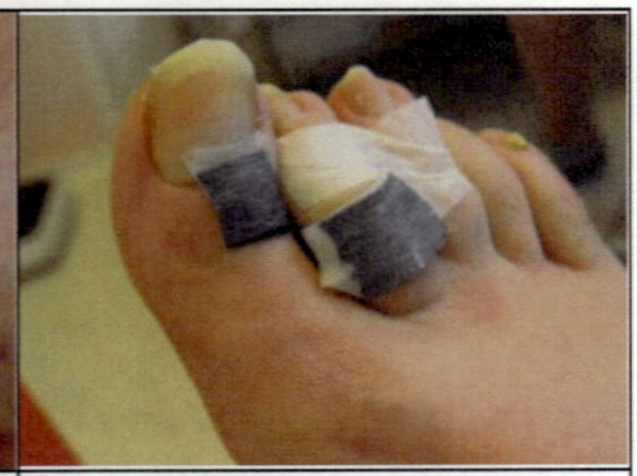
H-1: On May 13th 2004. First corrective Hapla Band TO and one inter-digital felt TO.	H-2: On May the 27th 2004. Fifteen days later.	H-3: Actisorb Ag+ application used all the treatment long.

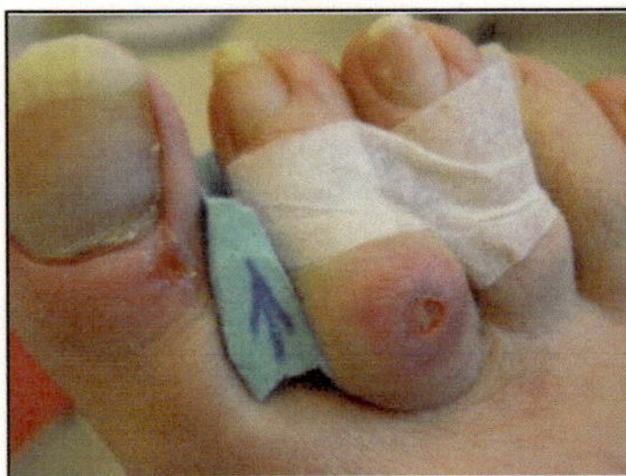	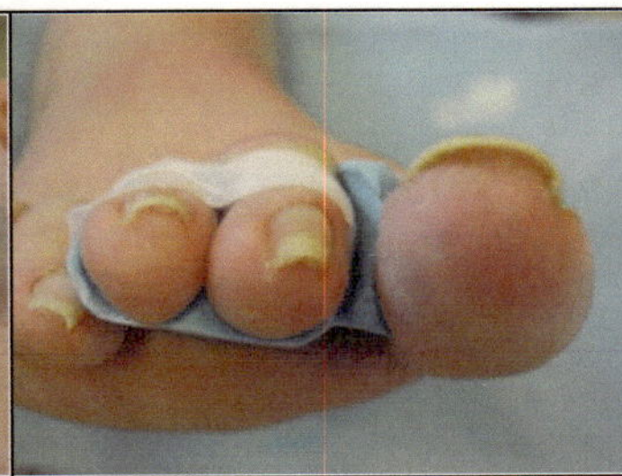	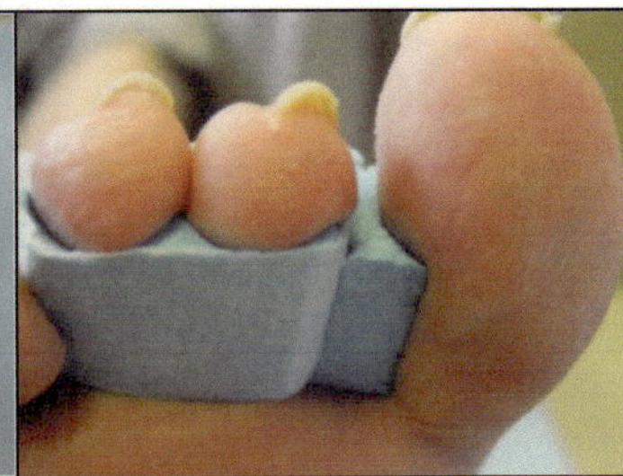
H-4 : On June 24th 2004, corrective thermoformable latex foam TO allowing to treat wounds et corrective sub-digital latex foam and a inter-digital device (dorsal view).	H-5: Front view	H-6: Plantar view

Fig. 13.

The protective TO was possible to fit after the articulations softening obtained by the Hapla-Band TO installing. It is held with Micrope. The silicone permanent orthosis couldn't be made because the patient couldn't reach his own feet.

Only the TO was replaced every 2 or 3 weeks.

3.3.3 CASE I: TO for an ulceration in order to amputate the fifth toe

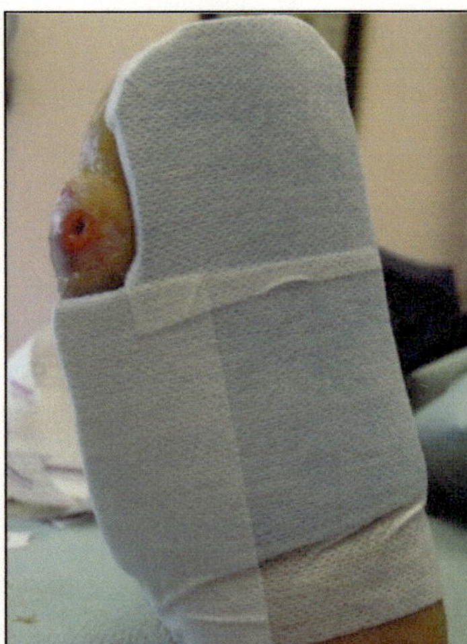	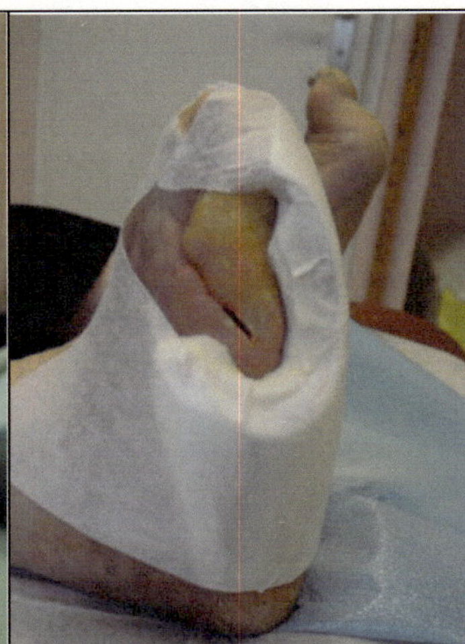	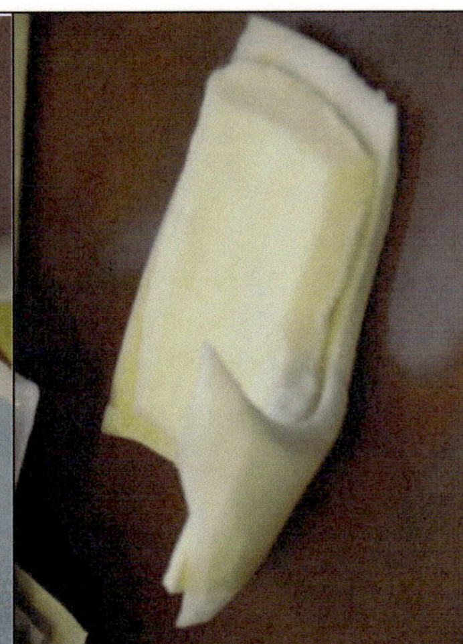
I-1 : Non-rigid thermoformed material TO.	I-2 : Thermoformed Plastazote TO, with felt inside.	I-3 : Offloading TO.

Fig. 14.

3.3.4 CASE J: Where creativeness is needed…

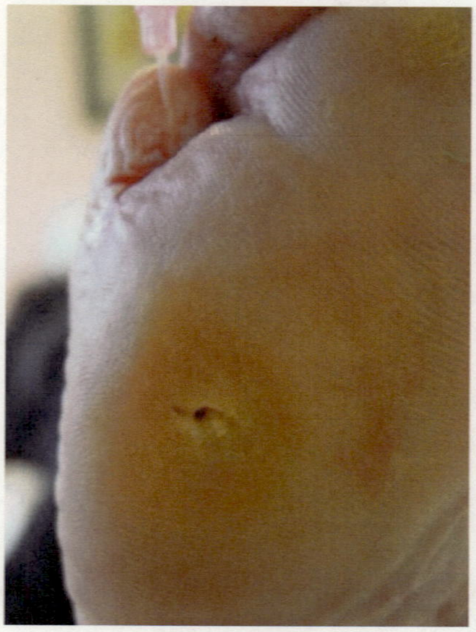	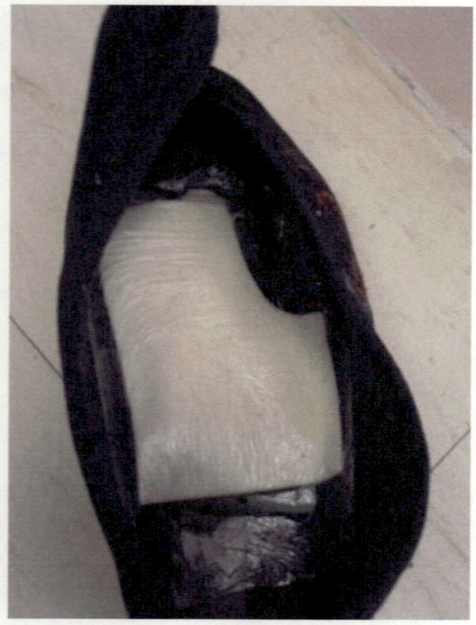
J-1: Fistulisation of a plantar ulceration in the inter-digital space of the fourth and fifth toes.	J-2: Offloading thermoformed TO, with felt inside, directly sticked in the shoe.

Fig. 15.

3.3.5 CASE K: Total transmetatarsal amputation

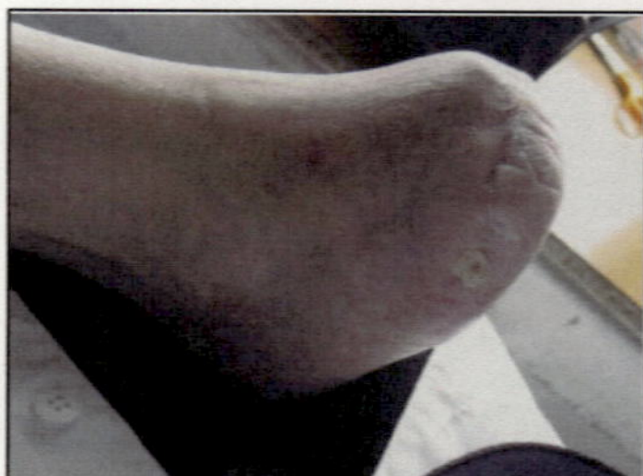	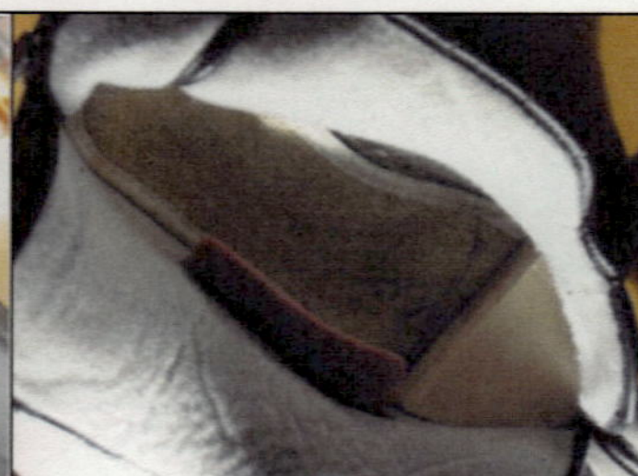	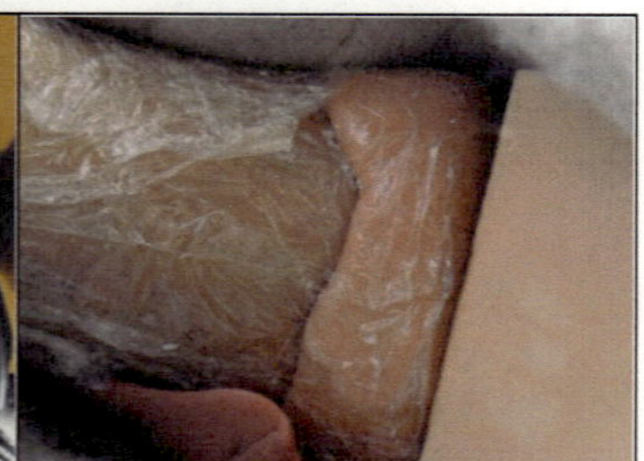
K-1 : Total amputation.	K-2: Inside shoe fitting : Plastazote has been used to fill in anterior part of the shoe. A silicone orthosis to avoid all stump frictions.	K-3: Offloading orthosis confection with Bland Rose ® from Fresco silicone, directly cast on the stump in the shoe.

Fig. 16.

The TOT used for this diabetic patient, helps us to understand the specialist's aim: he wanted to educate and hand-hold this patient in his decease's evolution.

The issues of protection and correction in this treatment are essential to make him accept the installing of a digital or plantar orthosis. The podiatrist helps his patient to have a therapeutic behavior to delay as long as possible the amputation.

4. What instances does the TOT method fail?

It is not the TOT method which presents a failure risk but the patient when he or she stops his or her treatment. When the work is properly done, there is no failure.

Precaution to be taken when installing a TO are those of any other treatment:

- The TO must not hurt, it is made to relief the patient.
- The TO helps scarring because of the offloading of the conflicted area.
- The TO is installed on safe areas and out of the irritated ones.
- The TO shape is adapted according to the recovery step.
- The TO opening will be as wide as the conflicted area requires.

Pressures repartition thanks to the TO installed on safe areas offloads the irritated area. Pressure is quite often the aggravating factor.

TOT is a very good therapeutic method in biomechanical pathology of foot.This is a quick technique aiming a immediate relief. This is the best treatment in severe pathologies.

The podiatrist will always try to correct but if it is impossible then, he will choose the TO and the silicone protection devices or the offloading plantar devices).

5. Conclusion

I hope this technique will be found essential to handle ulceration on a high-risk foot of a diabetic patient.

Having used this technique during twenty years now, I still discover the cleverness of this therapeutic methodology.

And as Mrs. Marie-José van Lith said: *"One has to be creative for each medical case he has to deal with"*. It is for me a real pleasure to do so.

During all his career, my teacher (Dr. Robert van Lith) tried to transmit this technique to our colleagues and students.

In 2001, I thought and I told to Dr van Lith that this would be possible by taking the diabetic foot treatment into account (we were on a world- congress of Podiatry in Paris and Dr Margreet van Putten and Mrs. Marie-José van Lith were there).

In 2010, during the Podiatrist International Federation world conference in Amsterdam, Dr van Putten wanted to pay tribute to my teacher, an exceptional man, and when his wife, Marie-José van Lith received this tribute, she announced that she had succeeded in launching TOT in several endocrinology departments; she said: *"This technique is based on medical laws which makes it a real treatment. To treat the wounds of the diabetic foot, this treatment is essential, before all permanent silicone or plantar orthosis which could be necessary after the complete wound recovery"*.

This therapeutic technique should be transmitted to all our foot specialists' colleagues.

In the near future, I hope that this technique will be part of the teaching curriculum for French Podiatrists. I wish the words *Temporary Orthesio-therapy* and *temporary orthosis* will find their definition in the medical terms dictionary (Garnier Delamare).

TOT should be officially recognized as beneficial to the public at large... to ensure a less harrowing future to the diabetic patients.

6. Definition

Temporary orthesio-therapy (Dr Robert van Lith): This technique is called erroneously *Padding* in France. This name was brought in France by Franklin Charlesworth. This is a very inventive technique to achieve an immediate relief, before the use of a permanent silicone or plantar orthosis.

7. References

[1] Van Lith Robert, July 2003, Podologie appliqué, Edition du Lau, ISBN : 2 84750 052 9. (page 67: ORTHESIOTHERAPIE TRANSITOIRE/ Une Thérapeutique de choix pour la suppression immédiate du Stress Mécanique.)

[2] Van Putten Margreet, van Lith Marie-José, van Lith Robert, The diabetic foot, Montelimar Seminary (Drôme, France), March 2002.

[3] The International Working Group on the Diabetic Foot, may 1999, International Consensus on the Diabetic Foot, Copyright by the International Working Group on the Diabetic Foot, ISBN : 90-9012716-x. (page 29: Pathways to diabetic foot ulceration.)

[4] The International Working Group on the Diabetic Foot, may 1999, Practical Guidelines on the Management and the prevention of the Diabetic Foot, Copyright by the International Working Group on the Diabetic Foot, ISBN : 90-9012716-x.)page 2 :Illustration of ulcer due to repetitive stress.)

[5] Richard Florence, L'orthésiothérapie transitoire. Conférence aux 28èmes Entretiens de Podologie à Paris 2003.

[6] Ha Van Georges (Paris), Equilibre N°197 1996 –Qu'est-ce qu'un mal perforant et comment le prévenir ?

[7] Sanders Joan, Goldstein Barry, Leotta Daniel, Journal of Rehabilitation Research and Development Vol. 32 N° 3. October 1995, Skin response to mechanical stress: Adaptation rather than breakdowm- A rewiew of the literature. (page 223).

[8] Boulton Andrew, Cavanagh Peter, Rayman Gerry, May 2006, The Foot Diabetes, Fourth Edition, Chapter 5, The Pathway to ulceration : Aetiopathogenesis. ISBN 9780470015049.

[9] Sanders, J.E., et al., skin response to mechanical stress : adaptation rather than breakdown – a review of the literature, University of Washington, Journal of Rehabilitation and Development , vol. N° 32, 1995.

[10] Granier-Delamare, Dictionnaires des termes de médecine ; 24èmes éditions, Maloine, 1995, ISBN : 2-224-02381-2.

[11] Richard, F., compte-rendu de séminaire de la journée de formation sur l'OTT, Nantes, septembre 1998.

7

The Biomechanics of the Diabetic Foot

Dennis Shavelson
The Foot Typing Center,NYC, Outreach Program, Surgical Attending, Department of Podiatry, Wyckoff Heights Medical Center, Member, New York Presbyterian Healthcare System, Brooklyn, New York USA

1. Introduction

The importance of the physician's role in examining and assessing the diabetic foot is hard to overstate.[1-2] Fifteen percent of the 16 million diabetic patients in the United States will develop foot ulcers.[3,4] The diabetic foot is responsible for more than half of the 67,000 annual non-traumatic lower extremity amputations in the developed world.[5] Lower extremity amputation is 15 times more likely to occur in a patient with diabetes.[6] The annual cost of amputations is $600 million and lost wages and morbidity are estimated at $1 billion, annually.[7] Finally, studies have shown that primary care physicians are rarely performing foot examinations on their diabetic patients during routine visits.[8]

The underlying reasons that the foot is the number one location for comorbidities in diabetes places peripheral neuropathy and its sequellae that include Loss of Protective Sensation (LOPS) and Loss of Proprioception atop the list[9] with Peripheral Arterial Disease (PAD) ranking a distant second. These risk factors magnify preexisting biomechanical risk factors that function in closed chain (Table 1) into often overlooked loss of balance, function, productivity and quality of life that precede or are adjacent to the more obvious presentations of wounds, infections, hospitalizations and amputations that are, in reality, end stage events for more and more diabetic patients.

1.	Ground Reactive Forces
2.	Hard, Unyielding Shoes
3.	Underlying Biomechanical Pathology
4.	Body Mass and Weight
5.	Activity Level
6.	Fitness Level
7.	Health State

Table 1. Underlying Biomechanical Risk Factors In Diabetes

Podiatry, as a profession and by degree, is the only profession armed with an underlying Functional Lower Extremity Biomechanics (FLEB) core· Three years of Undergraduate FLEB courses followed by up to three years of Residency that includes applying biomechanics to non operative and surgical decisions and the chief complaints of diabetic patients. This is then followed by Continuing Medical Education and most importantly, every Doctor of Podiatric Medicine (DPM) has an Evidence Based Practice Rooted in Biomechanics that includes orthotics and active and passive therapies that have been practiced for generations by the podiatric community.

It is my opinion that the medical community, weak in closed chain medicine, is not prepared to diagnose, treat and manage their patients biomechanically. This single fact is the reason that Podiatry plays such an important role in the medical community and the life of every diabetic.

2. Biomechanics of the foot

Definition: Biomechanics is the art and science of applying the scientific laws of Physics, Architecture, Engineering and Mechanics principles to living subjects. Although not a pure science and therefore, difficult to research and quantify, committed practitioners of Functional Lower Extremity Biomechanics (FLEB) have prepared themselves to conduct interpersonal practices by amassing foundational knowledge, professional experience and use the applicable evidence that has surfaced to produce, for each practitioner, his/her version of an Evidence Based Biomechanics Practice[10-13].

Unlike pure science that focuses on inanimate objects, living subjects often do not obey Primary Scientific Laws. This is offset by the Biomechanical Literature which contains over 200 additions providing evidence that foot orthotics work[14-18] in addition to continued research and study being called for and conducted but like other aspects of medicine, such as foot surgery, biomechanics remains as much an art as a science[19-20]. The Podiatry community has accepted as its responsibility, the closed chain foundation of our functional lives and in the case of the diabetic population, sits as educators, mentors and front line practitioners as no other specialist can when it comes to biomechanics and Closed Chain Medicine.

Understanding the biomechanics of the foot is an important component in the evaluation of the diabetic foot probably deserving greater focus than it has received. **The successful compensation of underlying foot type-specific biomechanical pathology cannot be underestimated as one of the most important adjacent preventive and treatment models in the health history of the diabetic.**

FLEB focuses on the human body from the low back down, in *closed chain* (standing [stance] or active [gait] and weighted upon the ground. Alternatively, Allopathic Medicine studies subjects in *open chain kinetics* (on an examining table or not weighted) [21].

The etiological forces that must be overcome in managing a patient biomechanically can be reviewed using Table 1. Since they differ for each individual, unless a patient encounter during which a biomechanical evaluation is performed as well as a historical interview to assess coexisting etiological factors is performed by a biomechanically oriented Podiatrist, the resultant orthotic and treatment plan may fall short of its potential benefits.

Removing pathological forces from the weightbearing surface of the foot, balancing and supporting the posture, leveraging the muscle-tendon units and training them to perform and providing functional and safe footwear for the diabetic foot are the biomechanical keys to preventing and treating foot ulcers, gait and balance problems and neuropathic foot syndromes. The use of straps, pads, foot orthotics, muscle strengthening and training programs and therapeutic footwear before considering surgery has been shown to reduce foot ulcers, foot infections, amputation and hospitalizations in a diabetic population while allowing the patient to maintain and improve walking and active functioning with a high level of efficiency and minimal injury and disability[22].

The Biomechanical Anatomy of the Foot. Biomechanically, the foot can be divided into functional segments in two main ways. The first divides it at the Midtarsal Joint into a rearfoot and forefoot and the second divides the foot at the second and third rays into medial and lateral arch segments (Figure 1).

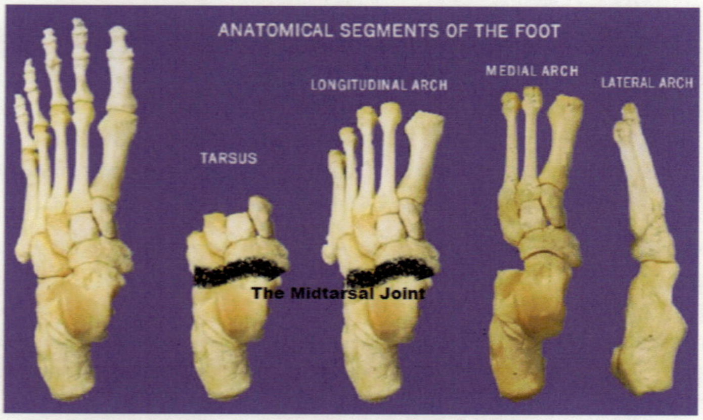

Fig. 1. Functional anatomy of the foot. (Adapted from Glick JB. Dynamics of the foot in locomotion. Pod Management 4:136, 2001, with permission).

The medial arch is composed of the calcaneus, talus, navicular, the three cuneiforms and the first, second and third metatarsals. The lateral arch is composed of the calcaneus, the cuboid and the fourth and fifth metatarsals.[9] These two arches are connected by a transverse roof of bone. The surface underneath these osseous supports, architecturally, is known as The Vault of The Foot (Figure 2).[23] This Vault, when centered and supported by healthy soft tissues, provides a lifetime foundation for upright weightbearing and function. In contrast if The Vault is allowed to become off-centered exhibiting excess stiffness, flexibility, collapse or arch, on a case to case basis, the resulting stressful compensations in pedal and postural bones, joints, muscles, tendons, ligaments and integumentary organs provides an ever increasing burden to society as we live longer and more active lives.

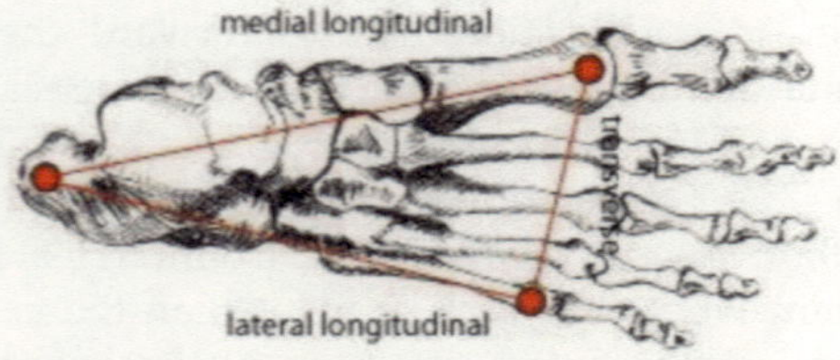

Fig. 2. The Vault of The Foot

The gait cycle

Human stance and activity is comprised of many patterns or cycles in order to maintain us erect and move us in all directions as we live our lives. Movement can be forward, backward, side-to-side or it may rock, sway or move us up or down. Each of these movements has a totally different Activity Cycle that makes different demands upon the body biomechanically. The Walking Cycle (moving forward) and The Backward Walking Cycle challenge the bones, muscles, tendons and ligaments very differently. The fact that we have so many different biomechanical tasks to accomplish combined with the variations in stress that each of them has on the structures performing them makes it impossible to present biomechanics in an understandable manner to inexperienced minds unless we focus on one specific Activity Cycle.

Historically, in order to understand biomechanics foundationally, educators, researchers and practitioners have universally chosen The Activity Cycle of Forward Movement (walking) as the cycle to use when demonstrating, researching and monitoring FLEB. This cycle is known as "The Gait Cycle".[24] It is important to note that there are variations in The Gait Cycle that include Midstance Contact Gait and Forefoot Contact Gait that impact the foot and posture differently than The Heel Contact Gait Cycle.

The Gait Cycle defines a complete step from heel contact to heel contact using one limb, either left or right. The gait cycle is first divided into a Stance Phase (60%), when the foot is in contact with the ground, and a Swing Phase (40%), when the foot is free floating. The stance phase is further divided into a contact phase (10%), a midstance phase (40%) and a propulsive phase (10%) (See Figure 3). Since pathology develops most when the foot is touching the ground, FLEB concentrates on the stance phase of gait.

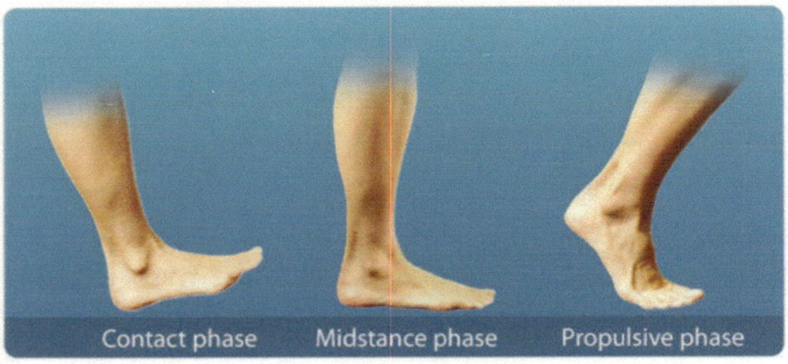

Fig. 3. The Stance Phase of Gait

Because the tendo Achilles is medially inserted on the calcaneus, it places the foot in an inverted position when the stance phase of gait begins and so the heel strikes the ground on the lateral side of the vault. As foot function cascades forward, the heel everts (pronates) in order to place the medial surface of the foot upon the ground. Because of pronation, the ball of the foot contacts the ground (midstance) with the metatarsals hitting in order of 5,4,3,2 and finally 1 as the medial side of the vault begins to support weight. Then, as the leg moves forward over the planted foot, the heel comes off the ground (Heel Rise) and when muscular power leverages to the point where they are stronger than the ground reactive forces and the metatarsal heads are firmly planted, the foot pushes off the ground (Propulsion) beginning the Float Phase of Gait. That is then repeated as we move from point A to point B.

The supporting structure of the lateral side of The Vault of The Foot, composed of bones that when healthy, has an architecture that allows it to lock when weighted without the need for much muscular and ligamentous support. This enables the lateral Vault to be primarily strong, stable, supportive and capable of assuming an Optimal Functional Position (OFP) without much ligamentous and muscular primary or compensatory assistance in both the rearfoot and the forefoot that is different for all individuals. When the lateral column functions from Optimal Functional Position, there is little compensatory tissue stress of the bones and supporting structures or compensatory muscle engine energy on both a microscopic or macroscopic level.

In opposition, the bony architecture of the medial side of The Vault of The Foot lacks the ability to lock on its own when weighted without the assistance of a large number of primary muscle engines and ligamentous systems. This means that without strong and trained muscle engines and a well developed and conditioned ligamentous supporting system, the medial Vault of the Foot is not capable of maintaining its Optimal Functional Position and so it serves as the anatomical location for much of the biomechanical pathology that exists in both the rearfoot and forefoot (figures 4) for most feet. Collapse of the bony position of the medial side of the foot from its OFP results in stretching and reduced leverage of the ligaments and muscles that are mandated to lock and support the vault in OFP (figure 5). This creates a subclinical vicious closed chain biomechanical cycle early on that stresses the tissues on a cellular level that when repeated over and over as we live our lives eventually rises to clinical events like pain and overuse syndromes, foot and postural deformities and irreversible degenerative changes. **Summarily, inherited medial vault weakness serves as the biomechanical etiology for FLEB and unless diagnosed and treated, guarantees compensatory degeneration, overuse, deformity and structural and functional breakdown in the feet and throughout the posture, in closed chain**.

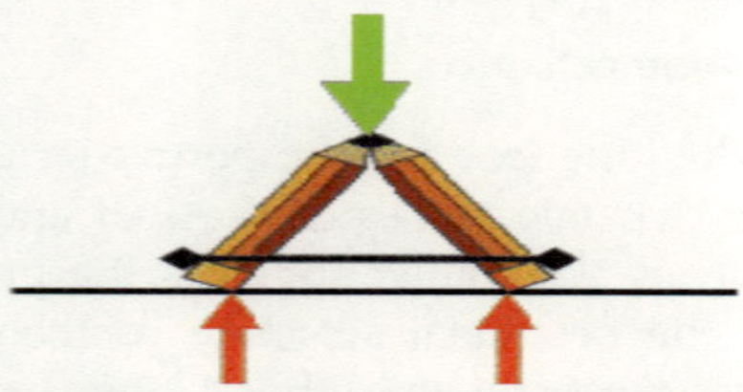

Fig. 4. The Ligamentous Tie Beam Supports The Bony Truss in the Medial Column

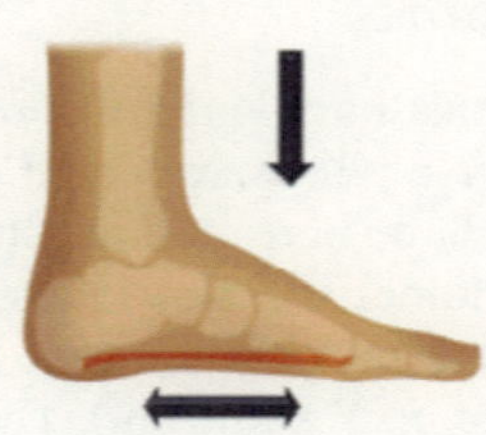

Fig. 5. The Longitudinal and Vertical Collapse of The Medial Column Deforming the OFP

The current gold standard, known as Subtalar Joint (STJ) Neutral Examination was developed thirty years ago by Podiatrist Merton Root et al.[25] In this system, all feet are cast for orthotics in subtalar joint neutral position to develop orthotic shells which are then modified using Orthotic Reactive Postings and Modifications such as suggested by McPoil and Hunt[27] in order to reduce tissue stress in areas of complaint. Rootian Biomechanics evolved what was known as orthopedics and the prescribing of custom arch supports in the colleges of podiatry into the current biomechanics and custom foot orthotics in the 1970's. Low level research proving that STJ Neutral casted shells and prescription orders for rearfoot and forefoot corrections when ordering custom foot orthotics were beneficial are difficult to deny[14-18]. Unfortunately, Rootian Biomechanics is being shown to lack scientific merit and a lack of reproducibility and evidentiary proof.[28-30] This may be because research is showing that in reality, most of the problems facing us in daily life involve lengthening, widening and collapse of the fore part of the foot on the sagittal and transverse planes and not the subtalar joint as Root and his followers preach.[30-33]

In response to this fact, modern theories are surfacing that when practiced by a new wave of biomechanically committed podiatrists are returning the podiatrist to the top of a Biomechanical Pyramid and exposing the claims of others to be exaggerated.

The doctor-patient relationship that only exists between a podiatrist using modern biomechanics to diagnose and treat the diabetic foot biomechanically using custom casting and prescribing techniques as well as individually tailored "Boot Camp" type training of the patient expands care beyond the "get sick and come to me" model of Kirby and Scherer[34] and Fuller[35] into more of a wellness model offered by Dananberg[31], Glaser[33] and Shavelson[38] that includes prevention, intervention and quality of life expansion as part of care using varied casting techniques and treatment for underlying pathology that includes prevention, intervention and quality of life expansion as part of care using varied casting prescribing and training techniques, not just complaints. One such theory gaining in popularity is called The Foot Centering Theory of Biomechanics or Wellness Biomechanics invented and U.S. Patented by this author[38-42]

The foot centering theory of biomechanics

When it comes to understanding the foot as a supportive structure, in The Foot Centering Theory of Biomechanics, the dynamic arches of the foot and The Vault of the Foot are compared to architectural arches and vaults applying the principles and terminology of architectural engineering to the positional structure of the foot (figure 6). The use of architectural language reduces the previous difficult language of physics and mechanical engineering that has distanced practitioners, patients and the foot suffering public investigating and applying biomechanics.

The architectural arches as structures have one function and that is to support. They are symmetrical (no back or front). Their pillars are equal in size, their component bricks are equal or proportional in size and shape and their keystones are centered. They resist wear and tear but fail as adaptive, functional and shock absorbing entities because they cannot provide leverage to ropes and pulleys trying to move it when attached. In opposition, pedal arches are assymetrical (they have a back and front). Their pillars are disproportional, their bones are of different size and shape and their keystones are off-centered. This means that pedal arches and vaults, in order to succeed as an adaptive, shock absorbing and mobile entities, are destined to fail as supporters (figure 6).

In Foot Centering, rather than treat all feet from a Subtalar Joint Neutral platform, feet are profiled into subgroups or types that share common characteristics called Functional Foot

Types or FFT's. These shared structural, functional and compensatory tendencies for those that test a particular foot type provide a platform from which to provide improved custom care for every patient. Within each subgroup, each subject shares similarities with respect to weightbearing position, segmental ranges of motion, predictable areas of strengths and weaknesses and certain precursor signs and symptoms that can help predict past, present and future foot and postural breakdown and performance issues.

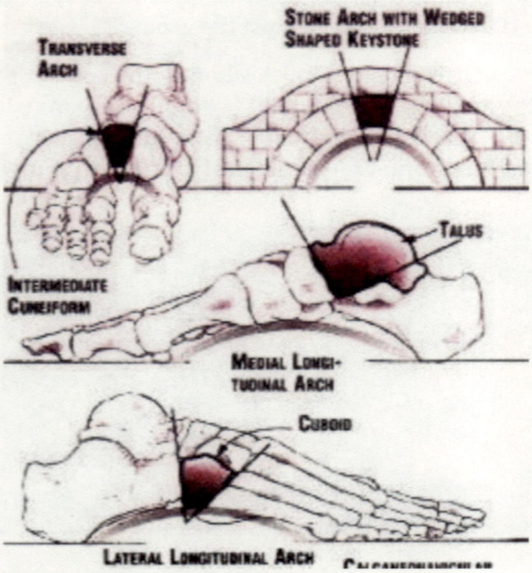

Fig. 6. Architectural vs. Pedal Arches

Starting from Root's well defined position of pedal neutrality (Figure 7) [43], two simple open chain tests are performed for the rearfoot and two tests for the forefoot determine

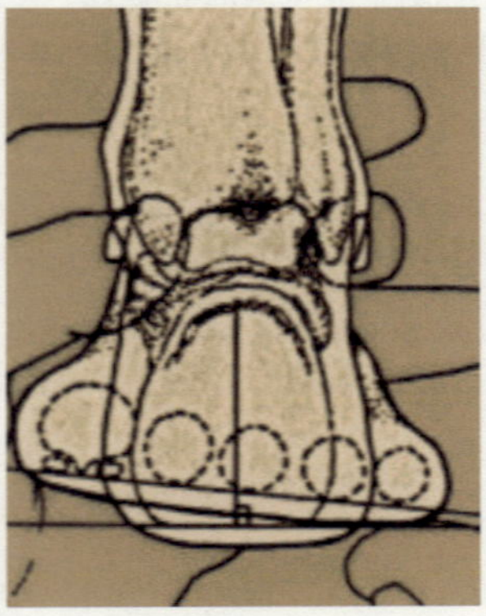

Fig. 7. Root's Neutral Position.

the Supinatory End Range of Motion (SERM) and Pronatory End Range of Motion (PERM) of each segment defining a rearfoot type and forefoot type for every foot. These two segmental foot types then combine to produce a Functional Foot Type (FFT) that serves as a starting platform to develop a plan of biomechanical care in the hands of a skilled professional.[37]

The functional foot typing system

In The Functional Foot Typing system, the total range of motion and the positional relationships within the rearfoot (the subtalar joint) and the forefoot (the midtarsal joint) gathered in open chain can be used to describe specific foot types and how they will compensate when placed in closed chain against the ground.

The RF SERM Test represents subtalar joint position in the contact phase of The Gait Cycle and the RF PERM Test represents subtalar joint position in the midstance phase of gait. The FF SERM Test represents the first ray position at the midstance phase of The Gait Cycle and the FF PERM Test represents the first ray at the heel lift phase of propulsion (figure 8).

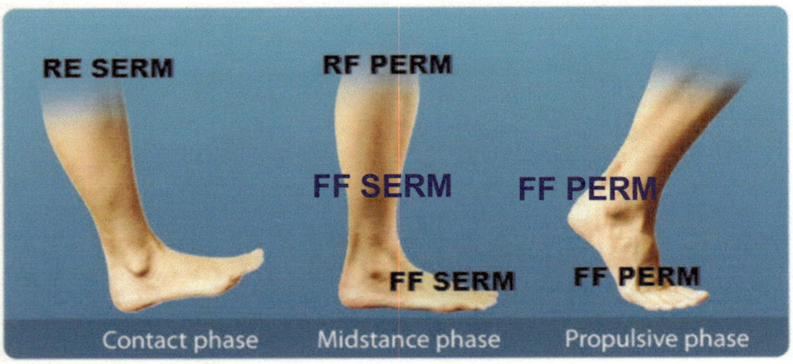

Fig. 8. The SERM-PERM Positions in Gait

The Rearfoot SERM-PERM and the Forefoot SERM-PERM tests each have four possible types that are designated Rigid, Stable, Flexible and Flat.

In trying to present functional foot typing in three paragraphs, we will begin by defining the four possible functional rearfoot types and four functional forefoot types.

The rearfoot foot types

In the **rigid rearfoot type**, the rearfoot total range of motion is less than 15 degrees with the calcaneus inverted to the lower leg at both SERM and PERM.

In the **stable rearfoot type**, the rearfoot total range of motion is 15 degrees with the calcaneus inverted to the lower leg at SERM and perpendicular to the lower leg at PERM.

In the **flexible rearfoot type,** the rearfoot total range of motion is greater than 15 degrees with the calcaneus inverted to the lower leg at SERM and everted to the lower leg at PERM.

In the **flat rearfoot type**, the rearfoot total range of motion is greater than 15 degrees in both SERM and PERM.

The forefoot foot types

In the **rigid forefoot type**, both the SERM and PERM position of 1st met horizontal bisection is plantarflexed to the 5th met horizontal bisection.

In the **stable forefoot type**, the SERM position of the 1st met horizontal bisection plantarflexed to the 5th met horizontal bisection and the PERM position of the 1st met horizontal bisection is online with the 5th met horizontal bisection.

In the **flexible forefoot type,** the SERM position of the 1st met horizontal bisection is plantarflexed to the fifth metatarsal head horizontal bisection and the PERM position of the 1st met horizontal bisection is dorsiflexed to the 5th met horizontal bisection.

In the **flat forefoot type**, both the SERM and PERM position of the 1st met horizontal bisection is dorsiflexed to the fifth met horizontal bisection.

Every pair of feet can be profiled as a specific rearfoot type and forefoot type. After a subject has been diagnosed with a Functional Rearfoot Type and a Functional Forefoot Type the Functional Foot Type is determined by combining both entities. The Functional Foot Typing System allows every foot to be classified into one of sixteen possible FFT's.

		Functional Forefoot Type			
Functional Rearfoot Type		**Rigid**	**Stable**	**Flexible**	**Flat**
	Rigid	**Rigid/Rigid (cavus)**	**Rigid/Stable**	**Rigid/Flex (bunion)**	**Rigid/Flat**
	Stable	**Stable/Rigid**	**Stable/Stable (normal)**	**Stable/Flex**	**Stable/Flat**
	Flexible	**Flex/Rigid**	**Flex/Stable**	**Flex/Flex (pronated)**	**Flex/Flat**
	Flat	**Flat/Rigid**	**Flat/Stable**	**Flat/Flex**	**Flat/Flat (flat)**

Fig. 9. The Functional Foot Typing Matrix

When the four functional rearfoot types are plotted horizontally and the four functional forefoot types are plotted vertically, a matrix composed of sixteen boxes is created, each box representing a possible functional foot type (figure 7). This means that there are 16 possible FFT's, however for the purposes of this chapter, 90% of all feet classify into one of five Common Foot Types (see figure 9)

After diagnosing a subject's foot type, a podiatrist can fabricate a positional prop in the form of a foot orthotic casted in the Optimal Functional Position (OFP) replacing his/her existing footbeds, foot type-specific. This reduces the need for the muscles to overcome pathological collapse allowing them to concentrate on balance and movement. Stress risers within the foot are reduced or eliminated due to healthy redistribution of weight, preventing biomechanical sequelae and preparing each patient to be trained for a better performance, efficiency and quality of life. The goal for success is strong feet and posture that performs efficiently with an end goal of reducing or eliminating the prop orthotic.

This means that by knowing the foot type of a diabetic, the location of future ulcerations and infections can be predicted and prevented utilizing biomechanical treatment to balance and distribute weight, pressure and shear away from areas these predictable areas while expanding the functional quality of life so important to the longevity and fitness of the patient.

The common functional foot types

As stated previously, we are going to focus on The Five Common Functional Foot Types that 90% of all feet profile into (Figure 10) and the forefoot biomechanics that leads to most of the biomechanical pathology seen in practice, including many ulcers and wounds that develop in the feet of diabetics.

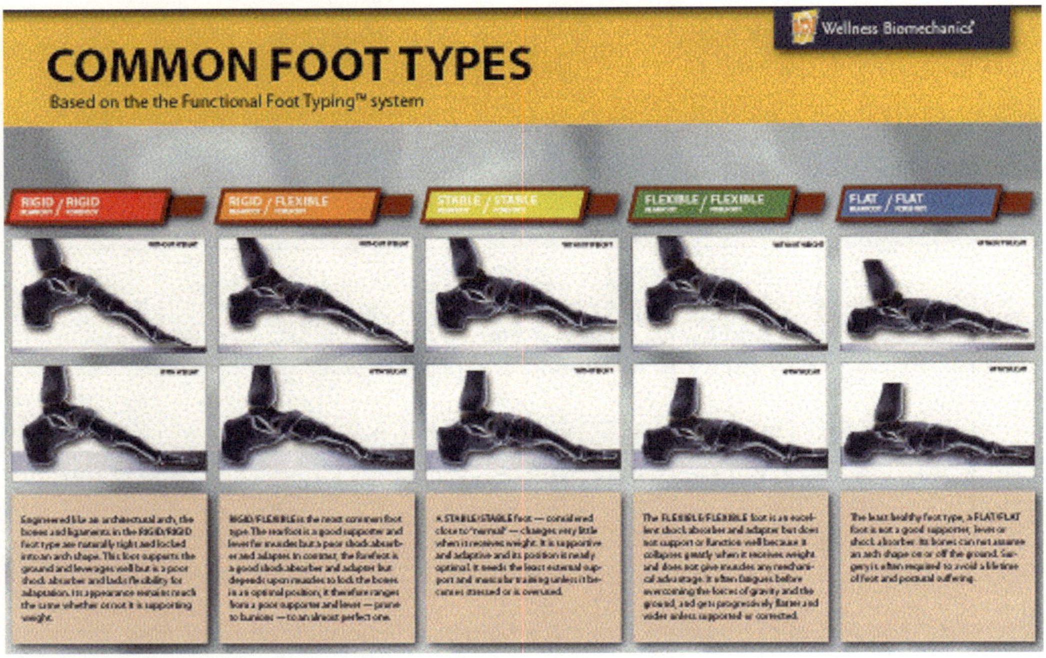

Fig. 10. The Common Functional Foot Types

The goals for success in Foot Centering are strong feet and posture that perform efficiently with reduced deformity, degeneration and suffering. In the case of the diabetic patient, we add the prevention, improved healing, reduction of invasive procedure needed and improved functional life when dealing with closed chain ulcers, wounds and infections.

The characteristics of the Functional Foot Types (FFT's) [44]

Each FFT is associated with a certain profile of features that as a whole unite the members of that FFT. These include lesion pattern, x-ray presentation, shoe wear pattern, foot deformities, foot pain and postural pain and fatigue symptoms.

This means that if given the characteristics of a given patient, a biomechanically practiced podiatrist can place that patient into one of the FFT's.

Since some foot type characteristics are shared by more than one type, some patients may resemble each other and not be in the same FFT but when profiled, the foot type can be confirmed by its overall characteristics. For example, the presence of a range of motion of the 1st ray to fifth of lets say, 35 degrees in a patient diagnosed as a rigid forefoot type probably reflects poor typing since that would definitely place that subject into the flexible forefoot subgroup.

Since they are foot type specific, pathological foot type characteristics, even if not yet evident for a given patient can be reduced or prevented by introducing OFP and compensatory threshold training as part of care.

As an example, please review the characteristics of The Rigid Rearfoot/Rigid Forefoot FFT (figure 11).

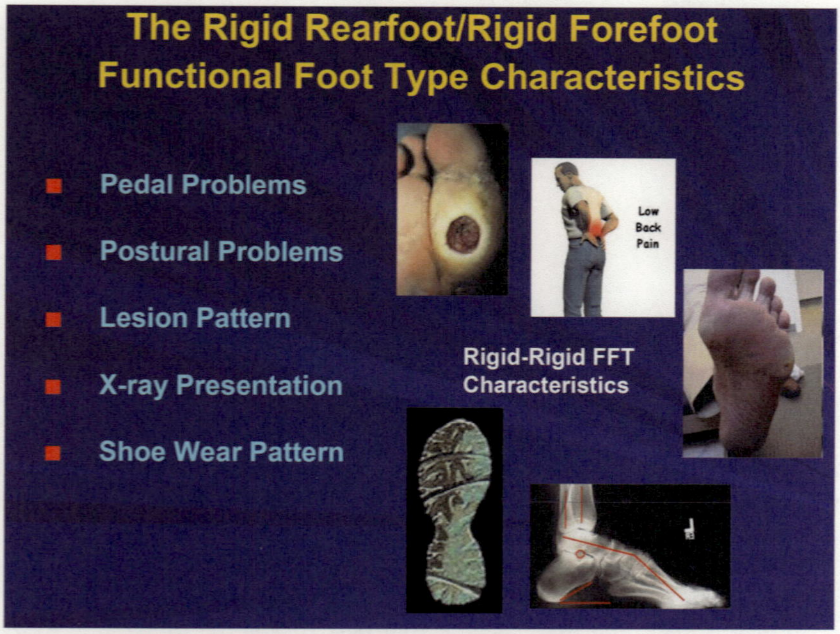

Fig. 11. The Rigid Rearfoot/Rigid Forefoot FFT Characteristics

Protective callus formation[1,39]

In closed chain, when an area of the foot is overloaded with weight, shear or torque, there are two possible reactive occurrences in the skin.

The first results from an overwhelming acute force that gives the skin no time to protect itself from injury. This acute injury is known as blistering. The skin separates into two layers, a base and a roof that then fills up with body fluid or blood depending on which organs are involved.

The second event occurs when there is subclinical repetitive microtrauma in the form of shear, pressure or torque to a weightbearing area of the foot and this results in reactive compression and thickening of the epidermal layers in that area presenting itself as a cascade of changes that occur ranging from protective callus (figure 12) to ulceration and wounding (figure 13). The level of change depends on how strong and how long the microtrauma continues.

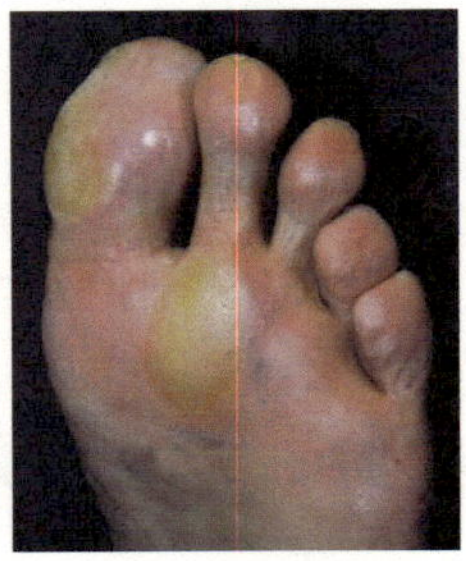

Fig. 12. Protective Callus

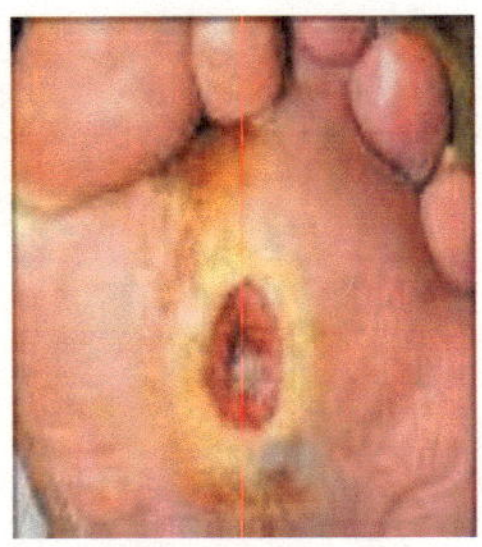

Fig. 13. Pressure Ulcer with Deep Wound

This means that if protective callus develops Functional Foot Type-Specific due at least in part to underlying, inherited biomechanical pathology, then foot typing diabetic patients, monitoring their protective calluses and treating them biomechanically utilizing Foot Centering so that they don't advance into ulcers and wounds defines the important role of The Podiatrist as an integral part of the health care team of every diabetic.

Ulcer, wound and amputation prevention in diabetics utilizing foot typing

The application of Functional Foot Typing that best serves the diabetic is to look at the functional forefoot type and state the location of forefoot callus for each of the Common Foot Types. Whether these calluses exist or not on a patients biomechanical timeline, these areas are accepting greater than normal tissue stress which will cascade to ulceration unimpeded in the face of diabetic neuropathy and must be decompensated biomechanically. [45-49]

The common functional foot type/ callus-ulcer patterns

Figure 14 introduces the reader to the predictable sites of excess closed chain weight forming callus. Although the body's desire is to protect these areas from injury, like the fingertips of a guitar player, continued ground and shoe reactive forces cascades the clinical picture to that of the very injury it is attempting to prevent .

After diagnosing a subject's foot type, a podiatrist can fabricate a positional prop in the form of a foot orthotic casted in the Optimal Functional Position (OFP) for that type. This reduces the need for the muscles to overcome pathological collapse allowing them to concentrate on balance and movement. Stress risers within the foot are reduced or eliminated preventing biomechanical sequelae and preparing each patient to be trained for a better foundational positioning and muscle engine performance. In addition, the need for protective callus formation reduces or is eliminated[42].

Functional Foot Type	Callus/Ulcer Pattern
Rigid/Rigid FFT	**First Met Callus, 5th Met Callus** 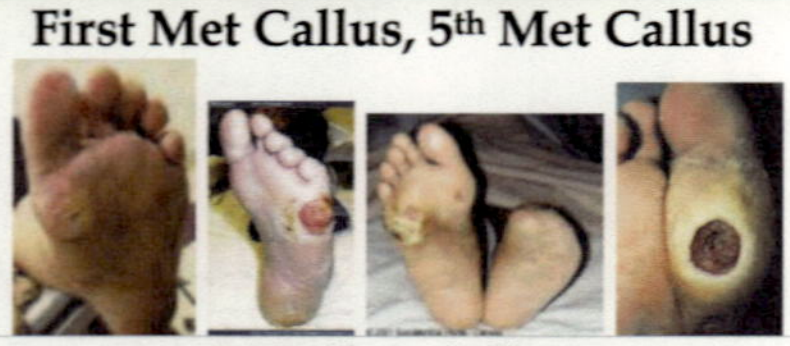
Rigid/Flexible FFT	**IP Hallux Callus, 2nd Met Callus** 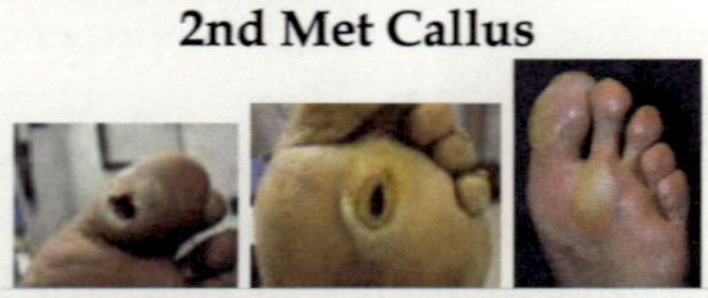
Stable/Stable FFT	**Callus Hallux IP Joint, 2nd Met If Stressed, No Ulcer or Wound Formation**
Flexible/Flexible	**Medial First Met Callus, Rolloff Hallux IP Callus, 2nd,3rd, 4th met callus** 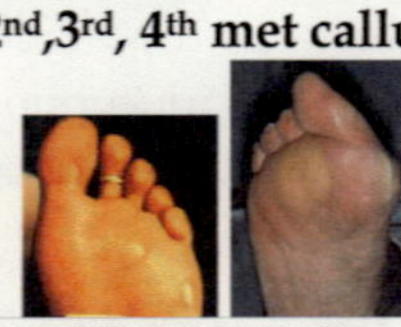
Flat/Flat	**Fifth Met Callus** 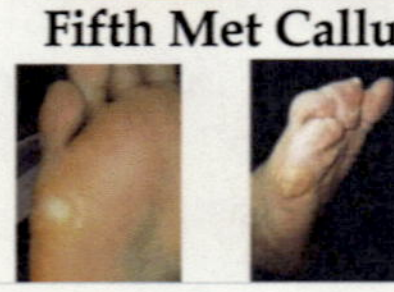

Fig. 14. Callus-Ulcer patterns of the Common FFT's

Why is the diabetic foot so prone to problems?

All of us inherits a functional foot type and are prone to accept its strengths and weaknesses. This inevitably leads us to suffer predictable quality of life issues due to biomechanical wear and tear and inefficient compensatory mechanisms that are impacted by concomitant factors such as weight, body type, age, activity level, health state, ground surfaces, equipment and vocation.

However, **no one factor is so overwhelmingly important to consider when rating the importance of podiatry care in the form of functional lower extremity biomechanics than Diabetes Mellitus.** This is because diabetics inheriting these very same FFT's end up with greater quality of life issues including ulcerations, infections, deformities and amputations than their non diabetic counterparts due to the devastating comorbidities of peripheral neuropathy and PAD. The most devastating component comorbidity of DM relates to the fact that neuropathic diabetics lose what is known as proprioception or the ability to "feel and react to the road and navigate through it".

Walking and many other tasks require daily closed chain sensory input to adapt and modify motor patterns and muscle output to carry out the desired task. Fully functioning joints and bones, combined with adequate muscle strength, are needed. The result of this activity is also coupled with local soft tissue compensations affecting the foot–ground interface. These can be affected by the frictional properties of the sole, internal muscle activity as well as the inherited underlying biomechanics of each subject that can be improved with foot orthotics.[50]

Proprioception

Proprioception is defined as "sensing the motion and position of the body. Knowing where we are in space and judging how we should navigate that space is a biological quality that when combined with our intelligence, elevates us from the rest of the animal kingdom.

Specialized nerve endings called Proprioceptors are present throughout the soft tissues of the musculoskeletal system. They interact with the central nervous system and coordinate our body movements, our postural alignment, and our balance. We rely on this delicately controlled and finely-tuned system of receptors and feedback loops and the validity and reliability of the information which is sent into the spinal cord tens of thousands of times every day.

Proprioceptive health allows us to "read" our environment in order to generate appropriate motor responses to perform the motions, actions, tasks and functional skills that we must perform. A reduction of Proprioception impacts our ability to stand weighted without sway as well as our ability to perform artistic and athletic physical activity efficiently and to move from point "A" to point "B".

Over time, areas of the body without adequate proprioception are exposed to increased tissue stress that weaken, deform, degenerate and eventually break down the skin, connective and supportive soft tissue, ligaments, tendons, muscles, bones and joints in those areas as well as in other areas of the body that must compensate secondarily in order keep the body performing.

The current scientific literature supports the following changes in the diabetic foot as a result of peripheral neuropathy: limited joint range of motion, glycosylation of tendons and soft tissue leading to restriction of motion, diminished plantar fat padding, and intrinsic muscle wasting with resultant clawing deformity of toes and contractures of the forefoot.[45-51]

Although it cannot be stated with certainty in all cases, there is evidence to state that underlying biomechanical pathology results in reductions in joint range of motion (functional hallux limitus, functional hallux extensus and ankle equinus to name a few) in the lower extremity. This results in stress in ligaments and tendons and joints such as the tendo Achilles, plantar fascia and great toe joint, especially in those foot types that are hypermobile such as the rearfoot and forefoot stable and flexible types. This in turn produces enlargement and fibrosis as well as subsequent contractures and weakness in the foot due to the sum of the repetitive micro injuries to the soft tissues, ligaments, muscles, tendons, joints and bones. [52-55]

Examples of where functional foot typing predicts locations for wounds, infections and ulcers would be the 2nd toe hammertoe prevalent in the rigid rearfoot-flexible forefoot FFT, The fifth met head lesions and wounds of the flat rearfoot-flat forefoot foot type, the hallux IP Rolloff Ulcers that cause hallux amputations are allied to the flexible rearfoot-flexible forefoot functional foot type and the severe ulceration of the plantar 1st metatarsal head that often leads to osteomyelitis of that area is linked to the rigid rearfoot-rigid forefoot FFT.

In diabetes, Loss of Protective Sensation (LOPS), the end stage of proprioceptor pathology, by eliminating the pain protection response from the equation, leads to overwhelming integumentary tissue stress that is not decompensated due to the fact that the body cannot recognize its existence. This leads to pressure callus, pressure ulcers and wounds, amputations and limb loss because of a lack of proprioceptive warning. Proprioceptive pathology is an early and common finding in the polyneuropathy peripheral neuropathy associated with the disease and may even precede the presence of high fasting blood sugars (prediabetics).

Summarily, insufficient information supplied by Proprioceptive Sensors reduces efficiency of movement, causes pathologic tissue stress, injury, problems with postural coordination and/or joint alignment and chronic, un-resolving pain in sensate areas as well as skin and soft tissue wounds and ulcers in advanced cases.

Locations of nerve receptors

The most important sensory nerve organs for controlling the muscular system are the muscle spindle fibers and the Golgi tendon organs.

Muscle spindle fibers are found interspersed within the contractile fibers of all skeletal muscles, with the highest concentration in the central portion (belly) of each muscle. Muscle spindles respond to changes in muscle length and stress. Without this basic "wiring," proper joint alignment can't be maintained and closed chain stance is almost impossible. [58-59]

Golgi tendon organs are located in the junctions of muscles and their tendons. These protective nerve endings exert an inhibitory effect on contraction of muscle fibers (figure 15).

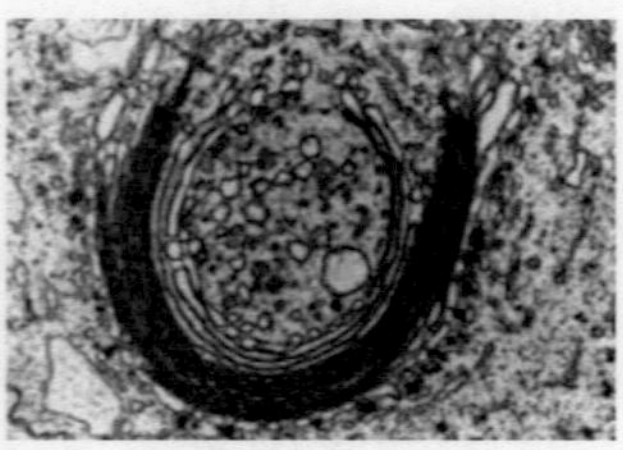

Fig. 15. A Golgi Tendon Organ

Joint mechanoreceptors (Table 2)

Surrounding and protecting all joints are tough, fibrous tissues that contain a variety of sensory nerve endings. The input from these specialized sensors keeps the nervous system informed as to the location of the joint, and also their degree of stress they are under by monitoring stretch, compression, tension, acceleration, and rotation.

Type I mechanoreceptors are found in higher densities in the proximal joints. They sense the position of a joint by signaling the joint angle through normal ranges of motion. These help determine postural (tonic) muscle contractions.

Type II nerve endings adapt to changes in position, and are most active at onset and termination of movement. These are more densely distributed though the distal joints, and affect phasic muscle actions.

Type III mechanoreceptors are high-threshold, which means they require considerable joint stress at end ranges before firing. These receptors serve a protective function similar to the Golgi tendon organs.

Type IV receptors are free nerve endings located in the ligaments, joint capsules, and articular fat pads which respond to pain stimulus. They can generate intense, non-adapting motor responses in all muscles related to a joint, resulting in the protective muscle contractions that restrict joint movement.

muscles and tendons	muscle spindle fibers Golgi tendon organs
joint ligaments and capsules (mechanoreceptors)	type I - low threshold, slow-adapting type II - low threshold, fast-adapting type III - high threshold, slow-adapting type IV - nociceptive (pain endings)

Table 2. Sensory Organs for Proprioception

In addition, stretch-sensitive receptors in the skin known as Ruffini ending, the Merkel cells in hairy skin and field receptors also signal postural and sensory information.

The biomechanics of proprioception in the diabetic foot

There are over 200 additions to the literature showing that custom orthotic support can help improve structural alignment, balance, gait, and athletic performance. [66-69] In addition, therapeutic shoes and orthotics have been shown to be effective in treating and preventing wound and ulcer formation and they are approved by U.S. Medicare for annual dispensing to diabetics as a cost saving to the health care budget.[70]

It has been suggested that this universe of improvements is due primarily to upgrades in the sense of proprioception.[66] A quick review of the mechanisms and components of proprioception will help us comprehend how patients can demonstrate such a large variety of improvements. Being able to explain this to patients (using simpler terms, of course) will help them understand the reasons you are recommending they wear in-shoe orthotics and train their muscle-tendon units to a higher fitness level.

Except for the spine, the foot is the anatomical region that contains the most proprioceptive sensory receptors. Because of the magnitude of sensory input, the feet are quick to produce problems when denied proprioception. These are magnified by the fact that the foot must additionally deal with ground reactive forces and hard, unyielding shoe boxes. Loss of balance, missteps, falls and a reduced ability to navigate efficiently and accurately are just some of the sequelae accompanying proprioceptive disease. Underlying foot type-specific biomechanical pathology impacts pedal posture, pedal muscle engine efficiency and the ability to perform tasks such as walking, lifting and recreational activities and when they exist in a diabetic, cause escalation of its musculoskeletal comorbidities.

Pedal involvement

The six specialized nerve sensors are found throughout the musculoskeletal system, in all skeletal muscles and in every ligament, joint capsule, and articular connective tissue. However, the feet are particularly well-supplied with proprioceptive nerve endings. Mechanoreceptors in the joints, along with the muscle spindles of the foot muscles are responsible for the positive support reflexes and a variety of automatic reflexive reactions[71]. These include the flexor/extensor reflex, which converts the lower limb into a firm, yet compliant pillar. Weightbearing compresses the joints and muscles, evoking reflexive activity in the extensors and inhibition of the flexor muscles.

The vicious cycle of proprioceptive loss and peripheral neuropathy

Second only to glucose control when it comes to managing diabetes is the need to be active and exercise. Increased metabolic disease via peripheral neuropathy causes a reduction in sensory perception of soft touch, pinprick, vibration, and pain eliminating a diabetic from recognizing and reacting to them. Proprioceptive deficits, on the other hand reduce a diabetics ability to know where they are, where they are going and how they are positioned in closed chain. It is the reduced proprioception causes diabetics to live their lives at a slower pace and reduced activity. This in turn allows the metabolic disease to become progressively worse causing advancement of the peripheral neuropathy.[72]

It is the job of the health care team to foster diabetics to increase their activity levels efficiently for the long term. In a foundational sense, this begins with pedal support, improved proprioception, healthy compensation of underlying biomechanical pathology and the incorporation of monitored training and exercise programs into the lives of all diabetics. Until this is accomplished, diabetes will continue to fester in greater portion when compared to the rest of the population and the economic and social drain that diabetes places on society will continue to mount[73].

Like other paradigms of functional lower extremity biomechanics and foot orthotic use, there is little high level evidence available for practitioners to apply in using foot typing as a starting platform. OFP casting and Foot Type-specific prescribing anecdotally allow for more organized and predictable diagnosis and treatment of underlying biomechanical pathology. By preventing postural collapse and reducing the need for primary muscle engines to participate in postural alignment and efficiency, they foster all other aspects of lifestyle upgrading and therefore it should be considered in the care of diabetics that suffer from underlying biomechanical pathology in the face of the dilution that has occurred for the current Rootian standard.

The biomechanics of Charcot Joint Disease

To site an example of the application of functional foot typing and Foot Centering Biomechanics to the ever-present factors in the development and progression of the comorbidities of diabetes and how podiatric closed chain diagnosis and treatment of these entities needs to be a part of the health care team one needs only to inspect Charcot Joint Disease (CJD).

Charcot Joint Disease (CJD)

Any physician treating patients with diabetes is aware that on any visit a patient can present with a foot or ankle that is red, hot, and swollen that is not infected. This presentation signals the beginning of a destructive process affecting the soft tissues and bone structure of the foot and ankle called Charcot Joint Disease (CJD). It leads to joint and osseous collapse and degeneration, functional disability, ulceration, infection and eventual loss of limb. Understanding the etiology and progression of this process should be one of the goals of all members of the diabetes health care team, especially those involved in primary care.

Although there is significant literature related to the diagnosis and treatment of Charcot joint once it develops[74,76], there has been little discussion as to the predisposing Biomechanical Risk Factors that precede the development of Charcot foot and the need for preventive biomechanical treatment once it exists.

The Precursors of Charcot Joint Disease (CJD) The pathophysiology of Charcot joint disease (CJD) remains unknown. One prevalent theory (Volkmann and Virchow) is named the neurotraumatic theory.[77] This theory proposes that the joint destruction of CJD is due to a neuropathic foot that leads to loss of proprioception and pain sensation, thereby permitting joints to be exerted to the point of collapse and destruction.[78] The neurotraumatic theory finds support in studies which demonstrate that plantar pressures are higher in the metatarsophalangeal joints of the forefoot in patients with acute CJD compared to patients with distal sensorimotor neuropathy or neuropathic ulceration.[75] In addition, the motor neuropathy in the diabetic lower extremity tends to precipitate a weakness of muscle groups in the lower extremity, creating dynamic and functional imbalances that either initiate or compound deformities within the foot.

Whether there is feeling the foot or not, the level of underlying biomechanical pathology that exists will determine the level and rate of progression of the cascade of degeneration, deformity, disuse and injury that an individual suffers.

We all suffer from subclinical injury that is of a biomechanical nature. Cellular and tissue stress that goes beyond physiological tolerance. These injuries repair and may even stimulate the development of stronger and more capable cells and tissues. However, once these stresses pass certain thresholds, clinical injury occurs accompanied by various signs and symptoms. These signs and symptoms alert one to address the injury so as to keep it from progressing. Pain, heat, pressure and pinching present early in injury and send a message to change ones lifestyle, environment or metabolism in order to prevent an injury from worsening. In the advanced stages of peripheral neuropathy, there is an absence of these cellular and tissue alarms allowing injuries to progress to a much higher level before becoming clinically evident. This phenomenon is known as Loss of Protective Sensation or LOPS.

This phenomenon, when present in a diabetic that has inherent underlying biomechanical pathology, instead of presenting with painful bunions, stress injuries or ligamentous stresses such as plantar fasciitis, presents with a pathological collapse of the foot, involving insensate joints that have lost proprioception in their end nerve organs that is The Charcot Foot.

In the Functional Foot Typing System, it is the stable and flexible rearfoot and forefoot foot types that are most commonly involved in Charcot Foot. The rigid and flat rearfoot and forefoot foot types, on the other hand resist collapse and the type of injury that may be a precursor of CJD.

More specifically, advanced flexible rearfoot types tend to lead to ankle CJD while moderate ones tend more towards a medial collapse under the navicular that leads to cuboidal ulcers and wounds. In contrast, the flexible forefoot foot types lead to 1st MP Joint neuroarthropathy and transfer ulceration under the 2nd metatarsal head, the IP Hallux and sub 5th metatarsal head.[94]

The pre-charcot foot[80]

When discussing the Charcot foot, the literature consistently points to the existence of peripheral neuropathy and a loss of protective sensation as necessary in order to develop a Charcot Foot and the presence of patent, healthy circulation in order for the hyperemia of CJD to occur. If ischemia is present, wet or dry gangrene, rather than CJD develops.

Finally, whether primary or secondary, trauma or repetitive micro-trauma is necessary in order for CJD to progress. This trauma is exacerbated by closed chain factors such as obesity and an active lifestyle that must be appreciated and overcome by the examiner in order to treat CJD successfully.

In summary we have defined the pre-Charcot foot as a clinical entity displaying the following quartet of signs and symptoms:

1. Loss of Protective Sensation (LOPS)
2. Patent Circulation
3. Underlying Pedal Biomechanical Pathology and Weakness (Functional Foot Typing)
4. Excessive Closed Chain Factors (obesity, over-activity, etc.)

Inherent pedal biomechanical pathology and weakness (see biomechanics)

The presence of inherited, underlying biomechanical pathology is almost universal in the development of CJD. It is indeed rare to find a foot with normal mechanics go on to develop CJD probably because those diabetics find it easier to navigate through lives more actively.

Excessive closed chain factors

The lifestyle and quality of life of each individual varies in many ways when in closed chain. A careful history revealing the existence and extent of closed chain factors will assist a practitioner to determine their impact on the need to actively treat a subject's functional foot type. A person who is morbidly obese, very active and wearing worn out athletic shoes may need treatment even if he/she has a stable foot type. Conversely, in the face of LOPS, patent circulation and biomechanical pathology, a healthy and fit, light weight person, who is not very active and wear well fitted shoes and socks that are not outworn has much less of a chance to develop a Charcot Foot.

3. Discussion

Biomechanically, we would like individuals to have a lifestyle that includes exercise along with varied daily activities that promote aerobic health and functional fitness. Our goal should not be to reduce patients from being active and living a healthy lifestyle but instead to promote an active lifestyle for all while supporting them and training them biomechanically, injury, deformity and wound free.

Even though podiatry has become more and more an acceptable part of the diabetes health care team, there remains a poor understanding of functional lower extremity biomechanics and the need for diagnosing and treating underlying biomechanical pathology before, during and after the devastating comorbidities of diabetes reveals itself clinically. It is the hope of the author that all readers will be stimulated to increase their knowledge base regarding the needs of the diabetic patient when it comes to their feet so that foot suffering diabetics can be better cared for.

The podiatrist, skilled in closed chain medicine, biomechanical pathology and the diagnosis and treatment of the functional foot types is a necessary part of the health care team involved in treating diabetics. An annual foot exam and necessary follow-up that includes functional lower extremity biomechanics should be a mandatory part of the care of every diabetic and capable of being delivered by all members of the health care team.

4. References

[1] Shavelson, D, Steinberg, J, Bakotic B. The Diabetic Foot, Chapter 25, The Principles of Diabes Mellitus, 2010, 6, 381-399 2nd Printing, DOI: 10.1007/978-0-387-09841-8_25, Springer International Publishing

[2] Arad Y, Fonseca V, Peters A; Beyond the Monofilament for the Insensate Diabetic Foot: A systematic review of randomized trials to prevent the occurrence of plantar foot ulcers in patients with diabetes; Diabetes Care, April 2011. vol.34 no 4, 1041-46

[3] Southern Arizona Limb Salvage Alliance patient information. Available at: http://diabetic-foot.net/CLEAR/Patients.html. Accessed August 31, 2010

[4] Manes J, Papazoglou J, Sossidou E, Soulis, K; D. Milarakis; Prevalence of Diabetic Neuropathy and Foot Ulceration: Identification of Potential Risk Factors—A Population-Based Study; Wounds, 14(1):11-15, 2002
[5] Boulton AJ, Vileikyte L, Ragnarson-Tennvall G, Apelqvist J. The global burden of diabetic foot disease. *Lancet* 2005;366:1719-1724.
[6] Moxey, P, Gogalniceanu, P, Hinchliffe, R; Lower extremity amputations-a review of global variability in incidence: Diabetic Medicine, vol 28 issue 10, p 1144-53, October 2011
[7] MacKenzie EJ, Jones AS, Bosse MJ, et al. Health-care costs associated with amputation or reconstruction of a limb-threatening injury. J Bone Joint Surg Am. Aug 2007;89(8):1685-92
[8] 16(11):1507-10, 1993.Kenny SJ, Smith PJ, Goldschmid MG, Survey of physician practice behaviors related to diabetes mellitus in the U.S: Physician adherence to consensus recommendations. Diabetes C:16(11):1507-10, 1993.
[9] Andrew J, Boulton M, Kirsner, M; Neuropathic Diabetic Foot Ulcers: New Eng Jour Med; July 1, 2004, 351;48-55
[10] Payne C; The Past, Present and Future of Podiatric Biomechanics; Jour Amer Pod Med Ass;Feb 1998;88-2;53-63
[11] Shavelson, D; The Tower of Biomechanics: The Foot in Closed Chain, Present Podiatry E-zine; 06/26/2009; http://www.podiatry.com/ezines/?pub_year=2009&section_id=51#ezine483
[12] Prior T; The practical application of biomechanical theory for patient assessment: J Foot Ankle Res, May 2011; 4 29-37
[13] Shavelson D; Current Mainstream Biomechanics: Part I The Science and Current Paradigms: The Foot in Closed Chain, present Podiatry E-zine; 08/02/10; http://www.podiatry.com/ezines/?pub_year=2010&section_id=51#ezine723
[14] Gross MT, Byers JM, Krafft JL, Lackey EJ, Melton KM: The impact of custom semirigid foot orthotics on pain and disability for individuals with plantar fasciitis. J Ortho Sp Phys Ther, 32:149-157, 2002.
[15] Powell M, Seid M, Szer IA: Efficacy of custom foot orthotics in improving pain and functional status in children with juvenile idiopathic arthritis: A randomized trial. J Rheum, 32:943-950, 2005.
[16] Kirby KA: Conservative treatment of posterior tibial dysfunction. Podiatry Management, 19:73-82, 2000
[17] Mundermann A, Wakeling JM, Nigg BM, Humble RN, Stefanyshyn DJ: Foot orthoses affect frequency components of muscle activity in the lower extremity. Gait and Posture, In Press, 2005.
[18] Dananberg HJ, Guiliano M: Chronic low-back pain and its response to custom-made foot orthoses. Jour Amer Pod Med Ass; 89:109-117, 1999
[19] Kemp M; Artists on Science: scientists on art; Nature 434, March 17, 2005;306-09
[20] Root-Bernstein, R, Root-Bernstein M; Artistic Scientists and Scientific Artists: The Link between Polymathy and Creativity: Jour Amer Psych Ass, Nov 2004, pp. 127-151

[21] Kelly G, Gitzgerald D; Open vs. closed chain exercise; Jour of Phys Ther, Dec 1997, 129-34
[22] Singh N, Armstrong D, Lipsky B, Preventing foot ulcers in patients with diabetes: JAMA, Jan 12, 2005, vol 292 no 217-28
[23] Kapandj, I; The Physiology of the Joints, Vol 2 Lower Limb, 5th Edition, 2002, Churchill-Livingstone Publishing
[24] Inman V, Ralston H, Todd F: Human Walking. Baltimore: Williams & Wilkins; 1981
[25] Root M, Orien W, Weed J; Clinical Biomechanics, Vol II Normal and abnormal function of the foot, Clinical Biomechanics Corporation, Los Angeles, CA, USA
[26] Kennedy S: Casting for foot orthotics…What works best? O&P.com http://www.oandp.com/articles/2004-08_08.asp
[27] McPoil, T, Hunt, G: Evaluation and Management of Foot and Ankle Disorders: Present Problems and Future Directions. Jour Ortho &Sports Phys Ther, Vol 21, Number 6, 1995, pp381-88
[28] Lee, W; An historical appraisal and discussion of the Root Model as a clinical system of approach in the present context of theoretical uncertainty: Clinics id Pod med & Surg, vol 18 no 1, Oct 2001 555-684
[29] Kirby K: Are Root Biomechanics Dying? Podiatry Today, Apr 1, 2009, p126-31
[30] Payne C, Miller K: Variability of neutral position casting of the foot; Jour Amer Pod Med Ass, 93 1, 1-5, 2003
[31] Dananberg H; Saggital Plane Biomechanics: Jour Amer Pod Med Ass, vol 90 no 1, p 292-98, Jan 2000
[32] Dananberg H: Gait style as an etiology to chronic postural pain: Jour Amer Pod Med Ass; vol 83 no 6, p443-41 August 1993
[33] Glaser E, Bursch D, Currie S: Theory and practice combine for custom orthoses: Biomechanics; vol 12 no 9, p111-15, Sept 2006
[34] Scherer, P, Kirby K: Recent Advances in Orthotic Therapy: Improving Clinical Outcomes with a Pathology-Specific Approach; LER Publishing, USA, 2011
[35] Fuller,E: Center of pressure and its theoretical relationship to foot pathology; JAPMA, June 1999, vol 89, no. 6, pp278-91
[36] Kuhn DR, Shibley NJ, Austin WM, Yochum TR. Radiographic evaluation of weight bearing orthotics and their effect on flexible *pes planus*. *J Manip Physiol Ther* 1999;22(4): p 221-226
[37] Albert, S, Curran S, Lower Extremity Biomechanics: Theory and Practice Vol II, 139-42 BiPedMed Publishing, Denver USA (in press)
[38] Shavelson D: A closer look at Neoteric Biomechanics; Podiatry Today; vol20 issue 9, p142-49, Sept 2007
[39] Shavelson D: Current Mainstream Podiatric Biomechanics Part II: The Foot Centering Theory; Present Podiatry E-zines; 11/05/10 http://www.podiatry.com/ezines/?pub_year=2010&section_id=51#ezine730
[40] Shavelson D, Henry L: Aching Feet…Aching Back…Is there a connection?; Radius Magazine, p203-209, Winter 2008
[41] Shavelson D: Profiling the pedal snowflakes; Present Podiatry E-zines, 09/14/09 http://www.podiatry.com/ezines/?pub_year=2009&section_id=51#ezine509

[42] Shavelson, D: Foot Typing Method; U.S. Patent # 7938788, Issue Date: May 10, 2011

[43] Burns MJ: Non-weightbeaing cast impressions for the construction of orthotic devices. JAPA, 67(11): 1977.

[44] Shavelson D: Functional Foot Type Closed Chain Characteristics; Present Podiatry E-zines, 05/05/2011, http://www.podiatry.com/ezines/#ezine810

[45] Spink M, Menz, H, Lord S: Distribution and correlates of plantar hyperkeratotic lesions in older people; Jour Foot Ankle Research, 2:8, Feb 2009

[46] A, Sanjari,M, Haghdoost A: Common foot features of 247 Iranian patients with diabetes, International Wound Jour, Apr 21, 2009

[47] Frykberg R: Diabetic Foot Ulcers: Pathogenesis and Management; Amer Fam Physician, vol 66 no, p 1159-62, Nov 9, 2002

[48] Cavanagh P, Ulbrecht J, Caputo G. New developments in the biomechanics of the diabetic foot. Diabetes Metab Res Rev, 16:1, 2000

[49] Spencer SA. Pressure relieving interventions for preventing and treating diabetic foot ulcers. Cochrane Database of Systematic Reviews, Issue 3 2000

[50] Kim R, Edelman S, Kim D: Musculoskelatal complications of Diabetes :mellitus; Clinical Diabetes; 19:132-5 Aug 2001

[51] Yentes J, Perell K: Diabetic peripheral neuropathy and exercise; Jour Amer Kines Ass, p29-36, Fall 2006

[52] Zimny S, Schatz H, Pfohl M: The role of limited joint mobility in diabetic patients with an at-risk foot. Diabetes Care 27:942-946, 2004

[53] Wrobel J, Najafi B: Diabetic foot biomechanics and gait dysfunction; J Diabetes Sci Technol, 4(4), p833-45, July 1, 2010

[54] Tajaddini A, Scoffone HM, Botek G, Davis BL. Laser-induced auto-fluorescence (LIAF) as a method for assessing skin stiffness preceding diabetic ulcer formation. J Biomech. 40(4), p736-41, May 2007

[55] Bolton NR, Smith KE, Pilgram TK, Mueller MJ, Bae KT. Computed tomography to visualize and quantify the plantar aponeurosis and flexor hallucis longus tendon in the diabetic foot. Clin Biomech, 20 (5) p 540-, June 2005

[56] Sinacore DR, Bohnert KL, Hastings MK, Johnson JE. Mid foot kinetics characterize structural polymorphism in diabetic foot disease. Clin Biomech, vol 23 no 5, p 653-61, Jan 2008

[57] Christensen K: Adjunctive therapies to the adjustment improving proprioceptive balance with orthotic support; Jour North Amer Rehab Spec, Autumn 2011

[58] Metz-Schimmer S: Functional anatomy and biomechanics of the ankle joint; Radiologe, vol 35 no7, p425-28, Jul 1995

[59] Novachek T: The biomechanics of running, Gait and Posture, 7, p77-95, June 1998

[60] Bakotic B. Shavelson D: The Pathogenesis of dystrophic toenails; Podiatry Management, p133-140, August 2006

[61] Fabrikant J: Plantar faciitis (fasciosis treatment outcome study: plantar fascia thickness measured by ultrasound and correlated with patient improvement; Foot vol 21 no 2, p79-83, Mar 12, 2011

[62] Root ML, Orien WP, Weed JH. Normal and Abnormal Function of the Foot. Vol 2. Los Angeles, Calif: Clinical Biomechanics; 1977

[63] Kararizou E, Manta P, Kalfakis N, Vassilopoulos D: Morphometric study of the human muscle spindle. Anal Quant Cytol Histol, 27, p 1-4, june 2005

[64] Moore, M: Golgi Tendon Organs: Neuroscience Update with Relevance to Stretching and Proprioception in Dancers; Jour Dance Med & Sci, vol 11 no 3, p 85-92, Sept 2007

[65] Slosberg M. Effects of altered afferent articular input on sensation, proprioception, muscle tone and sympathetic reflex responses. J Manip Physiol Ther;11:400-408, Apr 1988

[66] MacLean C, Hamill J: Short and long-term influence of a custom foot orthotic intervention on lower extremity dynamics in injured runners. Annual International Society of Biomechanics Meeting, Cleveland, September 2005

[67] Saxena A, Haddad J: The effect of foot orthoses on patellofemoral syndrome; Jour Amer Pod Med Ass, vol 93 no4.p 264-71, July 2003

[68] Rome K, Brown C: Randomized clinical trial into the impact of rigid foot orthoses on balance parameters in excessively pronated feet; Clin Rehab, vol 18, p 624–630, Nov 2004

[69] Lobmann R, Kayser R, Kasten G: Biomechanical evaluation of foot pressure and loading force during gait in rheumatoid arthritic patients with and without foot orthoses; Kurume Med J, 47, p211–217, Jan 2000

[70] Woolridge J, Bergeron J, Thornton C: Preventing diabetic foot disease: lessons from the Medicare therapeutic shoe demonstration; Amer J Public Health, vol 86 no 7, p935-38, July 10 1996

[71] Ochsendorf D, Mattacola C, Arnold B: Effect of orthotics on postural sway after fatigue of the plantar flexors and dorsiflexors; Jour Athletic Training. Vol35 no 1, p26-30, Jan 2000

[72] Armstrong D, Lavery L, Holtz-Neiderer K, et al: Variability in activity may precede diabetic foot ulceration. Diabetes Care, vol 27 no 8, 1980-84, Aug 2004

[73] Mokdad A, Ford E, Bowman B, et al: The Continuing Increase in Diabetes in the United States; Diabetes Care; 10. 24.2, Feb 2001, pp207-11

[74] Sinacore D, Withrington N. Recognition and management of acute neuropathic (Charcot) arthropathies of the foot and ankle: J Orthop Sports Phys Ther; vol 29 no12, p736-46, Dec 1999

[75] Lamm B, Gottlieb H, Paley D. A two-stage percutaneous approach to charcot diabetic foot reconstruction: J Foot Ankle Surg vol 49 no 6, p517-22, Nov-Dec 2010

[76] Yu G, Hudson J: Evaluation and treatment of stage 0 Charcot's Neuroarthropathy of the foot and ankle; Jour Amer Pod Med Ass, vol 92, p 210-20, Feb 2002

[77] Kelly M, Kearsley R, Mitchell D: The neurogenic theory of arthritis. J Hist Med Allied Sci; vol 20, p151-57, June 1965

[78] Brower A, Allman R: Pathogenesis of the neurotrophic joint: neurotraumatic vs neurovascular; Radiology;139: 349, 1981

[79] Banks A, McGlamry E: Charcot Foot; J Am Pod Med Assoc. 79: 5, 1989

[80] Poretsky L, Shavelson D, Kline M, Levine P: The PreCharcot Foot, A New Clinical Entity; Practical Diabetology, vol 14 no 3, p139-43, September 2006

[81] Damodar R. Ambur and James H. Starnes, Jr., NASA Langley Research Center, Hampton, VA: Presented at the 39th AIAA/ASME/ASCEIAHS/ASC Structures, Structural Dynamics, and Materials Conference, Long Beach, California April 20-23, 1998

[82] Liu D, Schultz P: Dynamic failure and energy absorption of composites with topological control; 16th international conference on composite materials, Michgan State University, 2007

[83] Jobjes M, Heuschel G, Pretzel C: Repetitive training of compensatory steps: a therapeutic approach for postural instability in Parkinson's Disease; J. Neurol. Neurosurg Psychiatry, 75, 1682-87, 2004

[84] Shavelson D: The Future of Biomechanics; Present Podiatry E-zines, 05/15/09, http://www.podiatry.com/ezines/?pub_year=2009&section_id=51#ezine416

[85] Shavelson D: The Tower of Biomechanics; Present Podiatry E-zines 06/26/09, http://www.podiatry.com/ezines/?pub_year=2009&section_id=51#ezine483

[86] Shavelson D: The Common Functional Foot Types: Present Podiatry E-zines,12/05/09, http://www.podiatry.com/ezines/?pub_year=2009&section_id=51#ezine541

[87] Shavelson D: The Supine Biomechanical Examination: Present Podiatry E-zines, 02/12/10, http://www.podiatry.com/ezines/?pub_year=2010&section_id=51#ezine567

[88] Shavelson D: The Functional Foot Typing Forefoot Exam: 03/28/10, http://www.podiatry.com/ezines/?pub_year=2010&section_id=51#ezine584

[89] Shavelson D: Biomechanics EBM Part I: Where Does Biomechanics EBM Stand; Present Podiatry zines: http://www.podiatry.com/ezines/?pub_year=2010&section_id=51#ezine603

[90] Shavelson D: Biomechanics EBM Part II: Biomechanics Evidence Based Practice (EBP): Present Podiatry E-zines, 06/28/10, http://www.podiatry.com/ezines/?pub_year=2010&section_id=51#ezine678

[91] Shavelson D: Biomechanics EBM Part III: The Levels of Evidence in EBM/EBP: Present Podiatry E-zines, 08/01/10, http://www.podiatry.com/ezines/?pub_year=2010&section_id=51#ezine692

[92] Shavelson D: Current Mainstream Podiatric Biomechanics Part 1: The Science and Current Paradigms; Present Podiatry E-zines, 10/18/10, http://www.podiatry.com/ezines/?pub_year=2010&section_id=51#ezine723

[93] Shavelson D: Rocker Bottom Shoes: A Position Paper, Present Podiatry Ezines, 12/09/10, http://www.podiatry.com/ezines/?pub_year=2010&section_id=51#ezine752

[94] Shavelson D: Wellness Biomechanics Kinesiology and Kinetics, Present Podiatry E-zines, 02/28/11, http://www.podiatry.com/ezines/?pub_year=2011&section_id=51#ezine780

[95] Shavelson D: Children's Shoes: A Position Paper, Present Podiatry E-zines, 08/05/11 http://www.podiatry.com/ezines/?pub_year=2011&section_id=51#ezine880

[96] Shavelson D: Plantar Fasciitis, the root of most heel pain; Radius Magazine, p 39-42, Spring 2010
[97] Shavelson D: Neoteric Biomechanics; Podiatry Management, p 123-26, Sept 2008
[98] Shavelson D: Barefoot'n…Did our ancestors have the right technique?; Radius Magazine, 132-34, Winter 2010
.podiatry.com/ezines/?pub_year=2011&section_id=51#ezine880

8

A Protocol for Primary Podogeriatric Assessment for Older Patients with Diabetes Mellitus

Arthur E. Helfand[1,2,3,4]
[1]*Temple University, School of Podiatric Medicine,*
Department of Community Health, Aging and Health Policy
[2]*Temple University Hospital, Thomas Jefferson University Hospital*
[3]*Temple University Institute on Aging*
[4]*Philadelphia Corporation for Aging*
USA

1. Introduction

The Pennsylvania Department of Health's Diabetes Prevention and Control Program provided a contract to develop a Comprehensive Podogeriatric and Chronic Diseases Podogeriatric Assessment Protocol (Helfand Index – Appendix A). The goal was to provide a methodology to assess foot, ankle, and related structural problems in older patients; stratify those patients most at risk to develop complications; develop a surveillance instrument for patient care: and to serve as a public health data collection outcome measurement. The information obtained would also provide a protocol to develop prevention (primary, secondary and tertiary) and management programs for individual patients, institutions, and their communities, augment geriatric and chronic disease assessment, as well as stressing the need for appropriate patient management, professional, and patient education.

Foot problems identified in older diabetic patients are the result of the aging process, disease, disability, deformity, and complications associated with other chronic diseases. They are related to societal, environmental, and life style issues. Foot discomfort and pain or podalgia represent some of the most distressing, disabling, and known quality of life limiting conditions. Diabetic foot problems in the older patient are a major cause of morbidity, disability, and hospitalization and contribute to a lessening of the quality and independence of life, thus contributing to an earlier and higher mortality. The high prevalence of chronic diseases in the older population, such as, diabetes mellitus, arthritis, peripheral arterial disease as well as those conditions that produce sensory, peripheral vascular, musculo-skeletal, dermatologic, onychial, and neurologic deficits, lead to serious complications that increase morbidity, mortality, and health care costs. (1, 2, 3, 4, 5, 6)

Other life altering issues in the older patient include constipation, weakened muscle and bone structure, social isolation, mobility deficits, reduced Activities of Daily Living and

Instrumental Activities of Daily Living, sleep problems, agitation and compulsive disorders, increased perspiration, self mutilation and excoriation. The immobility that results from a local foot problem or as the result of a complication of a systemic disease can have a significant negative impact on the patient's ability to maintain a productive quality of life as member of society and to live life, to the end of life with dignity. The senior years should not become a period of "waiting for GOD". (17, 18, 19, 20, 21)

Diseases and disorders of foot and their related structures in the older patient and in particular diabetes mellitus and its neurovascular complications are a significant public health concern. The changes in the individuals' ability to maintain their independence become financial concerns for the individual, their families, and society in general. Two important factors involved in the older patient's ability to remain as a vital part of society are a keen mind and the ability to retain their mobility through ambulation. (5) There are many other factors, which also contribute to the development of foot problems of the adult population including the aging process itself as well as abuse and neglect. Some of these considerations include: the degree of ambulation, the duration of prior hospitalization, limitation of activity, prior institutionalization, episodes of social segregation, depression, prior care, emotional adjustments to disease and life in general, polypharmacy and drug interactions, and the complications and residuals associated with risk diseases. Other focused issues include a loss of tissue and joint elasticity; atrophy of fat and protective tissue; a weakening of the intrinsic muscles of the foot; a loss of balance and range of motion; an increase in foot size due to tissue laxity; a decrease in arch height; dry skin; and onychial dystrophies. (16, 18)

High risk factors for older diabetic patients include age itself, elevated blood sugar, hypertension, a history of a stroke, retinopathy, nephropathy, a history and duration of diabetes for more than ten years, delayed treatment, failure of diabetic foot health education, visual impairment , the inability to bend, living alone, a history of tobacco use, cognitive impairment, dementia, risk taking behavior, sensory loss, a loss of protective sensation, structural abnormalities, altered gait, ambulatory dysfunction, abnormal or excessive foot pressure, subkeratotic or subungual hematoma, a history of foot ulcers, decreased peripheral arterial pulses, peripheral arterial and vascular disease, diabetic neuropathy, soft tissue and plantar fat pad atrophy and/or displacement, deformities (limited joint mobility, hallux valgus, hallux limitus, hammer toes, prominent metatarsal heads and prolapse), xerosis, fissures, obesity, and other related chronic diseases, such as degenerative arthritis, rheumatoid arthritis, and gout. (9, 10, 22)

Additional systemic and/or life changes contributing to the development of high risk foot problems include impaired cardiovascular function, chronic constipation and incontinence, weakened muscle and bone structure, impaired cardiovascular function, diabetes mellitus, peripheral vascular and lower extremity arterial and venous disease, reduced interest and/or participation in social activities, decreased and/or loss of mobility, weakened muscle and bone structure, a reduction in independent activities of daily living and/or instrumental activities of daily living, sleep disorders, agitation, compulsive activities, increased foot perspiration, neurological and sensory deficits, neurotic excoriation, changes in mental status, and cognitive impairment. Self-mutilation, untreated and/or under treated hyperkeratosis, onychauxis, onychomycosis, ulcers, tinea pedis, xerosis, abrasions and/or lacerations are also contributing factors. (25, 26, 27)

Older patients, especially those with chronic diseases, such as diabetes mellitus are usually taking more than one therapeutic drug at any given moment and may have increased sensitivity and they are usually more susceptible to infection because of the anatomic location of the foot itself. Associated avascularity, atrophy of soft tissue, muscle wasting, neuropathic changes, and a lack of concern for foot health, is associated with the aging and our society. They are concerned about life, as life in a sense is a terminal illness and they have a lower threshold of physical and emotional stress. They may have ambulatory limitation and usually have one or more chronic diseases. They are more prone to injury involving the lower extremity that additionally limits ambulation and mobility. And, they are prone to present with delayed or non-healing tissues. (12)

2. General information

The Assessment Protocol (Appendix A) reviews information related to demographics; primary medical facilities and management; a history of present problems; pertinent past medical history; a systems review; current medications; visual evaluation, foot dermatologic, foot orthopedic, peripheral vascular, and neurologic evaluation; neurologic risk stratification; peripheral arterial risk stratification; footwear evaluation; a primary assessment; an initial management plan; and referral direction; Medicare's class findings; risk stratification of onychomycosis, plantar pressure keratotic patterns, pre and ulcer classification, and the classification of mechanical or pressure hyperkeratotic lesions. (22, 23, 24)

The evaluation process is enhanced by the use of accessible instrumentation such as a C –128 Hz Tuning Fork; Neurologic Hammer; Percussion Hammer; Babinski Hammer; Neurothesiometer or similar instrumentation (Biothesiometer) to determine the Vibration Perception Threshold (VPT); Monofilament Sensory Testing (MST) devices such as the Semmes - Weinstein 5.07 nylon monofilament (SWM), Norton Monofilament, or the West Enhanced Sensory Test; Two Point Discriminator, Pinwheel, Tip-Therm, Tacticon; Doppler; Pulse Volume Recordings (PVR), Pressure-Stat, Temp-Stat, Radiometer - infrared surface temperature scanner for skin perfusion assessment; Ankle and Toe Brachial Index; Oscillometer; Transcutaneous Oxygen (TCPO2); Radiography; MRI and CT Scans; and Contrast Arteriography as indicated.

The demographics, past medical history, system review, medications and therapeutic programs, current health conditions should be reviewed and noted from the medical record. Primary foot problems as well as their relationship to chronicity and activities, including; swelling, pain, hyperkeratosis, joint deformities, onychial diseases and disorders, infections, coldness, and other problems, as well as location, quality, severity, duration, context, modifying factors, and associated signs and symptoms, should also be noted from the institutional record.

The primary and secondary "at risk" diseases and disorders include complications associated with diabetes mellitus and metabolic disorders, peripheral vascular , lower extremity arterial and venous diseases, sensory and motor impairment, edema, degenerative joint changes and the residuals of arthritis and collagen diseases, ambulatory dysfunction, obesity, and cognitive impairment. (28)

In 1971, Medicare Regulations identified a number diseases and/or disorders that develop vascular insufficiency and neurological insensitivity and their complications as risk factors related to management. The primary examples include the following but are not exclusive:

- Amyotrophic Lateral Sclerosis
- Arteriosclerosis obliterans (A.S.O., arteriosclerosis of the extremities, occlusive peripheral arteriosclerosis)
- Arteritis of the feet
- Buerger's disease (thromboangiitis obliterans)
- Chronic indurated cellulitis
- Chronic thrombophlebitis
- Chronic venous insufficiency
- Diabetes Mellitus
- Intractable edema - secondary to a specific disease (e.g., congestive heart failure, kidney disease, hypothyroidism)
- Lymphedema - secondary to a specific disease (e.g., Milroy's disease, malignancy)
- Peripheral neuropathies involving the feet

Associated with malnutrition and vitamin deficiency

- Malnutrition (general, pellagra)
- Alcoholism
- Malabsorption (celiac disease, tropical sprue)
- Pernicious anemia
- Associated with carcinoma
- Associated with diabetes mellitus
- Associated with drugs and toxins
- Associated with multiple sclerosis
- Associated with uremia (chronic renal disease)
- Associated with traumatic injury
- Associated with leprosy or neurosyphilis
- Associated with hereditary disorders
- Hereditary sensory radically neuropathy
- Angiokeratoma corporis diffusum (Fabry's)
- Amyloid neuropathy

Peripheral vascular disease
Raynaud's disease

The secondary "at risk" list of diseases and disorders include the following as examples: Deficiency of B-complex components, Lipidoses, Amyloidosis, Peripheral autonomic neuropathy in disorders classified elsewhere, Hereditary and idiopathic peripheral neuropathy, Acute infective polyneuritis, Polyneuropathy in collagen vascular disease, polyneuropathy in malignant disease, Polyneuropathy in other diseases classified elsewhere, Alcoholic polyneuropathy, Inflammatory and toxic neuropathy, Inflammatory and toxic neuropathy, unspecified, Atherosclerosis of native arteries of the extremities, Generalized and unspecified atherosclerosis, Raynaud's syndrome, Other specified peripheral vascular diseases, peripheral vascular disease, unspecified, Stricture of artery, Other lymphedema, Postphlebitic syndrome, Compression of vein, Chronic venous hypertension (idiopathic), Venous (peripheral) insufficiency, unspecified, Unspecified circulatory system disorder, Unspecified intestinal malabsorption, Chronic renal failure, Cellulitis and abscess of the toe (s), foot (feet) or leg (legs), prior foot ulceration, Hereditary edema of legs, Edema, and Injury to the knee, leg, ankle, and foot.

Examples of other significant at risk diseases and disorders include as examples: old age and frailty, Alzheimer's Disease, Cognitive dysfunction, Osteoarthritis (Degenerative Joint Disease), Rheumatoid Arthritis, Gout, Coagulopathies, Hemophilia, Prior Amputation, Reflex Sympathetic Dystrophy, Hansen's Disease, Mental Illness, the Mentally Challenged, Paralysis, Parkinson's Disease, visual impairment, physical impairment, ambulatory dysfunction, . In addition, patients with a history of vascular grafts, joint implants, heart valve replacement, active chemotherapy, renal failure and on dialysis, anticoagulant therapy, hemorrhagic disease, chronic steroid therapy, and immuno - compromised states (HIV - AIDS), pose additional risks when considering assessment, treatment and prevention. (52)

On June 16, 2009, the Department of Veterans Affairs (VHA Directive 2009-030) expanded the Medicare primary risk categories to appropriately include the following conditions: (50)

- Documented peripheral arterial disease
- Documented sensory neuropathy
- Prior history of foot ulcer or amputation
- Visually impaired
- Physically impaired
- Neuromuscular disease, i.e. Parkinson's disease
- Severe arthritis and spinal disc disease
- Cognitive dysfunction
- Chronic anticoagulation therapy
- >70 years old without other risk factors
- Diabetes without foot complications
- Obesity

3. Dermatological and onychial physical findings

The dermatologic section provides a focus on skin integrity and multiple changes that affect pressure, mechanical keratosis, onychial changes, infections, and pre-ulcerative states. (7, 8, 14)

The primary clinical signs and findings include the following: hyperkeratosis; keratotic lesions without hemorrhage or hematoma; tyloma; heloma durum; heloma milliare; heloma molle; heloma neurofibrosuum; heloma vasculare; onychophosis; intractable plantar keratosis; sub-keratotic hematoma (pre-ulceration); xerosis; onychauxis; tinea pedis; bacterial infection; verruca; ulceration; onychomycosis; rubor; onychodystrophy; pre-ulcerative conditions; cyanosis; and discoloration.

Some examples of dermatologic symptoms and signs include the following: exquisitely painful or painless wounds, slow healing or non-healing wounds, trophic ulceration, necrosis, skin color changes such as cyanosis or erythema, changes in texture and turgor, inelasticity, tenting, pigmentation, hemosiderin deposition, pruritus, neurogenic, and/or emotional dermatoses, contact dermatitis, stasis dermatitis, atopic dermatitis, nummular eczema, scaling, dehydration, xerosis or dryness, excoriations, verruca, moles, psoriasis, fissures, hyperhidrosis, bromidrosis, diminished or absent hair growth, diabetic dermopathy (shin spots), necrobiosis lipoidica diabeticorum, bullous diabeticorum, granuloma annulare, acanthosis nigricans, and poroma. Other factors include swelling, redness, an increase or decrease in skin temperature, and maceration.

Some examples of common onychial clinical changes include onycholysis, subungual hyperkeratosis, diabetic onychopathy, onychauxis, onychogryphosis, onychocryptosis, onychomycosis, onychia, paronychia, subungual abscess, subungual heloma, subungual exostosis, onychomadesis, onychoschizia, onychophosis, subungual hematoma, splinter hemorrhage, periungual ulcerative granulation tissue, onychodysplasia, onychodystrophy, onychorrhexis, Beau's Lines, pterygium, diabetic onychopathy, and hypertrophic onychodystrophy.

Onychomycosis evaluation includes: documentation of mycosis/dystrophy causing secondary infection and/or pain, which results or would result in marked limitation of ambulation and includes discoloration, hypertrophy, subungual debris, onycholysis, secondary infection, and limitation of ambulation and pain. The primary clinical presentation of onychomycosis include distal subungual, lateral subungual, superficial (white), proximal subungual, endonyx, total dystrophic and candida (14). The onychial grades at risk, which was modified and adapted from Strauss, Hart and Winant and recognizes earlier risk and includes the following: Grade - 1, normal; Grade - 2, mild hypertrophy, Grade 3, evidence of hypertrophy, dystrophy, onychauxis, onychomycosis, infection, and/or onychodysplasia; and Grade - 4, evidence of hypertrophy, deformity, onychogryphosis, dystrophy, onychomycosis, and/or infection.

4. Hyperkeratosis classification

The major functions of the foot are static and dynamic. The foot is an organ of weight bearing, propulsion, and locomotion. The foot is relatively rigid and changes are related to the activities of daily living, excessive and repetitive stress, the normal aging process, degeneration, and disease, producing functional disability and ambulatory dysfunction. Repetitive stress, hard and flat surfaces, increased shock, tissue trauma, past occupational stress, and the environmental factors associated with ambulation that do not provide for a compensatory element for weight diffusion and/or weight dispersion. Examples of related complications include atrophy of the intrinsic foot muscles, atrophy, and anterior displacement of the plantar fat pad, morphologic changes, digital contractures and deformities, inflammation, pain, and the residuals of biomechanical, pathomechanical, and balance and gait change. The stress factors related to the development of hyperkeratosis include; force, compression, tensile stress, shearing, friction, elasticity, and fluid pressure. (29, 30)

The classification of mechanical or pressure keratosis is a modification of the program outlined by Merriman and Tollifield , includes the following grading descriptions as follows: 0 - no lesion; 1 - no specific tyloma plaque but diffuse or pinch hyperkeratotic tissue present or in narrow bands; 2 - circumscribed, punctate oval, or circular, well defined thickening of keratinized tissue; 3 - heloma milliare or heloma durum with no associated tyloma; 4 - well defined tyloma plaque with a definite heloma within the lesion extravasation, maceration and early breakdown of structures under the tyloma or callus layer; and 5 -complete breakdown of structure of hyperkeratotic tissue, epidermis, extending to superficial dermal involvement. The plantar keratoma pattern is identified if present.

5. Ulcer classification

The Ulcer Classification was adapted from Simms, Cavanaugh and Ulbrecht and provides an earlier identification of risk given its ten grade classification and better identifies pre-ulcerative changes as follows: Grade - 0 - absent skin lesions; Grade - 1 - dense callus but not pre-ulcer or ulcer; Grade - 2 – pre-ulcerative changes (such as evidence of hemorrhage or hematoma in the keratotic lesion; Grade - 3 - partial thickness (superficial ulcer); Grade - 4 - full thickness (deep) ulcer but no involvement of tendon, bone, ligament or joint; Grade - 5 - full thickness (deep) ulcer with involvement of tendon, bone, ligament or joint; Grade - 6 - localized infection (abscess or osteomyelitis); Grade - 7 - proximal spread of infection (ascending cellulitis or lymphadenopathy); Grade - 8 - gangrene of forefoot only; and Grade - 9 - gangrene of majority of foot. A key factor in managing the diabetic is to prevent foot ulceration by finding clinical signs prior to skin breakdown. (13, 41, 41, 43, 44)

Other classifications include the Wagner Classification System (Grades 1-5) , the Liverpool Classification System for diabetic ulcers (Primary – neuropathic, ischemic and neuroischemic and Secondary – uncomplicated or complicated i.e., with cellulitis, abscess, or osteomyelitis, and the University of Texas Foot Ulcer Wound Classification Systems with Stages A, B, C, and D and Grades 1, 2, and 3 that encompass pre or post ulceration, superficial, penetration to tendon or capsule or penetration to bone, with no infection or ischemia, infection, ischemia, and infection with and ischemia. (46)

6. Foot orthopedic (musculoskeletal) physical findings

The foot orthopedic section highlights altered biomechanics and the most common foot and joint deformities and syndromes identified in the older patient and patients with chronic diseases, such as arthritis; Hallux valgus (bunion); anterior imbalance (identifies inappropriate weight bearing and correlates with the plantar keratoma pattern noted later in the examination); digiti flexus (hammer toes and rotational deformities); prominent metatarsal heads; Morton's Syndrome; improper weight distribution and pressure areas; soft tissues inflammation is also noted. Other primary findings include; diminished joint mobility (flexion, extension, inversion, and inversion); pes planus, pes valgo planus; pes cavus (equinus); hallux limitus or rigidus; bursitis; Charcot joints (neuropathic arthropathy); drop foot; osseous reabsorption; rear and/or forefoot varus; plantarflexed first ray; digital and or partial foot amputation; B/K and A/K amputation; and other clinical findings. (31, 33)

Other examples of musculoskeletal findings that should be considered include: gradual change in shape or size of the foot, decreased ranges of motion, a sudden and painless change in foot shape with swelling and no history of trauma, drop foot, "Rocker Bottom Foot" or Charcot foot, neuropathic arthropathy, elevated plantar pressure, limited joint mobility, abnormal foot pressure, atrophy of plantar fat pad, plantar fat pad displacement, foot muscle atrophy, hallux limitus, hallux rigidus, tailor's bunion, plantar fasciitis, soft tissue inflammation, calcaneal spurs, decalcification, stress fractures, metatarsalgia, Morton's Syndrome, Haglund's, entrapment syndrome, neuroma, sesamoid displacement, joint deformities as residuals of arthritis, ambulatory dysfunction, pododynia dysbasia, biomechanical and pathomechanical variations, and footwear evaluation. Gait evaluation includes mobility, gait speed, and balance as it relates to fall risk that may be associated with foot deformity and inappropriate footwear. Ambulatory aids such as canes, walkers, etc, as well as physical activities are also a consideration. Mobility should consider independent activity, independence with assistance, homebound status, non-ambulatory status, and wheel chair use. The ranges of motion include dorsiflexion, plantar flexion, inversion, and eversion of the foot and ankle, flexion and extension of the great toe, and intrinsic foot muscles. (45, 47, 48, 49)

7. Peripheral vascular physical findings

The Vascular Evaluation identifies those symptoms associated with arterial insufficiency and ischemia. The primary findings include: coldness, trophic changes, diminished or absent pedal pulses, such as the dorsalis pedis pulse and posterior tibial pulses; night cramps; edema; claudication; varicosities; atrophy and amputation if present (noted as above the knee (AKA), below the knee (BKA), FF (forefoot), and T (toes), which are particularly important in patients with diabetes and arterial insufficiency. Other findings include: fatigue, rest pain, decreased skin temperature, burning, trophic changes, color and pigmentary changes, hemosiderin deposition, petechiae, hypoxia, cyanosis, rubor, absent or diminished digital hair, skin fragility, skin inelasticity (tenting), tingling, numbness, ulceration, history of phlebitis, cramps, edema, history of repeated foot infections, diminished or absent popliteal and/or femoral pulse change, femoral bruits, Ankle-Brachial Index (ABI < 0.90), Toe-Brachial Index, prolonged subungual capillary refill (> 3 sec), reduced claudication time, changes in skin perfusion, color changes (rubor, erythema, or cyanosis), temperature changes (cool and gradient), xerosis (atrophic and dry skin), atrophy of soft tissue, superficial infections, onychial changes, induration, blebs, delayed venous filling time, prolonged capillary filling time, femoral bruits, microcirculatory dysfunction, ischemia, telangiectasia, stasis, delayed and/or non-healing wounds and/or ulcers, necrosis, and gangrene. (15, 32)

The vascular and risk stratification includes the following as part of the initial assessment: 0, no change; 1, mild claudication; 2, moderate claudication; 3, severe claudication; 4, ischemic rest pain; 5, minor tissue loss; and 6, major tissue loss.

Medicare currently may provide payment for Therapeutic Shoes for patients with diabetes mellitus who meet specific criteria. The criteria include the following: a history of partial or complete amputation of the foot, a history of previous foot ulceration, a history of pre-ulcerative callus, peripheral neuropathy with evidence of callus formation, evidence of foot and/or osseous deformity, and evidence of poor circulation.

8. Neurological physical findings

The neurologic evaluation identifies primary reflex and sensory changes. Those findings include: the deep tendon reflexes – (DTR i.e. patellar and Achilles) and superficial plantar reflexes, joint position, testing vibratory sensation, vibration perception threshold (VPT), sharp and dull reactions, evidence of paresthesia and burning. Other findings include: sensory changes (burning, tingling, and/or clawing sensations), pain and hyperactivity, two point discrimination variation, motor changes (weakness and /or foot drop), ankle clonus, autonomic changes (diminished sweating or hyperhidrosis), sensory vibratory deficits and/or proprioceptive, loss of protective sensation, changes in pain and temperature perception, and high plantar pressure areas as demonstrated by marked digital contractures, hyperkeratosis, metatarsal prolapse, prominent metatarsal heads, and plantar fat pad atrophy and displacement, bowstring tendons, muscle wasting, and Charcot foot (including rocker bottom deformity, erythema, heat, edema, fractures, neuropathy, swelling, bounding pulses, absent or diminished pain and proprioception, deep tendon reflex loss, anhidrosis, subluxation, the minus foot, equinus, hypermobility, ulceration, hyperkeratosis, and infection) . The use of monofilament testing and response are essential to measure sensory loss. Pinching the Achilles tendon and/or placing vertical pressure on a nail plate should demonstrate pain. The absence of pain is also an indication of sensory loss. Palpation of the common peroneal, posterior tibial and sural nerves may also demonstrate enlargement and tenderness. (34, 35, 36, 37, 38)

Medicare also provides a process for the evaluation and management of a diabetic patient with diabetic sensory neuropathy, resulting in a Loss of Protective Sensation (LOPS) to include the following: 1) a diagnosis of LOPS; 2) a patient history of diabetes mellitus; 3) a physical examination consisting of findings regarding at least the following elements, 3 a) visual inspection of the forefoot, hindfoot, and toe web spaces, 3 b) evaluation of protective sensation, 3 c) evaluation of foot structure, pathomechanics, and biomechanics, 3 d) evaluation of vascular status, 3 e) evaluation of skin integrity, 3 f) evaluation and recommendation of footwear, and 4) patient education.

The neurological risk stratification includes the following classification: 0, no sensory loss; 1, sensory loss; 2, sensory loss and foot deformity; and 3, sensory loss, a history of ulceration, and deformity.

9. Class findings

Medicare also has a series of Class Findings that need to be evaluated and documented as qualifiers for primary foot care for those patients with primary risk diseases noted. Those findings include the following: A - 1, nontraumatic amputation of the foot or part of the foot; B - 1, absent posterior tibial pulse; B - 2, advanced trophic changes; B - 2 - a, hair growth (decrease or absent); B - 2 - b, nail changes (thickening); B - 2 - c, pigmentary changes (discoloration); B - 2 - d, skin texture (thin, shiny; B - 2 - e, skin color (rubor or redness); B - 3, absent dorsalis pedis pulse; C -1, claudication; C - 2, temperature changes (cold); C - 3, edema; C - 4, paresthesia; and C - 5, burning.

10. Other findings

Other assessment areas include footwear, hygiene, and the type of stocking (nylon, cotton, wool, other), or none. Stockings or socks should also be inspected for staining and excessive wear (friction).The shoe or footwear evaluation includes the type of shoe, fit, depth, size, last, flare, shoe-wear, patterns of wear, shoe lining wear, shoe wear pattern (outsole and upper counter distortion), foreign bodies, insoles, and orthoses. Where special shoes, such as those defined as "therapeutic" by Medicare, they should generally include a padded collar and tongue, laces, adjustable strap or "Velcro" closure, wide toe box to accommodate deformities, added depth in the upper section to accommodate deformities, orthotics, and /or padded inserts to evenly distribute plantar pressure, a steel shank for stability, cushioning, and a broad sole base for support and traction.

The mechanical factors leading to ulceration need to be reviewed and noted, such as: body mass; evidence of tissue trauma; weight diffusion; weight dispersion; pathomechanics (defined as structural change in relation to function); biomechanics (defined as forces that change and affect the foot in relation to function; imbalance (defined as the inability to adapt to alterations of stress); force (alteration in physical condition, either shape or position); compression stress (one force moves towards another); tensile stress (a pulling away of one part against another); shearing stress (a sliding of one part on the other); friction (the force needed to overcome resistance and usually associated with a sheering stress; elasticity (weight diffusion and weight dispersion); and fluid pressure (soft tissue adaptation and conformity to stress).

Given the fact that assessment and re-assessment should be completed on a regular basis, management can then be instituted to reduce the complications of chronic disease and subscribe to the principles of secondary prevention of disease. The plan for care includes the following, as an example: plan podiatric referral, patient education, medical referral, special footwear, vascular studies, clinical laboratory studies, imaging (including radiographs, sequential bone scans, computed tomography (CT), magnetic resonance imaging (MRI), and Duplex Ultrasound), prescriptions, and follow-up assessment and management. (39, 40)

11. Discussion

The evolution of this protocol began in 1959 as the number of older individuals and those with chronic diseases began to increase. Those diseases and disorders that presented with complications, such as diabetes mellitus, peripheral arterial disease, degenerative joint changes, collagen diseases, and neurosensory disorders were recognized as having a significant effect on the future quality of older citizens. A visit to the United Kingdom by the Commissioner and Deputy Commissioner of Health of the City of Philadelphia demonstrated a need for foot care that was a part of the British heral care system. A joint effort with the Philadelphia Department of Health and St. Luke's & Children's Medical Center in Philadelphia resulted in the first US Public Health Service funded program dealing with foot health for an aging population. "Keep Them Walking" provided a three years study involving information, education, screening, assessment and care for in excess of 16,000 citizens over the age of 65 in Philadelphia. The number of foot problems that were uncovered was so significant that Philadelphia established podiatric services as a part of it community health care program, that remain today as a vital part of providing care for older citizens.

About that same time, similar efforts were initiated at the Queensbridge Health Maintenance Program in New York, the ambulatory clinics of the Washington, DC Health

Department and by the Minnesota Department of Health for Long Term Care Programs. The data also demonstrated a similar high prevalence for diseases and disorders of the foot and related structures.

In 1963, the US Public Health Service and the Gerontological Society of America began to develop its first clinical geriatric practice guide that also included Podiatric programs. In 1966, the US Department of Veterans Affairs also identified a significant need for foot care programs, as a part of their long term care services, especially for older adults. It became clear that screening had to be replaced by Assessment, Identification, Risk Stratification, Education, and Treatment programs to enhance the concept of the secondary prevention of chronic diseases in older patients.

The presented Clinical Podogeriatric and Chronic Disease Protocol (Helfand Index) was developed through a coordinated effort by the Diabetes Control Program of the Pennsylvania Department of Health and Temple University School of Podiatric Medicine and provides a means to assess older patients with diabetes mellitus and other chronic diseases to develop proper and appropriate care prevention and care programs.

The most recent validation study of this protocol, Foot Problems in Older Patients - A Focused Podogeriatric Assessment Study in Ambulatory Care demonstrated the prevalence of foot conditions in older individuals and their association with chronic risk diseases such as diabetes mellitus, peripheral arterial disease, and arthritis, and to develop care plans to reduce complications from local foot problems and chronic diseases. One thousand individuals older than 65 years who were ambulatory and not institutionalized underwent a standardized and validated podogeriatric examination assessment protocol or index.

The Summary of the Data is attached as **Appendix B.** The findings demonstrated that foot problems in the older population result from disease, disability, and deformity related to multiple chronic diseases as well as changes associated with repetitive use and trauma. Older people are at a high risk of developing foot-related disease and should receive continuing foot assessment, education, surveillance, and care. (J Am Podiatric Med Assoc 94(3): 293-304, 2004). The data also demonstrated that 77% of all patients were deemed to be at risk for significant complications involving the foot and its related structures that could impair the quality of life and significantly increase the cost of care.

The development of this protocol (Helfand Index) provided a means to identify older and diabetic patients who were at risk for complications involving the foot and its related structures; to focus on educational needs for patients and professionals; to provide referral for the rapid treatment and management of foot problems; and to provide a forum to discuss the need for appropriate foot wear for patients at risk, as a means to secondarily prevent future diseases and disorders of the foot.

The protocol provided a focus on the current patients history, the past medical history, a system review, current and past medications, the assessment of skin and toe nail conditions, foot deformities, pathomechanical and biomechanical changes, vascular assessment, neurological assessment and sensory deficits, risk stratification (vascular, sensory, class finding, mycotic, hyperkeratotic, and ulcers), footwear and foot covering, assessment, and a management plan. Examples for the reasons to refer patients for podiatric medical include but are not limited to the following:

- Signs suggesting generalized diseases that include neuropathy, vascular disease, diabetes mellitus, infection, ulceration, deformity, degenerative joint changes, focal neoplastic diseases, collagen diseases, and other conditions as indicated involving the foot and related structures in those cases where concomitant therapy is indicated where initial management is not effective:
  - In the presence of skin lesions involving the foot:
  - In the presence of postural deformities of the foot and related structures:
  - In the presence of diabetes mellitus, neurosensory, peripheral vascular, and other risk diseases:
  - In the presence of foot problems combined with ambulatory and/or walking difficulty and/or a history of or risk of falls:
  - Where orthotics are indicated:
  - If the patient is unable to obtain and/or provide foot care:
  - If the patient complains of a foot problem or has specific questions about care including information on footwear.

The assessment protocol clearly provided a means to identify the most significant risk factors. Although vascular and neurosensory deficits are usually thought of as most significant as to their potential impact for ulceration and amputation, class findings, mechanical or pressure keratosis, onychomycosis, onychial grades at risk, and pre-ulceration, become equally important in relation to prevention and a means to provide rapid and early treatment for conditions noted. The protocol does provide a means to identify previous amputations; past foot ulcer history, peripheral neuropathy, foot deformity including Charcot's Foot, peripheral vascular and arterial impairment, visual impairment, podalgia, pododynia dysbasia, and diabetic neuropath, especially in patient on dialysis. All of these factors increase the amputation risk for diabetic patients (1, 2). In addition, the assessment protocol is not time consuming.

There are a number of ulcer classifications in the literature including the Wagner Classification for Foot Ulcers, The University of Texas Diabetic Wound Classification, the National Pressure Ulcer Advisory Panel (NPUAP) Classification for Pressure Ulcers, as well as the one selected and described by Sims, Cavanagh, and Ulbrecht (46). This ten (10 grade classification provide three stages prior to a superficial ulcer that permitted earlier justification for treatment programs, associated with this assessment protocol.

The Loss of Protective Sensation was initially developed by Dr. Paul Brand at the Leprosy Mission in London and then for the USPHS National Hansen's Disease Program in Carville LA. With the recognition that the same findings were equal predictors of amputation in patients with diabetes mellitus, the use of the Semmes-Weinstein (5.07 gage) 10-gram monofilament has been defined universally in a consistent fashion to measure of light pressure. Vibration perception with the tuning fork 128 Hz (cps) and measurement of vibration perception threshold (Biothesiometer) were also employed. Pinching the Achilles tendon also provided a means to measure pain. Temperature perception, deep tendon reflexes and two-point discrimination are added procedures that provide addition al assessment benefits.

By early recognition of foot and related problems, not as an initial assessment tool, but as a subsequent re-assessment tool, patient education and rapid treatment program can be instituted to prevent progressing complications and maintain a maximum quality of independent life for older diabetic patients.

Since this Protocol was introduced, it has been employed by a number of programs and institutions, included and identified in multiple presentations and publications. Examples include the following: Pennsylvania Department of Health; Pennsylvania Diabetes Academy; Temple University - School of Podiatric Medicine and Institute on Aging; University of Pennsylvania - School of Nursing; Griffin Hospital - Yale - Department of Veterans Affairs Health System; Geriatric Educational Resources for Residency Training in Family Medicine and Internal Medicine - The John A. Hartford Foundation Geriatric Education Consortium for Residency Training (Stanford University Geriatric Education Center, Baylor College of Medicine, Harvard University, Johns Hopkins University, Stanford University, University of California - Los Angeles, University of Chicago, University of Connecticut, University of Rochester, American Academy of Family Physicians); Pennsylvania Geriatric Education Center; Delaware Valley Geriatric Education Center; Thomas Jefferson University Hospital; American Medical Directors Association; American Podiatric Medical Association; as well as journals and texts; including the Geriatric Review Syllabus of the American Geriatrics Society, W B Saunders, Martin Dunitz, Elsevier, Wiley, McGraw-Hill, Health Professions Press, the American Public Health Association Press, Cambridge University Press, and Oxford University Press.

12. Concluding remarks

Much of the ability to remain ambulatory in the period of aging is directly related to foot health. In order to accomplish this aim, practitioners must think comprehensively, and recognize that team care must be an essential part of chronic disease management in the care of the older patient. Foot health education for patients and professionals should be employed. It is clear that adults with chronic diseases, such as diabetes mellitus, and older patients are a high risk for foot related disease and should maintain continuing foot assessment, education, surveillance, and care. The consequences of considering foot care for the older population as "routine" and a failure to prevent complications and maintain mobility and ambulation will result in ambulatory dysfunction, gait modification, podalgia, pododynia dysbasia, morbidity, mortality, increased health care costs, and will be reflected in the quality of life and the ability to remain mentally alert and active in their communities (51). For our future, the golden years must be more than aging in place, thinking of their residence as a waiting room, or waiting for God. We must recognize that aging is not a disease, that older individuals should be able to live life to the end of life with the dignity of age, and that we must protect what cannot be replaced.

13. Acknowledgment

The project which helped develop this Protocol was completed with the support of a Contract from the Pennsylvania Department of Health, in cooperation with the

Pennsylvania Diabetes Academy, Foundation of the Pennsylvania Medical Society, Temple University, School of Podiatric Medicine and Temple University, Institute on Aging.

14. Appendix A

Assessment protocol

Date Of Visit **MR#**

Patient's Name **Age**

DATE OF BIRTH			SOCIAL SECURITY #
ADDRESS			
CITY	STATE	ZIP CODE	
PHONE NUMBER ( )			
SEX M F	RACE B W A L NA		
WEIGHT LBS	HEIGHT IN		
SOCIAL STATUS	M S W D SEP		

Name of primary physician/health care facility

Date Of Last Visit

History Of Present Illness

SWELLING OF FEET	LOCATION
PAINFUL FEET	QUALITY
HYPERKERATOSIS	SEVERITY
ONYCHIAL CHANGES	DURATION
BUNIONS	CONTEXT
PAINFUL TOE NAILS	MODIFYING FACTORS
INFECTIONS	ASSOCIATED SIGNS &
COLD FEET	SYMPTOMS
OTHER	

Past medical history

HEART DISEASE	DIABETES MELLITUS
HIGH BLOOD PRESSURE	*IDDM
ARTHRITIS	*NIDDM
*CIRCULATORY DISEASE	HYPERCHOLESTEROL
THYROID	GOUT
ALLERGY	FAMILY AND SOCIAL HISTORY
	SMOKING
	ALCOHOL

System review

CONSTITUTIONAL		
ENT	CARD/VASC	GU
EYES	MUSCULO- SKELETAL	NEUROLOGIC

SKIN/HAIR	ENDOCRINE	GI
RESPIRATORY	GYN	IMMUNOLOGIC
PSYCHIATRIC	ALLERGIC	
HEMATOLOGIC	LYMPHATIC	

Medications

Dermatologic

*HYPERKERATOSIS		XEROSIS	
ONYCHAUXIS	B-2-B	TINEA PEDIS	
INFECTION		VERRUCA	
*ULCERATION		HEMATOMA	
ONYCHOMYCOSIS		RUBOR	
ONYCHODYSTROPHY		*PREULCERATIVE	
*CYANOSIS	B-2-E	DISCOLORED	

Foot orthopedic

*HALLUX VALGUS	*HALLUX RIGIDUS-LIMITUS
*ANTERIOR IMBALANCE	*MORTON'S SYNDROME
*DIGITI FLEXUS	BURSITIS
*PES PLANUS	*PROMINENT MET HEAD
*PES VALGOPLANUS	*CHARCOT JOINTS
*PES CAVUS	OTHER

Vascular evaluation

*COLDNESS	C-2	*CLAUDICATION	C-1
*TROPHIC CHANGES	B-2-A	VARICOSITIES	
*DP ABSENT	B-3	OTHER	
*PT ABSENT	B-1	*AMPUTATION	
*NIGHT CRAMPS		*AKA BKA FF T	A-1
*EDEMA	C-3	ATROPHY	B-2-D

Neurologic evaluation

*ACHILLES		SUPERFICIAL PLANTAR	
*VIBRATORY		*JOINT POSITION	
*SHARP/DULL		*BURNING	C-5
*PARESTHESIA	C-4	OTHER	
LOSS OF PROTECTIVE SENSATION			

Risk category - neurologic

0 = No Sensory Loss
*1 = Sensory Loss
*2 = Sensory Loss & Foot Deformity
*3 = Sensory Loss, Hx Ulceration, & Deformity

Risk category - vascular

0 - 0 No Change
*I - 1 Mild Claudication
*I - 2 Moderate Claudication
*I - 3 Severe Claudication
*II - 4 Ischemic Rest Pain
*III - 5 Minor Tissue Loss
*III - 6 Major Tissue Loss

Footwear Satisfactory YES NO

Hygiene Satisfactory YES NO

Stockings: NYLON COTTON WOOL OTHER NONE

YES NO

Assessment

Plan

Podiatric referral
Patient education
Medical referral
Special footwear
Vascular studies
Clinical lab
Imaging
Rx

Class findings

A1 Nontraumatic Amputation
B1 Absent Posterior Tibial
B2 Advanced Trophic Changes
B2A Hair Growth (Decrease Or Absent)
B2B Nail Changes (Thickening)
B2C Pigmentary Changes (Discoloration)
B2D Skin Texture (Thin, Shiny)
B2E Skin Color (Rubor Or Redness)
B3 Absent Dorsalis Pedis
C1 Claudication
C2 Temperature Changes (Cold)
C3 Edema
C4 Paresthesia
C5 Burning

Onychomycosis

Documentation of mycosis/dystrophy causing secondary infection and/or pain that results or would result in marked limitation of ambulation.

Discoloration
Hypertrophy
Subungual debris
Onycholysis
Secondary infection
Limitation of ambulation and pain

Classification of mechanical or pressure hyperkeratosis

Grade description

0. No lesion
1. No specific tyloma plaque, but diffuse or pinch hyperkeratotic tissue present or in narrow bands
2. Circumscribed, punctate oval, or circular, well defined thickening of keratinized tissue
3. Heloma milliare or heloma durum with no associated tyloma
4. Well defined tyloma plaque with a definite heloma within the lesion
5. Extravasation, maceration and early breakdown of structures under the tyloma or callus layer
6. Complete breakdown of structure of hyperkeratotic tissue, epidermis, extending to superficial dermal involvement

Plantar keratomata pattern

LT 5 4 3 2 1 RT 1 2 3 4 5

Ulcer classification

Grade - 0 - Absent Skin Lesions
Grade - 1 - Dense Callus But Not Pre-Ulcer or Ulcer
Grade - 2 - Preulcerative Changes
Grade - 3 - Partial Thickness (Superficial Ulcer)
Grade - 4 - Full Thickness (Deep) Ulcer But No Involvement of Tendon, Bone, Ligament or Joint
Grade - 5 - Full Thickness (Deep) Ulcer With Involvement of Tendon, Bone, Ligament or Joint
Grade - 6 - Localized Infection (Abscess or Osteomyelitis)
Grade - 7 - Proximal Spread of Infection (Ascending Cellulitis or Lymphadenopathy
Grade - 8 - Gangrene of Forefoot Only
Grade - 9 - Gangrene of Majority of Foot

Onychial grades at risk

Grade I Normal
Grade II Mild Hypertrophy
Grade III Hypertrophic
Dystrophic
Onychauxis

Mycotic
Infected
Onychodysplasia
Grade IV Hypertrophic
Deformed
Onychogryphosis
Dystrophic
Mycotic
Infected

15. Appendix B

Summary of clinical findings in 1,000 older people (31)

Patients Percentage (%) of Clinical Findings:	%
History of present illness	
Swelling of feet	382
Painful feet	746
Hyperkeratosis	510
Onychial changes	895
Bunions	240
Painful toenails	357
Infections (bacterial)	37
Cold feet	197
Other	480
Past history	
Heart disease	258
High blood pressure	367
Arthritis	421
Circulatory disease	229
Thyroid disease	94
Allergy	53
Diabetes mellitus	572
Insulin-dependent	175
Non-insulin-dependent	397
Hypercholesterolemia	362
Gout	71
Smoking	63
Alcohol abuse	94
Systems review	
Constitutional	84
Ears, nose, throat	87
Eyes	487
Skin/hair	642
Respiratory	279
Psychiatric	242
Hematologic	21

Cardiac/vascular	410	
Musculoskeletal	842	
Gynecologic	420	
Lymphatic	32	
Genitourinary	273	
Neurologic	124	
Endocrine	619	
Gastrointestinal	270	
Immunologic	22	
Dermatologic evaluation		
Hyperkeratosis	770	
Onychauxis	470	
Infection	42	
Ulceration	24	
Onychomycosis	590	
Onychodystrophy	942	
Cyanosis	42	
Xerosis	652	
Tinea pedis	137	
Verruca	9	
Hematoma	104	
Rubor	61	
Preulcerative	114	
Discolored	89	
Foot orthopedic evaluation		
Hallux valgus	527	
Anterior imbalance	429	
Digiti flexus	589	
Pes planus	174	
Pes valgoplanus	121	
Pes cavus	192	
Hallux rigidus/limitus	322	
Morton's syndrome, bursitis	107	
Prominent metatarsal head	642	
Charcot's joint	46	
Other	172	
Vascular evaluation		
Coldness	483	
Trophic changes	796	
Dorsalis pedis pulse absent	347	
Posterior tibial pulse absent	322	
Night cramps	473	
Edema	418	
Claudication	223	
Varicosities	181	
Amputation	15	
Above-the-knee		2

Below-the-knee	4
Forefoot	3
Toes	6
Atrophy	689
Neurologic evaluation	
Achilles	42
Vibratory	721
Sharp/dull	432
Paresthesia	684
Superficial plantar	32
Joint position	214
Burning	621
Other	384
Risk category—neurologic	
No sensory loss	360
Sensory loss	217
Sensory loss and deformity	340
Sensory loss, history of ulceration, and deformity	83
Risk category—vascular	
No change	183
Mild claudication	133
Moderate claudication	90
Severe claudication	52
Ischemic rest pain	473
Minor tissue loss	6
Major tissue loss	9
Class findings	
A-1: Nontraumatic amputation	15
B-1: Absent posterior tibial pulse	322
B-2: Advanced trophic changes	796
B-2-a: Hair growth (decrease or absent)	780
B-2-b: Nail changes (thickening)	942
B-2-c: Pigmentary changes (discoloration)	89
B-2-d: Skin texture (thin, shiny)	473
B-2-e: Skin color (rubor or redness)	61
B-3: Absent dorsalis pedis pulse	347
C-1: Claudication	223
C-2: Temperature changes (cold)	483
C-3: Edema	418
C-4: Paresthesia	684
C-5: Burning	621
Onychomycosis	
Discoloration	590
Hypertrophy	590
Subungual debris	483
Onycholysis	521

Secondary infection	104
Limitation of ambulation and pain	107
Classification of pressure keratosis	
Grade 0: No lesion	230
Grade 1: Diffuse or pinch	78
Grade 2: Circumscribed oval or punctate	147
Grade 3: Heloma milliare or durum	204
Grade 4: Tyloma with heloma	203
Grade 5: Extravasation or maceration	114
Grade 6: Tissue breakdown	24
Ulcer classification	
Grade 0: Absent skin lesions	230
Grade 1: Dense callus	632
Grade 2: Preulcerative changes	114
Grade 3: Partial-thickness (superficial)	22
Grade 4: Full-thickness (deep)	2
Grade 5: Full-thickness (deep) with involvement of tendon, bone, ligament, or joint	0
Grade 6: Localized infection (abscess or osteomyelitis)	0
Grade 7: Proximal spread of infection (cellulitis)	0
Grade 8: Gangrene of forefoot	0
Grade 9: Gangrene of majority of foot	0
Onychial grades at risk	
Grade I: Normal	58
Grade II: Mild hypertrophy	888
Grade III: Hypertrophy, dystrophy, onychauxis, mycosis, infection, onychodysplasia	355
Grade IV: Hypertrophy, deformity, onychogryphosis, dystrophy, mycosis, infection	235
Footwear satisfactory	
Yes	637
No	363
Hygiene satisfactory	
Yes	972
No	28
Stockings	
Nylon	587
Cotton	302
Wool	93
Other	12
None	7
Plan	
Podiatric referral	1,000
Medical referral	272
Vascular studies	104

Imaging	123
Patient education	1,000
Special footwear	425
Clinical laboratory evaluation	36
Medication	824

16. References

[1] American Diabetes Association, Standards of Care, Foot Care Recommendations, Diabetes Care 33: S11, 2010, Journal of the American Podiatric Medical Association, Vol 101, No 1, January/February 2011, pp 75-77

[2] American Diabetes Association, Preventive Foot Care in Diabetes, Diabetes Care, Vol 27, S 1, January 2004, pp S63-S64

[3] American Geriatrics Society, Geriatric Review Syllabus, Sixth Edition, New York, NY, 2006

[4] American College of Foot and Ankle Surgeons, Diabetic Foot Disorders - A Clinical Practice Guideline, Park Ridge, IL: American College of Foot and Ankle Surgeons, 2000

[5] Arenson C, Busby-Whitehead J, Brummel-Smith K, O'Brien J G, Palmer M H, & Reichel W, Reichel's Care of the Elderly - Clinical Aspects of Aging, Sixth Edition, Cambridge University Press, New York, NY, 2009

[6] Armstrong, David G and Lavery, Lawrence A, Clinical Care of the Diabetic Foot, American Diabetes Association, Alexandria, VA, 2005

[7] Baran R & Haneke E, The Nail in Differential Diagnosis, Informa Healthcare, Oxford, UK, 2007

[8] Birrer, R. B., Dellacorte, M. P. & Grisafi, P. J., Common Foot Problems in Primary Care, Second Edition, Henley & Belfus, Inc, Philadelphia 1998

[9] Bolton, Andrew J M, Et. Al., Comprehensive Foot Examination and Risk Assessment, Diabetes Care, Vol 31, No. 8, August 2008, pp. 1679-1685

[10] Boike A M & Hall J O, A Practical Guide for Examining and Treating the Diabetic Foot, Cleveland Clinic Journal of Medicine, Vol 69, No 4, April 2002, pp 342-348

[11] Bowker, John H. & Pfeifer, Michael A., Levin's & O'Neal's - The Diabetic Foot, 7th. Ed., Mosby-Elsevier, Philadelphia, PA 2008

[12] Capezuti E A, Siegler E L, & Mezey M D, The Encyclopedia of Elder Care - A Comprehensive Resource on Geriatric and Social Care, Second Edition, Springer Publishing, New York, NY, 2008

[13] Caputo, G M, Cavanagh, P R, Ulbrecht, J, Gibbons, G W, & Karchmer, A W, Assessment and Management of Foot Disease in Patients with Diabetes, New England Journal of Medicine, September 29, 1994, 33: 854-860

[14] Dauber, Rodney, Bristow, Ivan, & Turner, Warren, Text Atlas of Podiatric Dermatology, Martin Dunitz, London, 2001

[15] Banks A, Downey M S, Martin D E, & Miller S J, McGlamry's Forefoot Surgery, Lippincott, Williams & Wilkins, Philadelphia, 2004

[16] Edmonds, Michael E, Foster, Althea V M and Sanders, Lee J, A Practical Manual of Diabetic Footcare, Blackwell Publishing, Malden, MA, 2004, Second Edition, 2008

[17] Evans J, G, Williams F T, Beattie B L, Michel J P, & Wilcock G K, Oxford Textbook of Geriatric Medicine, 2nd Ed, Oxford University Press, England, 2000

[18] Foster A V M, Podiatric Assessment and Management of the Diabetic Foot, Churchill-Livingstone-Elsevier, Edinburgh, 2006
[19] Gabel, L L, Haines, D J, and Papp, K K, The Aging Foot, An Interdisciplinary Perspective, The Ohio State University, College of Medicine and Public Health, Department of Family Medicine, Columbus, OH, 2004
[20] Halter J B, Ouslander, J G, Tinetti M E, Studenski S, High K P, & Asthana S, Hazzard's Geriatric Medicine and Gerontology, McGraw - Hill, New York, NY, 2009
[21] Ham R J, Sloane P D, Warshaw G A, Bernard M A, & Flaherty R, Primary Care Geriatrics - A Case Based Approach, Fifth Edition, Mosby/Elsevier, Philadelphia PA, 2007
[22] Helfand, Arthur E. Ed. The Geriatric Patient and Considerations of Aging, Clinics in Podiatric Medicine and Surgery, W. B. Saunders, Co., Philadelphia PA Vol. I, January 1993; Vol. II, April 1993.
[23] Helfand, A. E. & Jessett, D. F., Foot Problems, Principles and Practice of Geriatric Medicine, 4th. Edition, Pathy M S John, Sinclair, Alan S, and Morley, John R., Eds. 2006, John Wiley & Sons, Chichester
[24] Helfand, Arthur E., Assessing the Older Diabetic Patient, CD, Pennsylvania Diabetes Academy, Pennsylvania Department of Health, Temple University, School of Medicine, Office for Continuing Medical Education, Temple University, School of Podiatric Medicine, Harrisburg PA, December, 2001
[25] Helfand, Arthur E, Disorders and Diseases of the Foot, Geriatric Review Syllabus, A Core Curriculum in Geriatric Medicine, Cobbs E L, Duthie E D, & Murphy, J B, Eds, 6th. Edition, Malden MA, Blackwell Publishing Co, 2006
[26] Helfand, Arthur E, Clinical Podogeriatrics: Assessment, Education, and Prevention, Clinics in Podiatric Medicine and Surgery, Vol. 20, No 3, W B Saunders Co - Elsevier, Philadelphia Pa, July 2003,
[27] Helfand, Arthur E, Ed, Foot Health Training Guide for Long-Term Care Personnel, Health Professions Press, Baltimore, MD, 2007
[28] Helfand, Arthur E., Ed, Public Health and Podiatric Medicine - Principles and Practice - Second Edition, APHA Press, American Public Health Association, Washington DC 2006
[29] Helfand, Arthur E, An Overview of Shoe Modifications and Orthoses in the Management of Adult Foot and Ankle Pathology, Turkiye Klinikleri Journal of Physical Medicine and Rehabilitation - Special Topics 2010 3 (2), pp107-114
[30] Helfand, Arthur E., Clinical Assessment of Podogeriatric Patients, Podiatry Management, February 2004, Vol 23, No 2, pp 145.152
[31] Helfand, Arthur E., Foot Problems in Older Patients - A Focused Podogeriatric Assessment study in Ambulatory Care, Journal of the American Podiatric Medical Association, May - June 2004, Vol. 94, No. 3, pp. 293-304
[32] Helfand, Arthur E., International Journal of Clinical Practice, Blackwell Publishing, Clinical Assessment of Peripheral Arterial Occlusive Risk Factors in the Diabetic Foot, Editorial, April 2007, Vol. 61, No 4, pp. 540-541
[33] Helliwell P, Woodburn A, Redmond A, Turner D, & Davys, H, The Foot and Ankle in Rheumatoid Arthritis - A Comprehensive Guide, Churchill-Livingstone-Elsevier, Edinburgh, 2007

[34] International Diabetes Federation, International Consensus on the Diabetic Foot and Practical Guidelines on the Management an Prevention of the Diabetic Foot, Amsterdam, The Netherlands, 2007

[35] Kesselman, P. The Comprehensive Diabetic Foot Examination Revisited, Podiatry Management, October 2009, pp 65-74

[36] Levy, L A and Hetherington V J, Principles and Practice of Geriatric Medicine, Second Edition, Data Trace Publishing Co, Brooklandville, MD 2006

[37] Lorimer, D., French, G., O'Donnell, M., & Burrow, J. G. Neale's Disorders the Foot, Diagnosis and Management, Sixth Edition, Churchill Livingstone, New York, NY, 2002

[38] Mayfield J A, Reiber, G E, Sanders, L J, Janisse, D, & Pogach. L , Preventive Foot Care in People With Diabetes, Diabetes Care, Col 21, No 12, December 1998, pp: 2161-2177

[39] Menz H B, Foot Problems in Older People - Assessment and Management, Churchill-Livingstone-Elsevier, Edinburgh, 2008

[40] Merriman, Linda M & Turner, Warren, Assessment of the Lower Limb, Second Edition, Churchill-Livingstone, Edinburgh, Scotland 2002

[41] Ogrin R, Foot Assessment I Patients with Diabetes, Australian Family Physician, Vol 35, No 6, June 2006, pp: 419-421

[42] Pyibo, S O, Jude, E B, Tarawneh, I, Nugyen, H C, Harkless, L B, & Bolton, A, A Comparison of Two Diabetic Foot Ulcer Classification Systems, Diabetes Care, Vol 24, No 1, January 2001, pp: 84-88

[43] Pathy, M. S., Sinclair, A. J., & Morley, J E, Principles and Practice of Geriatric Medicine, Fourth Edition, John Wiley & Sons, Chichester, England, 2006.

[44] Pinzur, M S, Slovenkai, M P, & Trepman, E, Guidelines for Diabetic Foot Care, Foot & Ankle International, Vol 20, No 11, November 1999, pp 695-704

[45] Robbins, Jeffrey M., Primary Podiatric Medicine, W. B. Saunders Co., Philadelphia PA. 1994

[46] Sims, D. S., Canvanagh, P., & Ulbrecht, J. S., Risk Factors in the Diabetic Foot, Recognition and Management, Physical Therapy, 68: 1988, pp. 1887- 1902

[47] Strauss MB, Hart JD, Winant DM. Preventive Foot Care: a user-friendly system for patients and physicians. Postgraduate Med. 1998; 103:223-245.

[48] Turner, Warren A & Merriman, Linda M, Clinical Skills in Treating the Foot - Second Edition, Elsevier, Churchill, Livingstone, Edinburgh, UK, 2005

[49] Tyrrell W & Carter G, Therapeutic Footwear - A Comprehensive Guide, Churchill-Livingstone-Elsevier, Edinburgh, UK, 2009

[50] US Department of Veterans Affairs, Veterans Health Administration, VHA Directive 2009-30, June 16, 2009, Washington, DC

[51] US Department of Health and Human Services, USPHS, NIH, Feet Can Last A Lifetime - A Health Care Provider's Guide & Preventing Diabetic Foot Problems, Bethesda MD 11/2000

[52] Yates, Ben, Merriman's Assessment of the Lower Limb, 3rd Ed., Churchill Livingstone, Elsevier, Edinburgh, UK, 2009

Part 3

Treatment of Diabetic Foot Ulcerations

9

The Pathogenesis of the Diabetic Foot Ulcer: Prevention and Management

F. Aguilar Rebolledo, J. M. Terán Soto and Jorge Escobedo de la Peña
Centro Integral de Medicina Avanzada (CIMA), National Institute of Social Security: National Medical Center XXIst Century, National Institute of Social Security, "Gabriel Mancera" General Hospital Mexico

1. Introduction

The most important complications of diabetes mellitus are neuropathy and diabetic foot. Manifestations of resulting complications range from simple to highly complex, including limb amputations and life–threatening infections. Foot infections in people with diabetes are common; this creates complex social problems owing to the financial burden resulting from the high cost of treatment and healing (Aguilar, 2009). In addition to severe morbidity, foot infections cause prolonged hospitalization and psychological and social problems for the patient and his family. Even though foot pathology in diabetic patients entails high medical costs, it also causes loss of productivity in patients (Ramsey et al, 1999)

Predictions regarding the prevalence of DM have failed because the expected 300 million people worldwide with diabetes in 2025 were exceeded in 2011, some authors figure the rising to 347 millions (Goodarz et al, 2011), but in Lisbon, Portugal the International Diabetes Federation (IDF) said that the prevalence of DM around the world is 366 millions (Mbanya JC, 2011). Moreover, it is predicted that within 15 years (2025) there will be 500 million people worldwide with diabetes if we do not take the necessary measures to prevent the spread of this disease. On the other hand, the most common cause of non-traumatic amputations is diabetes mellitus, and 80% of these could be averted through adequate prevention and early intervention. For example, in 2002 the medical cost for treating patients with DM was 92 billion USD. Loss of productivity could represent an additional 40 billion. Projections for the cost of treatment will rise to approximately 160 billion in 2010 and close to 200 billion in 2020, or even higher (Hogan P et al, 2003). Therefore, complications arising from diabetic foot represent an important medical challenge in growing proportions. The cost of treatment of ulcerations without surgical interventions approaches several thousand dollars, and in some cases even more, compared to ulcers that are treated through amputation (Kruse & Edelman 2006). Foot ulcerations represent 85% of all amputations. Hence, the association between ulcers and lower extremity amputations is patently obvious. Taking into account that the major risk factor leading to amputation is ulceration, around 15% of all foot ulcers will ultimately require amputation at some point. Other risk factors for amputation include a long history of diabetes, peripheral neuropathy and structural changes of the foot, peripheral vascular disease, poor glycemic control, a prior history of foot ulcers, previous foot surgery and/or amputation, retinopathy and nephropathy. (Clayton et al, 2009, Aguilar & Rayo 2000)

The management of wounds requires meticulous care and early treatment by a multidisciplinary foot care team. This management team may include: infectious disease specialists, microbiologists, podiatrists, nurses specializing in diabetes and physicians with knowledge of DM, all striving to provide quality care and good metabolic control. Optimal care and early detection of diabetic ulcers can greatly reduce the occurrence of infections. We think that all specialists who treat diabetic foot need to remember this important message: *"Neuropathic symptoms correlated poorly with sensory loss, and the absence of sensory loss must not be equated to no risk of foot ulcers. Therefore, the assessment of foot ulcer risk MUST ALWAYS include a careful foot examination, with the removal of shoes and socks, regardless of the patient's neuropathic history."* (Boulton et al, 1998).

Unfortunately, diabetic foot ulcers (infected or not), are quite often treated improperly. Amputation rates have shown a variation of both gender and ethnicity. Males are at higher risk than females. Hispanics -particularly Mexicans- and African-Americans have been associated with higher risk of amputation (Velasco Mondragon et al, 2010). Difficulty of access to continuing medical education for physicians, especially in emerging countries exhibiting high prevalence, has caused many difficulties in providing early care for patients and in establishing preventive care routines. Another worrisome matter is the propagation of erroneous beliefs regarding treatment of DM (for example, insulin being linked to blindness) and wound healing (for example the inappropriate use of honey, spider webs, gelatin, herbal preparations, etc. as cures) and also poor involvement of the Federal Government in health programs. These factors all lead to a rise in the disease, and consequently increased risk of amputation (Tentolouris 2010). Many scientific studies have led to the establishment of programs designed to prevent and promote awareness on diabetic foot complications. As a result, the rate of amputations dropped by nearly 50% (Li R et al, 2010).

The underlying causes of risk factors leading to the onset of diabetic foot ulcers have recently been identified. The afore-mentioned conditions, together with peripheral neuropathy, contribute to a lack of sensation in poorly vascularized lower extremities that are prone to the development of chronic wounds. Lack of sensation leads to exacerbation of the injury. Dry, stiff skin cracks easily and causes splits or fissures. A fissure in the protective epidermal covering (stratum corneum), can become infected, resulting in localized cellulitis or even small longitudinal ulcerations that can potentially become infected and frequently lead to the spread of infection and the ultimate loss of the lower limb, either partial or full. Poor circulation occurs in conducting vessels, consequently affecting microcirculation, which in turn affects the basement membrane, thickening and diminishing vascular reparative capacity (Tanenberg RJ & Donofrio PD 2008). The most important risk factors for the development of diabetic foot ulcers are: peripheral neuropathy (motor, sensory and autonomic), structural and anatomical deformities, environmental factors, peripheral vascular disease, a compromised immune system and poor metabolic control, in addition to social influences such as emotional, psychological and behavioral problems (Lyons 2008).

The purpose of this chapter is to help gain an understanding of different types of management strategies, ranging from general through specific strategies, starting with the initial examination of the patient who comes in for examination of a foot injury all the way through the final diagnosis. The clinical exam begins with a complete examination, classification of the ulcer, basic measures, treatment with antibiotics (if the wound is infected) in order to establish the appropriate intervention and follow-up treatment to avert major complications, including amputation.

We hope that better insight of the pathogenesis of diabetic foot complications will contribute to creating improved, effective and successful preventive strategies in order to save lower limbs.

2. Pathogenesis of the wounds

Risk factors for the development of foot ulcers in diabetic patients should be evaluated from 3 different dimensions:

1. Physiopathology
2. Anatomical and structural alterations
3. Environmental influences

2.1 Physiopathology

These changes occur at a biomolecular level and are caused by hyperglycemia, which leads to the development of neuropathy, as described in Fig 1.

Over the past two decades considerable evidence has been accumulated to support the potentially pathogenetic role of a number of mechanisms that lead diabetic persons to develop wounds. The major mechanisms are: (Aguilar F, 2009a)

- Nerve hypoxia/ischemia
- Auto oxidative stress
- Polyol pathway overactivity
- Increased advanced glycation end-products
- Deficiency of gamma linolenic acid
- Protein kinase C, especially B-isoform increase
- Cytokines dysfunction
- Disorders of collagen molecules (elastin, proteoglycans)
- Endothelial dysfunction
- Mitochondrial dysfunction
- Growth factors deficiency
- Alteration of the immune mechanism
- Increased secretion of proteases
- Others

Under normal circumstances, wound repair is a highly orchestrated event that involves the interaction of the elements described above. Each stage of the healing process entails this orchestrated effort. The damaged tissue quickly releases tissue factor and other stimuli, such as expulsed collagen, to activate a variety of physical mechanical, biological or chemical events. These changes cause damage to the nerve fiber and even peripheral vascular disease, which in turn takes its toll at the molecular level. Endothelial dysfunction is the most serious impairment affecting microcirculation, owing to changes in the proliferation of endothelial cells, thickening of the basement membrane, decreased synthesis of nitric oxide, increased blood viscosity, alterations in microvascular tone and decreased blood flow. On the other hand, the immune system is compromised by lowered leukocyte activity, inappropriate inflammatory response and the disruption of cellular immunity (inhibition of fibroblast proliferation and impairment of the basal layer of keratinocytes, reducing epidermal cell migration). (Aguilar F, 2005, Boulton AJM, 2003)

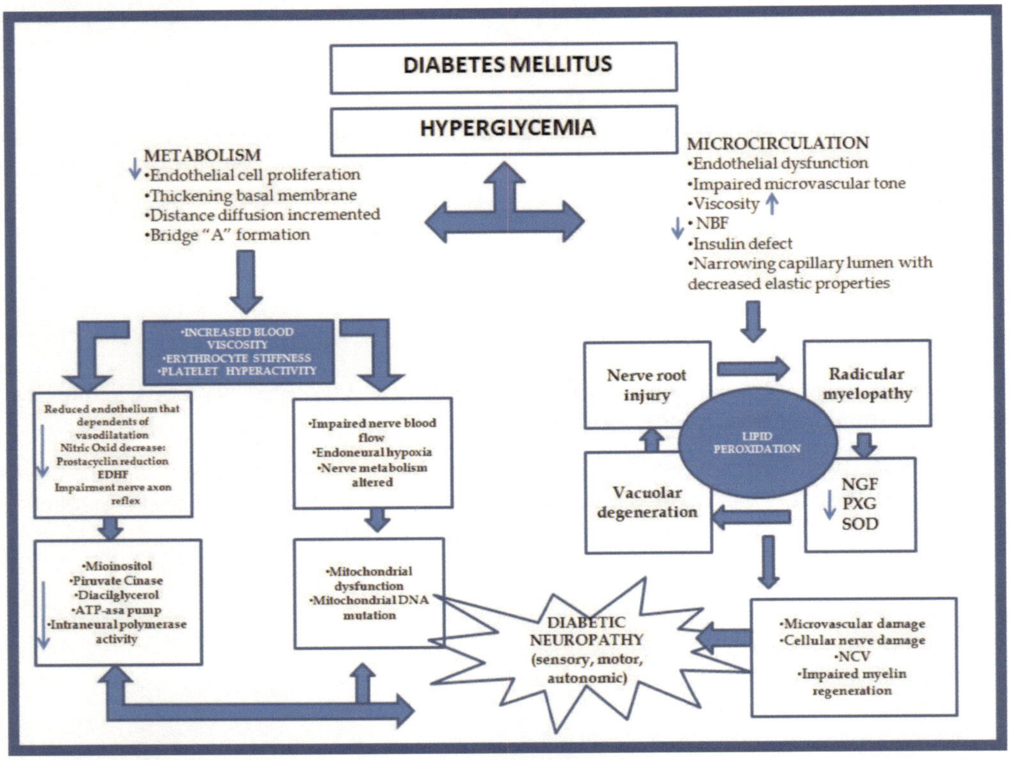

Fig. 1. Role of different mechanisms in neuropathy. The most important are oxidative stress and endothelium dysfunction; these mechanisms produce disorders in metabolism and microcirculation. EDFH= Endhotelium derived hyperpolarizing factor, NBF=nerve blood flow, NGF=nerve growth factors NVC= Nerve velocity conduction, PXG= Glutathion Peroxidase, SOD= Superoxide Dismutase **(Modified from Aguilar R, 2009a).**

Another important factor that affects neuropathic foot microcirculation is the disability of the nerve axon reflex. The stimulation of the C-nociceptive fibers produces retrograde stimulation of adjacent fiber (Caselli A, et al, 2003). These fibers instantly secrete a vasomodulator, such as substance P (SP), a calcitonine gene-related peptide (GCRP), neuropeptide Y (NPY), and histamine. These peptides produce vasodilation (this response is known as Lewis Triple Flair Response) (Lyons 2008). The Lewis response mechanism is: red spot due to capillary dilation, flare due to redness in the surrounding area, in turn due to arteriolar dilatation mediated by axon reflex and wheal due to exudation of fluid from capillaries and venules, drawn up in Fig 2 for normal and diabetic patients.

The main substances are histamine and peptides. In the absence of this response the skin blood flow is affected when the injury occurs and this is one of the major factors related to impaired wound healing (Parkhouse N, 1988).

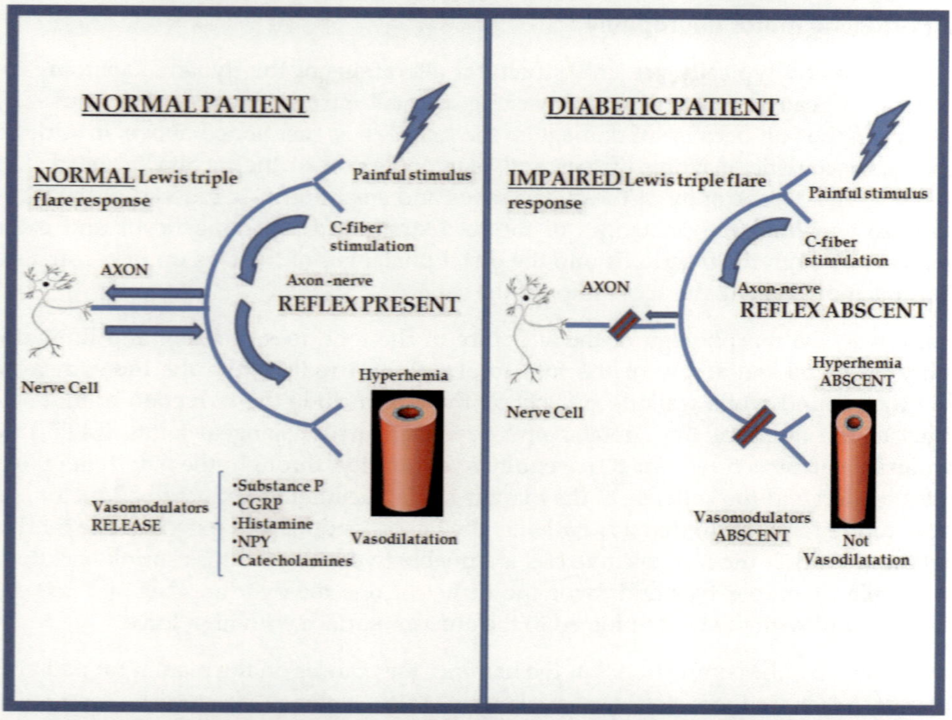

Fig. 2. **Injury and inflammation in normal subjects and diabetic patients.** The nerve axon reflex. Stimulation of C-nociceptive fibers produces retrograde stimulation of adjacent fibers to release vasomodulators. The results are hyperemia during injury or inflammation. The Lewis Triple Flare Response is absent in diabetic patients affecting wound healing. **(Modified from Lyons 2008a)**

2.2 Anatomical and structural alterations

The anatomical and structural alterations that are the result of diabetic neuropathy are divided into three types: sensory, motor and autonomic.

2.2.1 Peripheral sensory neuropathy

Close to 30-50% of all diabetic patients present peripheral sensory neuropathy. Sensory neuropathy is the most common predictor of foot ulceration in a patient with diabetes (Nather et al., 2011). The development of foot ulceration reported in sensory neuropathy occurs in 78% of cases. Peripheral sensory neuropathy initiates a series of events that together with peripheral motor and autonomic damage eventually result in foot ulceration. In a normal situation, treatment centers would tell the patient to continue walking or walk some with changes in gait. The recipients of this information are the sensory nerves. In diabetic foot, sensation is affected and the stimulus to refrain from ambulation does not exist. These are the causes that lead the patient to continue walking even when no sensation of pain is present, which in turn prolongs affectation and delays healing of the traumatized area. The damage to sensation that provides protection is the key element in the development of ulcers (Reiber GE., et al 1999).

2.2.2 Peripheral motor neuropathy

Motor neuropathy typically presents structural alterations of the dynamic anatomy of the foot and joints, causing weakness and wasting of small intrinsic muscles. This causes a loss of balance in the gait because of damage to the muscles, as mentioned above, in addition to another characteristic: clawing of toes and plantar flexion of the metatarsal head (Carine HM et al 2004). The atrophy of the interosseous and small intrinsic muscles of the foot acts to stabilize and hold the phalanges of the toes straight, as the long flexor and extensor tendons act through the insertions into the distal phalanges of the toes up into dorsiflexion, similar to a foot pressing the accelerator of the car.

Alterations in the morphology of the structure of the foot, toes, forefoot and limited joint mobility impaired the ability of the foot to absorb and redistribute the forces relayed to impact the ground while walking. Effects on the foot include the reduction of motion and changes to the angle of the subtalar and first metatarsophalangeal joints **(MTPJ)**. Vital musculoskeletal structures, such as equinus deformity through the shortening of the Achilles tendon and the collapse of the plantar fascia, facilitating abduct to adductor equine changes to the forefoot. In diabetic patients, the flexor tendons and extensor tips tend to be straight and rigid. If the intrinsic muscles are unable to do this, the toes shrink back to form what is called hammer toes and favor the thrust of one toe over another or a toe on the metatarsal head with the weight forced to the anterior surface with high force.

On the other side, the contraction that the hammer toes causes on the plantar fat pad and the metatarsal heads reduces soft tissue plantar MTPJ, making them more susceptible to fracture of the skin, including the bone next to the formation of traumatic ulcers, owing to inappropriate weight loads. The mechanism is related to the high pressure exerted on the foot that occurs during the gait, in turn caused by motor neuropathy, which itself in turn causes structural changes in the anatomy and sliding of the fat pads of the foot, in addition to occasional blows received.

Fig. 3 presents three different images at different stages of changes in architecture of the foot, allowing us to better understand the condition. In addition to the shortening and thickening of the joints, the decreased capacity of distribution of plantar pressure in DM patients contributes to the development of high foot pressure and ensuing ulcerations. Excessive pressure and structural deformities in individuals with neuropathy is a prerequisite for the development of wounds. Consequently, structural changes and offload pressure favors the formation of calluses on various prominent parts of the foot, including the plantar region, the heel, the big toe, etc.

The structure of the foot is a major determinant of plantar pressure. Although some structural factors are independent of the DM, others are predisposed to high pressure and appear to be a consequence of the disease. Obviously, the major collapse is seen in Charcot neuroosteoarthropathy in which foot fractures lead to increased pressure. (Lyons et al., 2006). A significant reduction of plantar soft tissue thickness is seen in diabetic patients with a form of neuropathy such as rheumatoid arthritis. Metatarsalgia is a common, frequent symptom of offloading of MTPJ with pressure on the head of the first metatarsal **(MTT).** It could explain almost 70% of the variation in plantar pressure in the joint on the thickness of soft tissue (Schie CHM, & Boulton. 2006).

It is necessary to clarify the concepts that influence structural and biomechanical abnormalities (Fryckberger RG, et al 1998, Lawrence L, et al 2008) as shown schematically in Fig 3.

Clawing toes: hyperextension of MTT phalange joints, usually accompanied by cavus foot and calluses on the dorsal surface of the fingers and the plantar surface of the metatarsal head or the tip of fingers.

Cavus Foot: under normal conditions the foot is shaped convexly due to the longitudinal medial arch that is extended from the head of the first MTT and the calcaneus; if this arch is abnormally high it produces an abnormal distribution of weight loads, favoring the formation of calluses in the forefoot and rearfoot .

Equinus Deformation: shortening of Achilles tendon (three muscles: *lateral, internal gastrocnemius* and *soleus*), falling of plantar fascia and facilitating abduct or adduct in the forefoot, beside the lost at the long flexor and extensor tendons that produce dorsiflexion.

1st toe rigid: it is due to hardening of the first MTT phalange joint with loss of dorsiflexion, resulting in excessive weight forces on the plantar surface and callus formation.

Joint stiffness: The limitation of joint movement is produced by the glycosylation of collagen and thickening of periarticular structures (tendons, ligaments, joint capsule, etc.) which favors deformities and plantar pressures, upsetting the biomechanics of the foot during walking by limiting plantar flexion and promoting equinus foot.

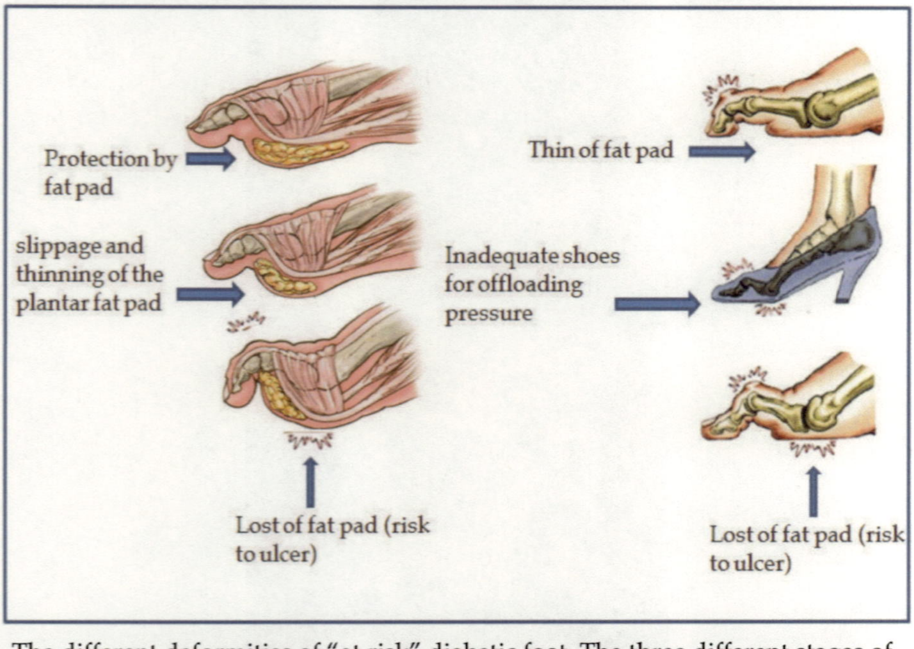

Fig. 3. The different deformities of "at risk" diabetic foot. The three different stages of changes in the architecture of the foot which causes hammer toes and contraction of the plantar fat pad (look arrow). Above: normal foot. Middle: beginning of deformation. Bottom: Complete deformation. **(Modified from Levin & O´Neal 2008. Right images courtesy from Ramos F, MD)**

Deformity of the nail: Thickening or deformity of the nail atrophies the nail plate with convex deformity, causing pressure on the ridge tissues and, in turn, ingrown nail. The nail flange forms a callus in response to pressure and inflammation. As a result the tissue of the trauma may become ulcerated and infected and penetrate the nail flange.

2.2.3 Autonomic neuropathy

Autonomic neuropathy is common in longstanding DM. In the lower extremities, autonomic neuropathy may result in arteriovenous shunting, resulting in the dilation of small arteries and producing distension of the foot veins, not alleviated through elevation of the foot. Consequently, neuropathic edema hinders treatment through diuretic therapy. Neuropathic feet have a tendency to swell and to feel warm as a result of arteriovenous shunting. Autonomic neuropathy results in decreased autonomic nerve roots that innervate the sweat skin glands with appendage tissue, causing dryness of the skin and decreased elasticity, especially from the middle third of the leg down, where there is also discoloration of the skin shown in Fig 4. Dry, stiff skin produce cracks more easily forming splits, fissures or fractures of the skin and callusing around the foot injury, more frequently in the heel rim, plantar medial and first MTP -especially during the dryer months, as observed in both images of Fig 5. The first one (A) shows the first stages and the second one depicts the final stages. These fractures or skin fissures can become infected, resulting in local cellulitis and then on to small longitudinal ulcerations. (Aguilar R, 2009)

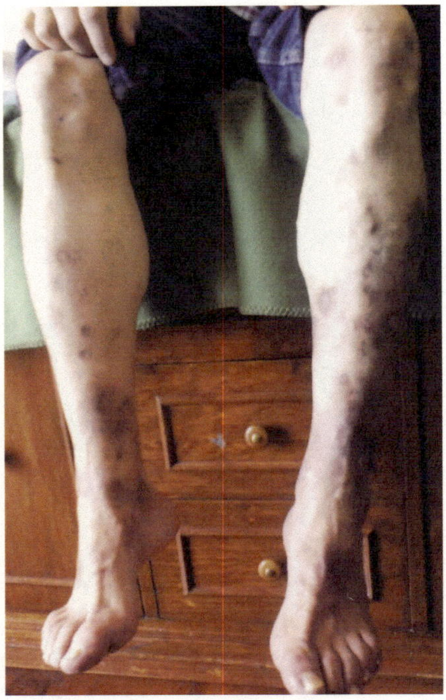

Fig. 4. Lower extremities of a patient with DM presenting the 3 types of neuropathy: sensitive (pain, burning, disesthesias, numbness), motor (cavus foot and claw toes) and autonomic (dry skin, absence of hair, changes in skin color). **(Courtesy of Aguilar F & Terán JM, 2011)**

2.3 Environmental influences

Environmental influences acutely and chronically accelerate ulceration, starting with lesions in the soft tissue followed by stratum corneum of the skin, subcutaneous tissue, muscle and fat pad.

2.3.1 Limited joint mobility

Restriction of joint mobility is a part of diabetic neuropathy, related mainly to collagen glycosylation that results in thickening of the periarticular structures such as tendons, ligaments and joint capsules. At the foot level, all joints may be involved –ranging from the talar, subtalar, MTPJ, to flattening of the arch or pronation. These structures absorb the shock of gait, and reduce and attenuate ground reactive forces. In diabetic patients the absence of this mechanism impairs the ability of the foot to adapt to the ground surface and absorb the shock that develops when the heels make contact with the ground during walking. High pressure develops more in the forefoot area, consequently becoming an additional factor in the development of foot wounds (Pham HT et al., 2000).

The footwear designed in diabetic patients reduces the risk of foot ulcerations. We recommend the design and manufacturing of footwear and other items designed to potentially reduce foot pressure in neuropathic feet and offloading, thus redistributing and reducing foot pressure in areas that are prone to ulceration. Shoes are an important consideration for patients that are at risk for foot ulcerations (Sicco A, et al 2011).

2.3.2 The gait

Diabetic ulcers can occur anywhere on the foot but clinically the most frequent presentation is on the plantar surface. This predilection of diabetic ulcer on the plantar surface is related to the trauma that is developed in this area due to increased discharge pressure on the plantar surface during walking. Under normal conditions the foot has the ability to distribute the load equally over the entire surface -the forefoot, middle foot and rear foot- consequently preventing the development of ulcers. This capability is lessened in diabetics, first of all because of changes in the architecture of the foot related to the fundamental motor neuropathy that produces disorders in the mobility of joints, limited both by neuropathy as well as by the metabolic changes producing glycosylation of the collagen structure through a covalent bonding process which increases the rigidity of the ligament structures, tendons, and the joint capsule of both the subtalar and metatarsal region. Additionally, there is decreased mobility of the Achilles tendon, in turn creating an equinus deformity that directs plantar forces to the region of the forefoot. As a result of these changes, the pressure of certain areas of the foot is considered at high risk for producing a tissue injury, even after walking short distances. It is important to note that the presence of sensory neuropathy in a patient at risk and using inappropriate shoes will induce injury of the subcutaneous cellular tissue during the gait, compromising the integrity of skin tissue; this, together with the absence of pain, is conducive to the onset of foot ulceration (DÁmbrogi E et al., 2003).

These 3 dimensions (physiopathology, anatomical and structural alterations, and environmental influences), contribute to the formation of ulcers. The dimensions are integrated by 2 mechanisms:

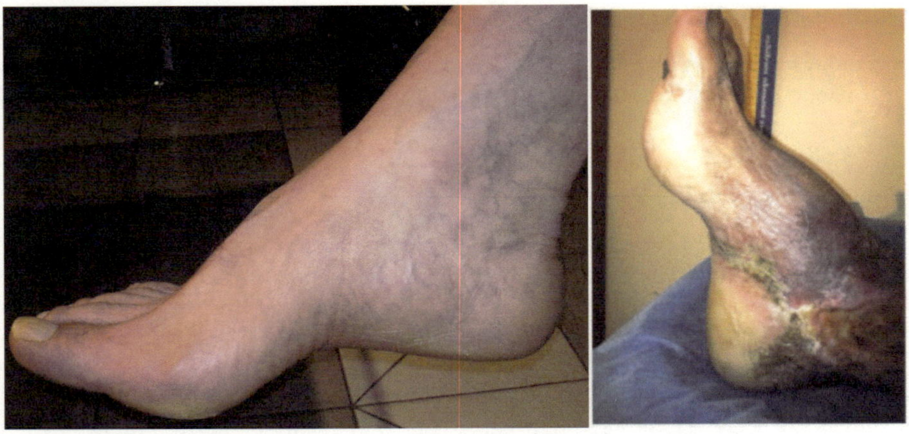

Fig. 5. Two different feet with "cavus foot". (A) Cavus foot with skin hydrated (first stages). (B) Cavus foot wit dry skin, fissures, peripheral vascular disease and ulcered ankle. **(Courtesy of Aguilar R & Terán JM, 2011)**

CRITERIA	RISK FACTORS	MECHANISM OF INJURY	INFLUENCE IN THE ULCER DEVELOPMENT
NECESSARY	**NEUROPATHY** • Motor • Sensorial Periphery • Autonomic	• Impaired foot anatomy (hammer toes or claw toes) cavus foot, subluxation of metatharsophalangeal joints. • Lost of protective sensation. • Impaired sweating, dry skin.	Are undoubtedly necessary for the formation of an ulcer in a diabetic patient.
COMPLEMENTARY	**METABOLIC DESCONTROL** • Hyperglycemia • Immune compromise **STRUCTURAL AND ANATOMIC ALTERATION** • Charcot neuroosteoarthropathy • Limited joints mobility **VASCULAR COMMITMENT** • Vascular disease (arterial or venous)	• Immune affectation • Abnormal anatomy and biomechanics mainly for the high pressure in the middle foot • Affectation in the viability of tissue and health of wound plus neutrophylia.	Can or not be presents, but frequently are necessary factors, having and important influence in the development of the ulcer
POSSIBLE	**DISCAPACITIES** • Limited vision, limited mobility, previous amputations **MALADAPTATIVE BEHAVIOR OF PATIENTS** • Bad attitude • Bad adherence to treatment • Bad hygiene • Inadequate shoes **FAIL IN THE HEALTH SYSTEM** • Inadequate education to patient • Poor glucose control and skin care	• Inadequate adherence to the precaution measures of foot and hygienically measures, poor compliance to the medical indications.	Can or not be presents but his presence it's transcendental for the progress of the ulcer.

Table 1. Risk factors for the development of ulcers **(Modified from Lipsky 2004).**

- **Internal mechanism**: Associated with structural deformities of the foot anatomy which are favored by sensory, motor and autonomic neuropathy disorders. Together, limited joint mobility and structural alterations are caused by glycosylation of collagen and thickening of the periaarticulares structures that are produced for a disorder in the production of elastin (tendons, ligaments, articular capsule and, etc.), at subtalar, metatarsal and metatarsophalangeal head levels. Because the diabetic condition invariably involves hyperglycemia, non-enzymatic glycation of collagen and a deterioration of elastin, fibronectin, proteoglycans, epithelial cells and other proteins are noteworthy in wound healing during repair sequence (Ahmed N 2005, Huijberts MS 2008).

- **External mechanism:** Related to chronic trauma of the soft tissues of the foot that precipitate the onset of an injury on the same structures that later produce the wound.

These mechanisms, together with risk factors, do not act independently to cause ulcers. They require the combination of numerous events (sometimes fewer than others) to produce wounds in different areas of the foot, different sizes and different components. In fact, the most important factors that produce foot injury and lesion of the extracellular basement matrix of the skin are: neuropathy, deformity, trauma, peripheral circulation failure, inflammation, dryness and calluses on the foot (Boulton AJM 2006).

The accumulation of the principal components corresponds to the causal pathways that result in diabetic foot ulcer when applying the Rothman model of causation (Reiber GE 1999). These factors that are insufficient on their own, combined will ultimately result in the formation of a diabetic foot ulcer; the interaction of a number of component causes may result in sufficient cause for ulceration, as shown in Fig 6. The most common causes interact between one another to result in ulceration in the diabetic foot. These risk factors are: neuropathy, deformity, trauma and impaired healing (present in 63% of cases) (Pecoraro RE, 1990).

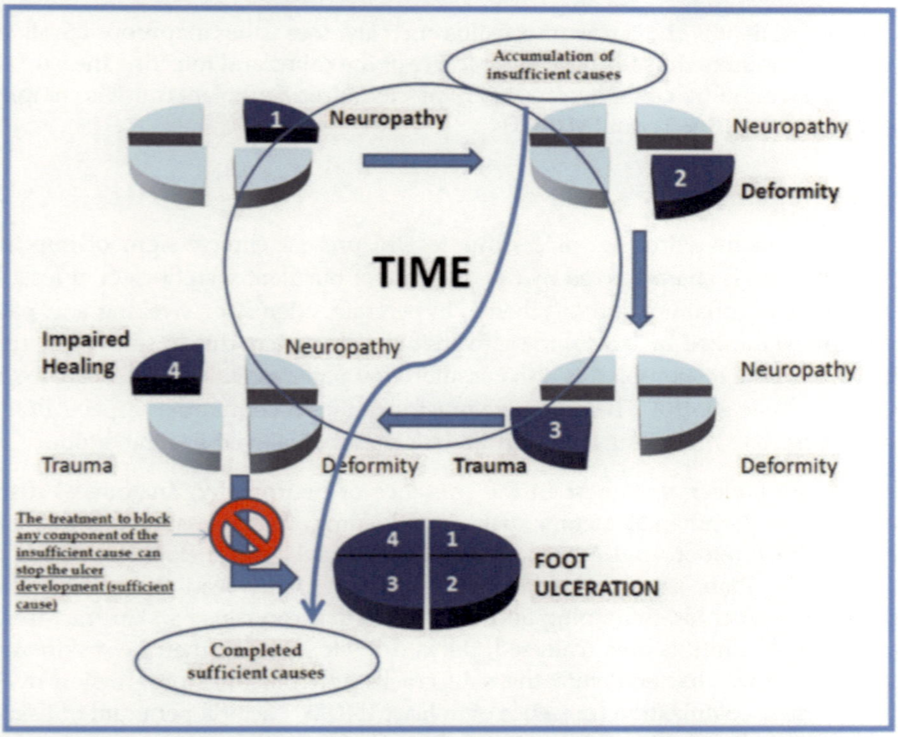

Fig. 6. **S**ufficient cause. The factors that comprise sufficient cause for ulceration are: neuropathy, deformity, trauma, and impaired healing. It is imperative that the 4 factors be present to create sufficient cause. If any of the factors is absent, the ulcer cannot be formed **(Modify for, Lyons 2008, Boulton 2006, Ziegler 2003)**

The classical example is a patient with insensitive feet who buys shoes too small that traumatize the feet with maximum pressure exerted on different points caused by the tight fit, as shown in Fig 7. In our experience, neuropathy was the first component cause (present in 100% of patients with ulcers), and the ischemia was a component cause in 35% of ulcers. Another independent component of the triad is the difficulty of healing the ulcer that is related with alterations in the immune response, decreased blood flow to the wound area, cellular components of the inflammatory system, abnormal expression of growth factors, cytokines and their receptors that are involved in the healing process; it is usually the combination of the various components that leads to chronic ulceration and amputation.

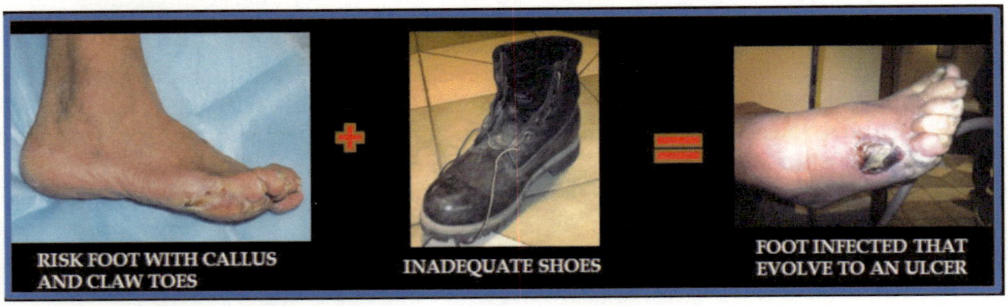

Fig. 7. Diabetic patient with neuropathy, callus and claw toes using inappropriate shoes that cause repetitive trauma, thus forming the fracture of the callus and infecting the skin. The final result is a wound that later evolves to an infected ulcer. Sufficient cause is complete. **(Courtesy of Aguilar F & Terán JM 2011)**

3. Clinical presentation

About 50% of patients with foot ulcers due to DM present clinical signs of infection. By definition, infection is characterized by the presence of purulent secretions or at least two of the classic signs of inflammation (erythema, hyperemia, edema, or swelling and pain) but these data can be masked by lack of the sensitivity in the patient due to sensory neuropathy or impaired immune response. It is also common that patients with infection are associated with poor metabolic control. Therefore, we must take into account other aspects of infected ulcers due to diabetes, including lack of granulation tissue, delayed healing or odor.

The prevalence of ulcer is highest in the presence of neuropathy, anatomical disorders, structural and environmental factors such as offloading, high-pressure processes on the plantar foot, the forefoot, midfoot, rearfoot and especially the metatarsals heads. These overloads on the limb associated with limited joint mobility lead the plantar fascia to undergo changes, such as shortening and thickening that can cause a skin fracture due to poor quality of skin in this area (callused, thick, dry, etc) causing their own skin germs to progress or introduce bacterial into the skin cracks and potential progression over time resulting in critical colonization (presence of at least 100,000 bacteria per gram of tissue) and finally culminating in infection (Lipsky BA, & Berendt AR 2006).

It's important to consider that pain is not a prominent sign in patients with infected diabetic foot owing to the loss of sensitivity caused by affected short and long fibers (A-beta and A-delta) secondary to hyperglycemia. In the same way, we have to consider a possible infection in any patient with DM who presents a fever, leukocytosis, or recent metabolic uncontrolled. (Pataky Z, & Assal JP, & Conne P, et al 2005)

The molecular pathways that are involved in the ulcer formation are:

1. The ulcer develops because structures of connective tissue fail.
2. Absence of an important matrix of cellular organization resulting in deterioration in the protection of normal epithelial growth.
3. Reduced angiogenesis and fibroplasia.
4. Persistence of inflammatory cells, neutrophils or macrophages, which act in an appropriate immunological environment.

NUMBER OF ULCERS	1	1 ulcer
		>2 ulcers in the limb
		>2 ulcers in both limbs
SIZE	2	< or = to l a 2cms
		>2 cms but < of 10 cms
		>11 cms
DEEP	3	Skin and cellular subcutaneous tissue (Wagner I)**
		Muscles and joints exposed (Wagner II)**
		Bone exposed (Wagner III)**
SKIN INSIDE THE WOUND	4	Epithelial Islands (+ 3)
		Granulation tissue
		Fibrin /scars (+50%)
		Necrosis (+50%)
EXUDATES	5	Without exudate (dry wound) or minimal exudate
		Minimal exudates with or without serous to blood serous material
		Mild to severe exudates with serous to blood serous material or purulence serous to purulent
EDGES	6	Present edge (like beach)
		Adhered edge (like gulch)
		Inflammatory or undermined edge (hole)

ADJACENT SKIN	Edema	7	Minimal (< 2 cms)
			Mild(All foot)
			Severe (foot and leg)
	Colour		Pink (normal)
			Erythematosus
			Pale , ocher, dark
	Inflamation		Minimal or without inflammation (around the ulcer but less of 5 cms)
			Mild (more than 5 cms around ulcer)
			Severe (more than 50% of the limb, foot and lower middle third of tibia)
MACERATION		8	Without maceration or until 25% (don't includes adjacent skin)
			26 a 50% (adjacent skin includes)
			>50%
PAIN		9	Without or occasional minimal pain
			Mild (continuous or quasi continuous)
			Severe (unsupportable and continuous)
INFECTION		10	Minimal or without infection (San Antonio I B*** or PEDIS 2*)
			Mild (San Antonio II-B to III-D*** or PEDIS 3*)
			Severe (systemic) (PEDIS 4*)

Table 2. Record the characteristics of the wound in every exam of diabetic foot (every week). This decalogue helped to evaluate ulcer evolution, prognosis and the healing process. PEDIS (*): see table 3, Wagner (**): see table 4 and San Antonio (***): see table 5. **(Courtesy of Aguilar R & Terán JM).**

The elements listed above persist and lead to deterioration in the integrity and restoration of tissue, resulting in a chronic ulcer with persistence of bacterial infection, which alone stimulates an inappropriate inflammatory cellular response. There is also a chemical injury that leads to loss of oxygenation with absence or decrease of tissular perfusion, local cellular ischemia and tissue necrosis or death.

If the trauma persists and overload pressure continues, the healing of the ulcer is delayed due to failure in the formation of granulation tissue and to the development of epithelial tissue. At this point proteolytic degradation surrounding the injury is the most important cause of secretion of proteins, including elastase, protease and metalloproteinase, capable of degrading not only the adhesive substrate for cell migration but also signaling molecules that would promote wound healing, such as development of growth factors and cytokines.

In conclusion, the accelerated proteolysis can cause a high level of breakdown products of connective tissue cellular processes that activate inappropriate inflammation. That's why the necrotic tissue should be debrided extensively and aggressively from the start of ulcer treatment, as this tissue is a negative factor in the wound healing, with difficulty due to the high content of substances mentioned above (Davidson JM, & Di Pietro L 2006; Cooper DM et al 1994; Sheehan P et al 2006).

4. Diabetic foot infections

In diabetic patients with foot wounds, the physician should perform a systematic examination to determine if the wound is infected and the degree of severity of said infection. The examination should start with vital signs, consciousness, complete review of the limb to the foot end, **always removing the patient's shoes and socks**, and should include a neurological, vascular, dermatological and musculoskeletal examination to determine the external characteristics of the skin, the shape and structure of the foot and alterations in the fingers, protruding metatarsal, heel, etc. The physician should also perform an instrumental exploration, neurological reflex hammer, tuning fork 128 cycles, 10 gm monofilament, thermograph, etc, Table 6. A clinical vascular examination will focus on the search for foot pulses. All this will determine the stage of neuropathy with or without ischemia. Fig 8 (American Diabetes Association (ADA) 2011)

After locating the ulcer, evaluate the wound characteristics, just as proposed in Table 2, (number of ulcers, depth, size, color, exudation, edges, adjacent skin, maceration, pain, infection, etc.). In most cases an x-ray should be taken to dismiss presence of gas, or a foreign body or osteomyelitis. During initial ulcer debridement, look for aerobes and anaerobe organisms. As concerns a blood test, we recommend a complete blood count, blood chemistry and if it is considered prudent speed glomerular sedimentation and reactive "C" protein (Eneroth M, & Larsson J, & Apelqvist J 1999; Kaleta JL, & Fleischli JW, & Reilly CH 2001)

This complete examination will help the doctor to draw up a clinical classification of the degree of infection (mild, moderate or severe), table 3, as well to evaluate the depth, extension, table 4, and ischemia with presence of infection, table 5. The severity ratings guide us to reference the patient to further hospital care, and start empirical implementation of antibiotics. The types of diabetic foot infections can start from a simple paronychia, onychomycosis, cellulitis, foot infection, deep tissue infection, septic arthritis, osteomyelitis, necrosis or gangrene. Infections can be painless, persist for days, weeks or months and progress rapidly even in a few hours. Bed debridement, incision and drainage of the ulcer will be necessary in most circumstances. (Lipsky et al 2004)

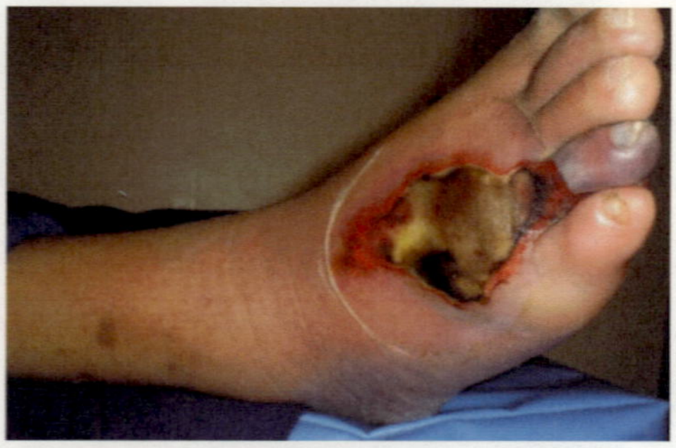

Fig. 8. Diabetic foot infection for insensitive repetitive trauma. The wound is close to deep tissues, involving bone as well. This patient need antibiotics and appropriate debridement **(Courtesy Aguilar F & Terán JM, 2011).**

Clinical manifestation of infection	Infection severity	PEDIS*	Wagner**	San Antonio***
Wound lacking purulence or any manifestations of inflammation**, ***	Uninfected	1	1**	A-1 ***
Presence of >2 manifestations of inflammation: • Purulence • Erythema • Pain • Tenderness • Warmth or induration But any cellulitis/erythema extends < 2 cm around the ulcer: • Infection limited to the skin or superficial subcutaneous tissues**, *** • No other local complications or systemic illness	Mild	2	1 or 2**	B-1 to B-2***
Infection (as above) in a patient who is systemically well and metabolically stable but which has > 1 if the following characteristics: • Cellulitis extending > 2 cms • Lymphangitic streaking • Spread beneath the superficial fascia • Deep tissue abscess *** • Gangrene ** • Involvement of muscle, tendon, joint or bone**, ***	Moderate	3	4**	B-3 ***
Infection in a patient with systemic toxicity or metabolic instability (fever, chills, tachycardia, hypotension, confusion, vomiting, leukocytosis, acidosis, severe hyperglycemia or azotemia)	Severe	4	——	——

Table 3. Table with PEDIS* grade of foot infection correlated with the most common classic scales for wounds (Wagner** and San Antonio***). Each item "asterisk and color" was selected according to the scale **(modified from Lispky BA 2004)**

Wagner Classification.
0: No ulcer (risk foot).
1: Superficial ulcer.
2: Deep ulcer (involve tendons but no bone involvement).
3: Deep ulcer with bone involvement (osteomyelitis).
4: Localized gangrene.
5: Gangrene of whole foot.

Table 4. Meggit-Wagner classification (Deep and Extension) **(Meggit B ,1977 & Wagner FW, 1981)**

Stage	**Grade**			
	0	**1**	**2**	**3**
A	**Prepost-ulcer lesion without skin break**	**Superficial Ulcer**	**Deep ulcer (tendo/capsule)**	**Wound penetrating bone/joint**
B	+infection	+infection	+infection	+infection
C	+ischemia	+ischemia	+ischemia	+ischemia
D	+infection and Ischemia	+infection and Ischemia	+infection and Ischemia	+infection and Ischemia

Table 5. San Antonio scale. (Infection and Ischemia) **(Armstrong et al, 1998)**

Level of evaluation, by area(s) to be assessed	**Relevant problems and observations**	**Investigations**
• **Patient** Systemic response to infection Metabolic state Psychological/cognitive state Social situation	Fever, chills, sweats, vomiting, hypotension, and tachycardia Hyperglycemia ,volume depletion, azotemia, tachypnea , hyperosmolarity, acidosis Depression, delirium, impaired cognition Self neglect, potential noncompliance, and lack of home support.	History and physical examination Serum chemistry and hematological testing Assessment of mental status Interviews with family and caregivers.
• **Limb or foot** Neuropathy Biomechanics Environmental influences Vascular status (arterial our venous)	Loss of protective sensation. Motor and autonomic exam. Pain (burning, shooting, stabbing pains like pins and needles) Deformities (Charcot foot, claw/hammer toes and callosities Gait, instability, limited joint mobility Ischemia, necrosis, gangrene/edema, stasis or thrombosis	Pin prick test, "Light touch, cotton wisp, vibration test (128 Hz tuning fork), pressure perception (10 g monofilament), ankle reflex, patellar and Achilles, thermograph . Muscle weakness. Dry skin. Clinical foot examination: architecture of the foot and radiography Inspection : walking, foot pulses, blood pressure (Ankle arm index), duplex ultrasonography. Angiograms.
• **Wound** Size Depth (tissues involved) Edges Presence, extent, and etiology of infection	Necrosis, gangrene, foreign body, and involvement of muscle, tendon, bone or joint Purulence, warmth, tenderness, pain, indurations, cellulitis, bullae, crepitus, fasciitis, osteomyelitis, gas, fetid odor..	Inspect, debride, and probe the wound deep; and X-ray foot. Gram staining and culture, ultrasonography or CT for detection of deep abscess, and radiography and/or MRI for detection of osteomyelitis.

Table 6. Evaluating the diabetic patient who has an infected foot **(Lipsky et al, 2004 modified for Aguilar & Terán 2011)**

4.1 Evaluating the diabetic patient who has an infected ulcer

All diabetic foot infections require antibiotic treatment. However, not all ulcers are infected from the beginning and therefore do not require antibiotics. The main premise is that antibiotic treatment will be used to clear up infection and not for wound healing, which takes longer (Lipsky BA, 1999). Take into account the following aspects to choose the right antibiotics:

1. Understand the microbiology of the wound, starting with broad-spectrum empirical therapy for moderate and severe infections and a relatively small range for moderate infections. We can't forget factors such as recent antibiotic use, exposure to hospital facilities and local antibiotic susceptibility.
2. The route of administration is of great importance for the success of treatment; for serious infections the recommended route is parenteral, and mild to moderate infections can start with oral or parenteral impregnation treatment for further oral treatment, adjusting to highly bio-available drugs like quinolones and the oxazolidinones.
3. The duration of antibiotic treatment should be determined according to the severity of the infection; mild infections only require 2 to 4 weeks, severe infections may require 6 to 12 weeks or more. Unfortunately in severe infections the amputation of part or the entire foot is a high probability.
4. The selection of a specific agent or combination of antibiotics is based on the considerations discussed above and the condition of each patient (renal failure, allergies, etc.), restrictions of presentation, convenience and monetary cost. (Lipsky BA, Berendt AR 2006)

5. Basics measures in the treatment of diabetic foot

The treatment of foot ulcers in diabetic patients varies constantly depending on the severity of the ulcer and the presence or absence of ischemia. However the basic points of treatment are:

- Debridement in case the ulcer presents thick edges or necrotic tissue.
- Reduction in overload pressure.
- Complete rest of the foot (orthotics).
- Treatment of the infection.
- Local wound care.

To start this care we require the knowledge of the patophysiology listed above in relation to wound healing. The care and products that have shown to improve wound healing are:

1. **Debridement** .- The goal is complete debridement of all necrotic tissue with impaired vascular and non-viable tissue, large incision and maintain good drainage when necessary in order to allow a granular bed and a better flow of the wound.
2. **Reduced offloading.** – Reduction of pressure is essential in the healing of foot ulcers; as has been said, ulcers occur in areas of high pressure on a foot without sensitivity or with damaged sensitivity. There are several methods to reduce the pressure; the most popular includes mandatory resting of the foot with a cast and other new light materials, special shoes, leg braces and bandages using felt and/or foam.
3. **Treatment of Infection**. - The ulcers that are already colonized with bacteria serve as a port of entry to further infection. The diagnosis of infection is first based on clinical

appearance and cardinal symptoms (erythema, edema, pain, tenderness and warmth). Meanwhile, care must be taken, aside from the bacteriological diagnosis, to treat cellulite, start antibiotics empirically and request the necessary x-rays employing the most advanced techniques available to reject the possibility of abscess with osteomyelitis (such as MRI or CT scan of the foot). **Tables 7 & 8.**

4. **Wound care**. -The effective use of bandages is essential to ensure optimal management of foot ulcers in diabetic patients, applying the concepts of cleanliness, humidity and proper environment for wound healing to prevent tissue dehydration and cell death, accelerate angiogenesis and facilitate the development of growth factors with the epithelial cells resulting in less discomfort for patients.
5. **Products for advanced wound care**: These products have been developed in response to an improved understanding of the holistic healing of injured tissue in diabetic foot ulcer. A greater knowledge of the patophysiology of wound microenvironment deficiencies decreased development, growth factors, inactivity, altered cell, to the development of products to correct these deficiencies. These include human growth factor platelet derived, Epidermal growth factor recombinant human DNA (Heberprot-P®), colony stimulating factor granulocytes, biological cultivate skin substitutes (Dermagraft®, Epifast®) hyperbaric oxygen, larva therapy, etc. (Boulton JM 2003)

Syndrome	Foot Infection	Pathogen Microorganisms	Duration of therapy
A.-Involved soft tissue only.	Cellulitis with/without open skin. Infected ulcer was previously treated with antibiotics therapy.	β- *hemolytic streptococcus, Staphylococcus aureus* and enterobacteriaceaes (groups A, B, C and G).	1-2 weeks; may extend up to 4 weeks if slow for resolve.
B.-Involved infected skin tissue, subcutaneous tissue, muscles, joints (but no bone.)	Ulcer that is macerated of soaking polimicrobials.	*Pseudomonas aeuroginosa* (often combinated with other organism) often polymicrobial.	3-4 weeks; sometimes may needed extend 6-8 weeks to resolve.
C.-Involved residual infected tissue (still viable), muscle, joints, ligaments (with or without bone)	Long duration non-healing wound with prolonged broad spectrum antibiotics therapy.	Aerobic gram- positive cocci (*Staphylococcus aureus* coagulase negative, Staphylococci and enterococci), diphteroids (*Corynebacterium species*), enterobacteriaceae, *Pseudomonas* species, non fermentative Gram - negative, rods** and possible fungi with possibly anaerobius species (more frequently *bacteroides fragilis**)	4-8 weeks; may extend 8-12 weeks if can resolve. High risk to partial amputation.
D.-Residual tissue and bone is death.	"Fetid foot" extensive necrosis or gangrene, malodorous.	Mixed (Gram positive cocci, Gram negative cocci) and including enterococci, enterobacteriaceae, non fermentative Gram negative rods and obligate anaerobes pathogens.	12 weeks or more with high risk to amputation (some part or entire foot)

*Gram negative: *Bacteroides fragilis, vulgatus, ovatus, distasonis, ureolyticus, gracilis*
**Antibiotic resistance species. For example: meticillin-resistent *S. aureus*, Vancomycin-resistent enterococci or extended-spectrum B-lactamase produce Gram-negative rods are common.

Table 7. Pathogens associated with various clinical foot-infection syndromes. (Modified from Lipsky 2004)

Severity	Mild	Moderate	Severe
Advised route	Oral for most	Oral or parenteral, base accord clinical situation and agent(s) selected	Intravenous, at least initially
• Amoxicillin/clavulanate	✓	✓	✓
• Dicloxacilin	✓		
• Trimethoprim-sulfamethoxazole	✓		
• Cephalexin	✓		
• Clindamycin	✓	✓	
• Levofloxacin	✓	✓	
• Cefoxitin	✓	✓	✓
• Ceftriaxone		✓	
• Ampicillin/sulbactam		✓	
• Linezolid (with or without aztreonam)		✓	
• Daptomycin (with or without aztreonam)		✓	
• Ertapenem, imipenem		✓	
• Cefuroxime (with or without metronidazole)		✓	
• Moxifloxacin*	✓		
• Moxifloxacin and Cefuroxime (with or without metronidazole)*	✓	✓	✓
• Levofloxacin or ciprofloxacin with clindamycin		✓	✓
• Moxifloxacin** and vancomycin (with or without ceftazidime)		✓	✓
• Ticarcillin/clavulanate		✓	
• Piperacillin/tazobactam		✓	✓
• Imipenem-Cilastatin		✓	✓

Table 8. Suggested empirical antibiotic regimens accord the severity of disease. *recommended by the authors **(Aguilar & Terán 2011)**. ** For patients in whom methicillin-resistant *S.aureus* infection is proven likely. **(Lipsky 2004)**.

6. Ulcer recurrence

The clinical evaluation of patients with diabetes, particularly in the assessment of the foot should be referred to the history of previous ulceration or amputation. A history with a record of ulceration or amputation increases the risk of a future return of ulceration, infection and amputation. Above 60% of diabetic patients with a history of foot ulcer may develop another ulcer within a year of healing ulcers. (Luca DP 2003)

There are 3 possible explanations:

1. Risk factors that caused ulceration in the first place in many cases will be still present.
2. The skin and soft tissue at the site of previous ulceration do not retain the same properties after healing compared with the conditions they had before the ulcer. Thus, the skin and soft tissue, after the ulcer is healed, are more fragile and break more easily, as shown in Fig 9.

3. Areas of previous amputation can leave residual deformities which in themselves are areas of increased pressure that may lead to ulceration. In addition, any previous surgery can alter biomechanics, leading to irregularities of the gait and imbalance where high pressure areas will develop new ulcers in the future.

A musculoskeletal examination will allow us to understand the structure and dynamics of the forces of the foot. The presence of foot deformities, joint mobility and their limitations must be recorded as both increased pressure and the cause of foot ulceration. Bone prominences can be observed on second plane as Charcot osteoarthropathy, motor neuropathy, foot deformities, hallux valgus limitus-rigiduz and hammer toes. Also, in the plantar region there may be callus formation, as we now know that many of these calluses are focal areas of increased pressure that can lead to a potential site of ulceration. Any area of erythema owing to the use of inappropriate shoes should be protected with padded patches and as soon as possible changed to proper shoes to relieve the pressure (Abbott CA & Carrington AL, & Ashe H, et al. 2002).

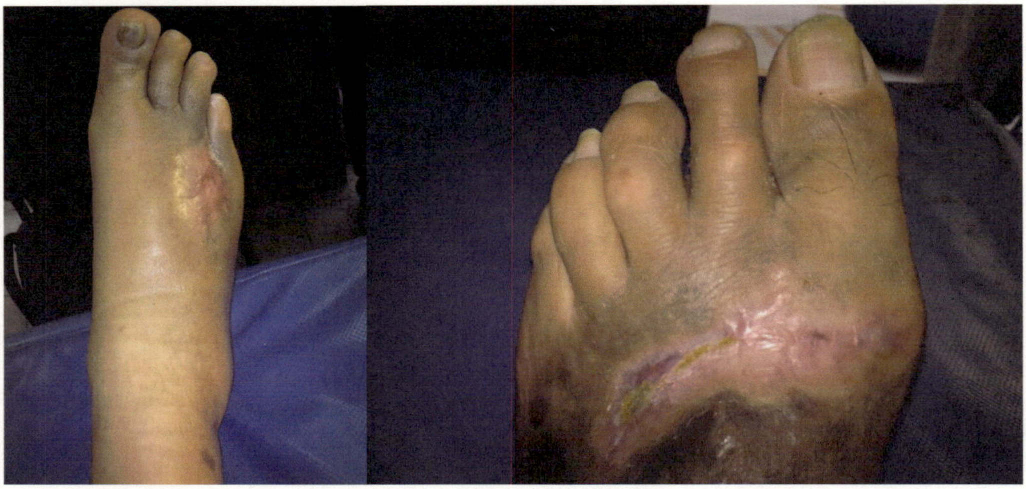

Fig. 9. After the wound is healed, the patient needs to protect the foot due to changes in the architecture and labile skin in order to prevent ulcer recurrence. The use of orthetics, correct shoes, special socks and rehabilitation of the foot is a priority **(Courtesy of Aguilar F & Terán JM 2011).**

7. Conclusions

Despite progress in knowledge regarding the pathophysiology of ulcers, the mechanisms involved nowadays are not completely clear. The main mechanisms: neuropathy, deformity and trauma along with physiopathogenic information at the molecular level and knowing the structural and anatomic alterations (clawing toes, hammer toes, cavus foot, equinus foot, etc), are all important to draw up strategies for treatment and prevention This information is summarized in Fig 10. On the other side, offloading increases pressure on the foot, thus leading to alterations in environmental factors such as gait, instability and limited joint mobility. All of this suffices to explain the changes in the architecture of the foot and this, in turn, allows for drawing up prevention policies. Changes in the microcirculation of the foot in patients with diabetes remains one of the major causes of difficulty in wound healing associated with thickening of the vascular endothelium, the release of vasodilator substances and the participation of endothelial cells in angiogenesis and reparative processes of the wound. These together represent the most advanced knowledge available at the molecular level. The vasodilatation depending on the endothelium cell reduces the expression of nitric oxide synthase which further deteriorates the microenvironment of the wound. More recent mechanisms, such as the knowledge of the deterioration on the nerve cell particularly the reflex nerve-axon, coupled with changes in the polymerase activity (ADP ribose) and the increase of the formation of nitrous tyrosine give us hope for the future of healing ulcers. A better understanding of cellular changes and the interplay between formation of connective tissue, collagen tissue formation (collagen is part of the skin, bone, tendons and ligaments) the expression of growth factors and cytokines are involved in tissue repair of wounds in people with diabetes as shown Fig 10. In addition, we proposed increased care in early injury or trauma and prevention of use of inadequate shoes and offload pressures to stop formation of ulcers. If ulcers do form, adequate treatment, foot care and complete rest for the foot could prevent amputation. Fig 10 (red)

It is clear that the spectrum of treatment of diabetic foot ulcers requires the participation of several specialists. Foot ulcers are not the responsibility of a single medical professional, they are the responsibility of a multidisciplinary team working for the care and healing of foot ulcers. On this team we can find first contact physicians, surgeons, orthopedic, vascular surgeons, podiatrists, neurologists, endocrinologists, orthotics, specialist nurses and all practitioners and specialists interested in the care and attention of the foot. In this chapter we have tried to give a clear, complete and current vision of the management of ulcers in diabetic patients by detecting and treating risk factors at an early stage, directing the entire team of health professionals as one would an orchestra in which the symphony focuses on sparing the patient with diabetic foot from dire consequences.

7.1 What is expected for the future?

There are various factors that will work together to improve wound care in the next few years. We must urge scientists, clinicians and even government regulators to get involved in the control of diabetes mellitus and wound healing. The problem is overwhelming worldwide and demands greater attention focusing on the occurrence of diabetes morbidity and mortality. Diabetic wounds continue to spiral out of control. New trends show interest and progress in the biology of healing and wound care. There is a great deal of exciting science and work done that has defined some of the basic pathogenesis of chronic wounds. This can be divided into the biological scientific and technical care of wounds.

7.1.2 Biological scientific

1. **Modulation of temperature.** Recently advances with modulation of temperature to control pressure of diabetic foot necrosis prevent cell death and progression of the ulcer formation in patient with DM. Cooling as well as pressure relief will be an important tool in the management of diabetic foot wound. With this measure we can to prevent the inflammatory changes due to the pressure and the flow-reflow phenomena.

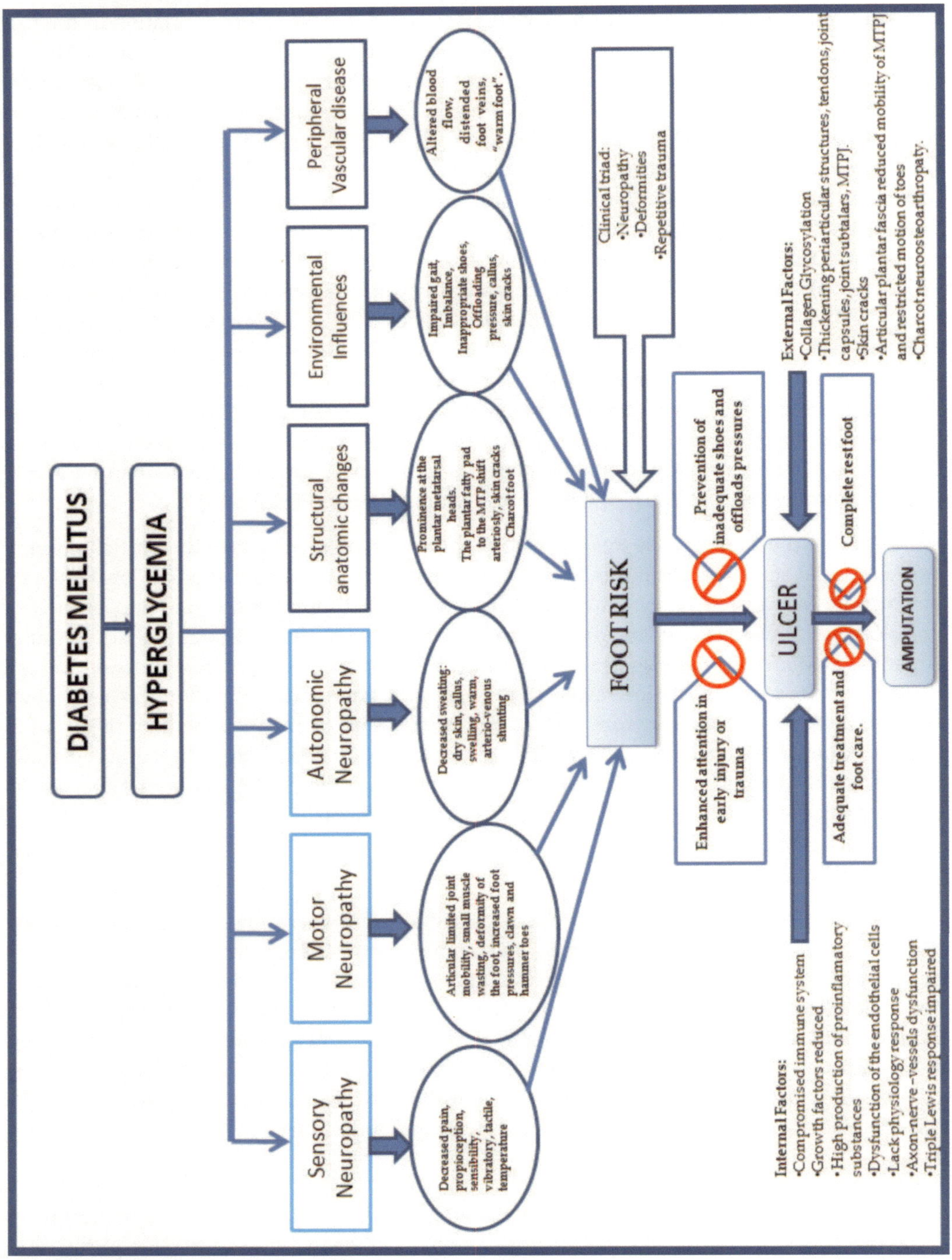

Fig. 10. This algorithm summarize all events that are at play in the development ulcers and potential amputations. Prevention is the key. (red block)

2. **Proteases.** The early inflammatory response of diabetic foot wounds produces excessive proteases. Although the protease issue is relevant, it is only the tip of the iceberg. The healing of the wound requires angiogenic factors and these are destroyed by proteases. New therapy would be enhancement of endogenous antiproteases in order to improve healing. Another important issue is the control of free radical production by polymorphonuclear leukocytes (PMNs) as free radicals stimulate inflammation and increase proteases.
3. **Oxidative Stress.** Although there are many metabolic disturbances that occur in DM, the oxidative stress (OS) play an important pathogenesis roll of a numerous mechanisms in DM and diabetic neuropathy. Diabetes contributes both directly and indirectly to increased oxidative stress. Thus, there is elevated production of reactive oxygen species (ROS) and a reduced endogenous capacity of free radical cell scavengers. Contributors to the increased oxidative stress include auto-oxidation of glucose and its metabolites, advanced glycation, mitochondrial abnormalities, ischemia reperfusion, microvascular damage, and enhanced flux through the polyol pathway. OS produce endothelium dysfunction, and diminishing nitric oxide release. Alpha lipoic acid in combination with arginine and citrulline increase nitric oxide, reduce OS by both benefits improved free radical scavenger and metal chelator. Besides, there is evidence that improved nerve functional deficit, endoneural perfusion and vascular bed perfusion and the microcirculation and capillary blood perfusion. Nevertheless antioxidant vitamins potentially improve healing of the wound.
4. **Gene therapy**. We are still grappling with this area of medical knowledge. On the other hand, this care is expensive, though we expect that we will see cost-effective gene therapy in the future. The focuses are: stimulating growth factor production and gene therapy to inhibit proteases to permit growth factors to work well.
5. **New drugs to treat diabetes.** The best option is to keep blood sugar within normal range; this produces less glycosylation of all sorts of tissues in the body, reducing diabetic complications.
6. **Education.** Continuing medical education (CME) is important to every professional to treat DM. CME needs to develop strategic projects to stimulate initiatives for early prevention and detection of complications in DM and neuropathy. Updated medical information needs to cover all news about nutrition, hypertension, obesity and dyslipidemia (metabolic syndrome).

7.1.3 Technical care

1. **Industry**. The relevant industry must listen to scientist and improve the quality of studies and on a scientific basis produce potential products for clinical application.
2. **Wound healing centers.** The concept of the wound healing center is excellent if we have evidence and monitoring of formal education for health care providers at these centers and implement frequent reviews and updates.
3. **Progress in communications.** We live in an era in which computerized communication is superb, yet we have not taken advantage of this benefit for our patients, especially for wound healing. Google®, PubMed®, Cochrane® and the American Diabetes

Association journals database are a big help for medical information and updates. The team of wound care health workers needs to have readily accessible information. Being a doctor is hard work, but part of this work is being updated through new technologies.

4. **Emotional aspects.** Every patient needs to be referred to psychological specialists so as to better handle their emotional problems, equally important as the physical aspects. Everyone on the team is involved in the pathological process and must heed details. The initial assessment of the DM patient with neuropathy and ulcer demands a thorough examination and MUST ALWAYS include a careful foot exam after removal of shoes and socks. Additionally, the exam includes: inspection of foot deformity, pressures, neurologic exam, vascular exam, monofilament, vibration and so on. It is surprising to note how many patients seek expensive, inadequate, quack or esoteric therapies in an attempt to save their leg.
5. **Federal Government Policies.** The federal government should be more involved in supporting scientific and clinical projects and encouraging medical prevention in all communities in countries with a high prevalence of this disease, such as Mexico.
6. **Education.** Many courses on wound healing it are necessary to disseminate and updated information, to offer clear ideas and give practical advice. Regrettably, there are even national conferences in which there is an absence of information about new concepts on wound healing, proper evaluation and treatment. There is a window of opportunity here.
7. **Offloading the diabetic foot:** New role of footwear. Several methods of measuring and reducing foot pressure include new advances but we need to be aware of their limitations. Extra-deep footwear, jogging shoes, hosiery, insoles, and orthotic hosiery have been shown to decrease plantar foot pressures. Furthermore these devices can prevent the occurrence and recurrence of foot ulceration. Research at present is still in the initial phase of developing methods and measuring shoe shear forces. Piezoelectric transducers are currently being evaluated; these may be able to measure both vertical and share forces in the near future.

8. New devices

Actually in some countries are available some systems to promote the support of wound healing such as the negative pressure wound therapy (V.A.C®), the wound cleansing and debridement system (Jetox®) and the infrared therapy system (Anodyne®).

The process in wound healing is a cascade of inflammatory reactions and cellular interactions. Modern technologies are focused on reversing this unfortunate complication. For that reason we propose the points mentioned above in technical care. The science, knowledge and practice are attempting to promote vascularization, devices and molecules of tissue growth and a better understanding of pathophysiology of the wounds; therapeutical approach and prevention.

9. References

Abbott CA, & Carrington AL, & Ashe H, et al. (2002); The North-West Diabetes Foot Care Study: incidence of, and risk factors for, new diabetic foot ulceration in a community-based patient cohort. *Diabetic Medicine,* 19, 5, (2002), pp 377–384.

Aguilar F, Rayo MD. (2000) Part 1, Diabetic Neuropathy: Classification, physiopathology and clinical manifestations. 38, 4, (2000), *Rev Med IMSS*, pp 257-266, ISSN 0443-5117.

Aguilar F , (2005), "Diabetic Neuropathy" for doctors, *Plast & Rest Neurol*, 4, 1-2, (2005), pp 35-47. ISSN 1665-3254

Aguilar F (2009a), Diabetic Foot; physiopathology and treatment, In: *Diabetic Neuropathy, Practical aspects, treatment, diagnostic and prophylactic measures*, Aguilar Rebolledo Francisco, pp 335-336, Alfil editorial, ISBN 978-607-7504-56-6, Mexico.

Aguilar F (2009b), Diabetic Foot; physiopathology and treatment, In: *Diabetic Neuropathy, Practical aspects, treatment, diagnostic and prophylactic measures*, Aguilar Rebolledo Francisco, pp 341-342, Alfil editorial, ISBN 978-607-7504-56-6, Mexico.

Aguilar F(2009c), Neurophysiology and physiopathology of pain , In: *Diabetic Neuropathy, Practical aspects, treatment, diagnostic and prophylactic measures*, Aguilar Rebolledo Francisco, pp 75-87, Alfil editorial, ISBN 978-607-7504-56-6, Mexico.

Ahmed N, (2005), Advanced glycation end products--role in pathology of diabetic complications, *Diabetes Research and clinical practice* (2005); 67(1):3-21., ISSN: 0168-8227

American Diabetes Association (2011), Standards of Medical care in Diabetes, *Diabetes care*, 34, supply 1, (2011); pp S1-S66, ISSN 0149-5992.

Armstrong DG, Lavery LA, Harkless LB (1998). Validation of a diabetic wound classification system: contribution of depth, infection, and vascular disease to the risk of amputation, *Diabetes Care*, 21, 5, (1998), pp 855-859, ISSN 0149-5992.

Boulton AJM, & Gries FS, & Jervell J. (1998), Guidelines for the diagnosis and outpatient management of diabetic peripheral Neuropathy, *Diabetic Medicine*; 15, 6 (1998) pp 508-14 ISSN: 1464-5491

Boulton AJM, (2003a), The diabetic Foot, In: Textbook of diabetic neuropathy Ziegler D, & Gries A, & Low P et al, Thieme editorial, pp 297-298, ISBN 1-58890-005-3

Boulton AJM, (2003b), The diabetic Foot, In: Textbook of diabetic neuropathy Ziegler D, & Gries A, & Low P et al, Thieme editorial, pp 300-305, ISBN 1-58890-005-3

Boulton AJM, (2006), The pathway to ulceration: Aetiopathogenesis. In: *The foot in diabetes*, Boulton, Cavanagh, Rayman, pp 61-79 John Wiley & Sons Ltd, ISBN 978-0-470-01504-9, UK

Carine Hm, et al., (2004), Muscle Weakness and Foot Deformities in Diabetes: relationship to neuropathy and foot ulceration in Caucasian diabetic men, *Diabetes Care 27: 7* (2004), pp 1668-1673, ISSN 0149-5992.

Caselli A et al, (2003), Role of C-nociceptive fibers in the nerve axon reflex-related vasodilatation in diabetes, *Neurology*, 60, (2003); pp 297-300, ISSN 0028-3878

Clayton W & Elasy & Tom A, (2009) A review of the patophysiology, classification, and treatment of foot ulcers in diabetic patients, *Clinical Diabetes*, 27, 2, (2009), pp 52-53. ISSN: 0891-8929.

Cooper DM et al, (1994), Determination of endogenous cytokines in chronic wounds. *Annals of surgery* 219, 6 (1994); pp 688-692 ISSN 0003-4932

D´Ambrogi E et al, (2003), Contribution of Plantar Fascia to the Increased Forefoot Pressures in Diabetic Patients, *Diabetes Care* 26 , 5 *(2003)*, pp 1525-1529, ISSN 0149-5992.

Davidson JM, & DiPietro L, (2006), The wound-Healing Process, In: The Diabetic Foot, Veves A & Giurini JM & LoGerfo F, Humana Press editorial, pp 59-82, ISBN, 1-59745-075-8 USA

Eneroth M, Larsson J, Apelqvist J (1999), Deep foot infections in patients with diabetes and foot ulcer: an entity with different characteristics, treatments, and prognosis, *Journal of Diabetes and its Complications* 13, 5-6, (1999), pp 254-263 ISSN 1056-8727

Fryckberger RG, Lavery LA, et al,(1998) Role of neuropathy and high foot pressures in diabetic foot ulceration, *Diabetes Care*, 21,5 (1998): 1714-1719.

Goodarz D. et al, (2011), National, regional, and global trends in fasting plasma glucose and diabetes prevalence since 1980: systematic analysis of health examination surveys and epidemiological studies with 370 country-years and 2·7 million participants. *The Lancet*, 378, 9785(2011), pp 31– 40, ISSN 0140-6736.

Gries FA, Cameron NE, Ziegler D, (2003), *Textbook of Diabetic Neuropathy*, Thieme Editorial, pag 380 ISBN 3-13-127581-2, Germany

Hogan P, & Dall T, & Nikolov P. (2003), Economic costs of diabetes in the US in 2002. *Diabetes Care*, 26, 3, (2003), pp 917-932. ISSN 0149-5992

Huijberts MS,et al (2008): Advanced glycation end products and diabetic foot disease. *Diabetes Metabolism Research and Reviews* 24, Suppl 1, (2008) pp S19–S24, ISSN: 1520-7560

Kaleta JL, Fleiischli JW, Reilly CH, (2001), The diagnosis of osteomyelitis in diabetes using erythrocite sedimentation rate: a pilot study *Journal of the american podiatric medical association* , 91, 9, (2001), pp 445-450 ISSN 8750-7315

Kruse I, & Edelman S. (2006), Evaluation and treatment of diabetic foot ulcers. *Clinical diabetes,* 24, 2 (2006), pag 91. ISSN: 0891-8929

Lawrence L, et al., (2008), Reevaluating the Way We Classify the Diabetic Foot: Restructuring the diabetic foot risk classification system of the International Working Group on the Diabetic Foot , *Diabetes Care , 31, 1* (2008), pp *154-156,* ISSN 0149-5992.

Levin & O´Neal (2008), The Diabetic Foot (7 th edition), Mosby Elsevier, pag 35, ISBN 978-0-323-04145-4, USA.

Li R, et al, (2010) Cost-Effectiveness of Interventions to Prevent and Control Diabetes Mellitus: A Systematic Review, *Diabetes Care*, 33, 8 (2010), pp 1872-1894, ISSN 0149-5992.

Lipsky BA, (1999), Evidence-based antibiotic therapy of diabetic foot infections, *FEMS immunology & medical microbiology*, 26, 3-4, (1999), pp 267-276

Lipsky et al, (2004), Diagnosis and treatment of diabetic foot infections, *Clinical Infectious Disease*, 39, 1, (2004), pp 885-909

Lipsky BA, Berendt AR (2006a), Infection of the Foot in persons with diabetes: Epidemiology , Patophysiology, Microbiology , Clinical presentation, and Approach to therapy, In: The foot in diabetes, Boulton, Cavanagh, Rayman, pp, 187-197, John Wiley & Sons Ltd, ISBN 978-0-470-01504-9, UK

Lipsky BA, Berendt AR (2006b), Infection of the Foot in persons with diabetes: Epidemiology, Patophysiology, Microbiology , Clinical presentation, and Approach to therapy, In: The foot in diabetes, Boulton, Cavanagh, Rayman, pag 192, John Wiley & Sons Ltd, ISBN 978-0-470-01504-9, UK

Luca DP et al, (2003) Ulcer Recurrence Following First Ray Amputation in Diabetic Patients: A cohort prospective study, *Diabetes Care*, 26, 6, (2003), pp 1874-1878, ISSN 0149-5992

Lyons et al, (2006) Foot pressures abnormalities in the diabetic foot, In: *The Diabetic Foot*, Veves A, & Giurini JM, & LoGerfo F, Humana Press editorial, pp 168-174, ISBN, 1-59745-075-8 USA

Lyons TE, (2008a) Management of diabetic foot complications, In: *Diabetic Neuropathy, Clinical management*, Veves A, Malik R, Humana Press editorial pp 480-82, ISBN 978-1-59745-311-0, USA

Lyons TE, (2008b) Management of diabetic foot complications, In: *Diabetic Neuropathy, Clinical management*, Veves A, Malik R, Humana Press editorial pp 475-76, ISBN 978-1-59745-311-0, USA

Mbanya JC (2011), Worlwide prevalence of diabetes. Presentation of Diabetes Atlas 2011 (International Diabetes Federation), Procedings of 47th EASD annual meeting Lisbon, Portugal, conference in Lisbon, September 2011.

Meggit B, (1976), Surgical management of the diabetic foot, *British Journal of Hospital Medicine*, 16, 2 (1976), pp 227-232 ISSN 0007-1064

Parkhouse N, & LeQueen PM (1988), Impaired neurogenic vascular response in patients with diabetes and neuropathic foot lesions, *New England Journal of Medicine* 318, 25, (1988), pp 1306-1309, ISSN 0028-4793.

Pataky Z, Assal JP, Conne P, et al (2005), Plantar pressure distribution in type 2 diqabetic patients without peripheral neuropathy and peripheral vascular disease. *Diabetic Medicine*, 22, 6, (2005), pp 762-767 ISSN 1464-5491.

Pecoraro RE & Reiber GE & Burgess EM (1990) Pathways to diabetic limb amputation: basis for prevention, *Diabetes Care*, 13, 5, (1990), pp 513-521, ISSN 0149-5992

Pham HT, et al (2000) Screening techniques to identify the at risk patients for developing diabetic foot ulcers in a prospective multicenter trial. *Diabetes Care, 23, 5, (2000)*, pp 606–611. ISSN 0149-5992.

Ramsey SD, &Newton K, & Blough D, et al. (1999), Incidence, outcomes and cost of foot ulcers in patients with diabetes. *Diabetes Care*, 22, 3, (1999), pp 382-387, ISSN 0149-5992.

Reiber GE, et al., (1999), Causal pathways for incident lower-extremity ulcers in patients with diabetes from two settings, *Diabetes Care*, 22, 1, (1999), pp 157-162, ISSN 0149-5992.

Schie CHM, & Boulton JM, (2006)The biomechanics of the diabetic foot, In: *The Diabetic Foot*, Veves A,& Giurini JM, & LoGerfo F, Humana Press editorial,pp185-191, ISBN, 1-59745-075-8 USA.

Sicco A, Haspels R, Tessa E, (2011), Evaluation and Optimization of Therapeutic Footwear for Neuropathic Diabetic Foot Patients Using In-Shoe Plantar Pressure Analysis , *Diabetes Care*, 34, 7 (2011), pp 1595-1600, ISSN 0149-5992.

Sheehan P et al, (2006), Percent Change in wound area of diabetic foot ulcers over 4-week period is a robust predictor of complete healing in a 12-week prospective trial. *Plastic and Reconstructive Surgery,* 7 Supply, (2006), pp 2395-2445, ISSN 0032-1052.

Tanenberg RJ, & Donodrio PD, Neuropathic problems of the lower limbs in diabetic patients, In: The diabetic foot, Levin & O´ Neal, Mosby Elsevier editorial , pp 33-74, ISBN 978-0-323-04145-4, USA.

Tentolouris N (2010), Introduction to diabetic Foot, In: Atlas of the diabetic Foot, Katsilambros et al, pp 1-10, Wiley-Blackwell editorial, ISBN 978-1-4051-9179-1, UK.

Velasco Mondragon HE, et al, (2010) Diabetes Risk Assessment in Mexicans and Mexican Americans, *Diabetes Care,* 33,10, (2010), pp 2260-2265, ISSN 0149-5992.

Wagner FW (1981), The dysvascular foot: a system for diagnosis and treatment. *Foot and Ankle* 2 , (1981), pp 64-122, ISSN: 1071-1007.

10

Role of Nitric Oxide in Extracellular Matrix Metabolism and Inflammation in Diabetic Wound Healing

Victor L. Sylvia[1], Audra D. Myers[1], Brandon M. Seifert[1], Eric M. Stehly[1], Michael A. Weathers[1], David D. Dean[1] and Javier LaFontaine[2]
[1]*University of Texas Health Science Center, San Antonio,TX*
[2]*Texas A&M Health Science Center, Temple, TX*
United States of America

1. Introduction

Diabetes and its subsequent complications present a significant challenge to our healthcare system. In particular, chronic diabetic wounds are a major cause of morbidity and use of healthcare resources in the U.S. Recent statistics reveal that 15% of diabetic patients develop foot and ankle chronic ulcers (Singh et al., 2005). Of these chronic wounds, 1 in 5 results in amputation. Further statistics reveal that 60% of nontraumatic lower-limb amputations occur in people with diabetes (Reiber, 2001). Chronic diabetic wounds result in a state of chronic inflammation about the wound site with decreased collagen and nitric oxide (NO) levels. The aims of these studies were to examine whether NO donor compounds will decrease inflammation and extracellular matrix destruction and simultaneously improve collagen production and wound healing. Specifically, we examined the effects of NO donors NOR-3 and SNOG on expression of matrix metalloproteinases (MMP)-1, -2. -8, -9 and -13, the inflammatory mediator interleukin-6 and collagen types I and type III by normal and diabetic fibroblasts under both normoxic and hypoxic states.

2. Methods

Prior studies by others have resulted in the development of a catalog of factors (altered MMP/TIMP ratio, decreased cell proliferation and migration, changes in growth factors [TGF-β, VEGF, PDGF-BB] and cytokines [IL-1β, IL-6, TNF-α], extracellular matrix, oxygenation, and nitric oxide) which are important in normal wound healing and demonstrate the dysregulation that exists in chronic wounds (Chen et al., 1999; Cook et al., 2000; Lobmann et al., 2002; Efron and Moldawer, 2004;Vandeberg et al., 2005). What was intriguing to us was the observation that a number of MMPs were known to be elevated in chronic wounds and that nitric oxide levels were quite low, but no one had drawn the connection that nitric oxide may regulate MMPs and promote wound healing by altering the MMP/TIMP ratio. By returning the MMP/TIMP ratio to near normal levels, matrix remodelling and growth factor regulation of the healing process could begin. The experiments described in this chapter were designed to examine these questions by testing short-acting and long-acting NO donor compounds in fibroblast culture and in an *in vivo* skin wound repair model. We chose to evaluate enhancement of matrix production by measuring type I and III collagen expression and amelioration of inflammation by measuring interleukin-6 (IL-6) production. We have previously demonstrated that long-acting NO donors significantly raise NO levels and reduce MMP gene expression in human diabetic skin fibroblast cultures (Burrow et al., 2007).

2.1 Diabetic ulcer model

Genetically diabetic, male C57BL/KsJ-*m*+/+*Lepr*^{db} mice and control parental strain C57BL/KsJ mice were obtained from Jackson Laboratories (Bar Harbor, ME). According to an IACUC-approved protocol, mice were anesthetized and a 10mm full thickness wound was created on the dorsum. Treated mice received a single topical application of vehicle or 500 nM (±)-(E)-ethyl-2-[(E)-hydroxyimino]-5-nitro-3-hexeneamide (NOR-3) or S-nitrosoglutathione (SNOG) applied to the wound. The rate of wound healing was compared throughout the experimental period and wound area was determined by tracing the edge of the wound onto a glass microscope slide and determining changes in wound area by use of Adobe Photoshop.

2.2 Cell culture and treatment

Primary dermal fibroblasts were isolated from normal and diabetic mice by mincing excised skin samples and digesting for 2 hours in 0.20% collagenase (type I, Worthington, Freehold, NJ) in serum-free Dulbecco's modified Eagle's medium (Mediatech Inc., Manassas, VA) at 37°C. The dissociated cells were cultured in Dulbecco's modified Eagle's medium with 20% FBS (Atlanta Biologicals, Norcross, GA) and 1% antibiotic/antimycotic supplement at 37°C with 100% humidity in 5% CO2 in air. Third passage fibroblasts were treated with control media, short-acting NOR-3, or long-acting SNOG NO donor compounds. Cells were incubated at 37°C in Dulbecco's Modified Eagle's Medium + 20% FBS + antibiotics for 1, 3 or 7 days. Similar experiments were carried out using human skin fibroblasts from age- and gender-matched non-diabetic and diabetic human subjects. Human diabetic and control fibroblasts (catalog no. GM00043, normal fibroblasts, and catalog no. GM01486, maturity onset diabetes fibroblasts) were obtained from the Coriell Institute for Medical Research (Camden, NJ). GM00043 cells were obtained at passage 11 and used for experiments at passages 14–16. GM01486 cells were obtained at passage 3 and used at passages 4–6. The cells were grown in T75 tissue culture flasks (Falcon BD, Bedford, MA) in minimal essential medium containing 15% fetal bovine serum (catalog no. 100-602; Gemini Bio-Products, West Sacramento, CA) and 1% penicillin-streptomycin at 37°C, following the recommended split ratios of 1:4 for the normal GM00043 cells and 1:3 for the diabetic GM01486 cells. For experiments, cells were plated in 24-well tissue culture plates (BD Biosciences, San Jose, CA) at a seeding density of 40,000 cells/well and cultured to confluence. The experiments were conducted under normoxic conditions (20% oxygen) and hypoxic conditions (2 % oxygen) using a Model NU-4950 CO_2 incubator with the ability to accurately regulate the oxygen level (Nuaire Corp., Plymouth, MN).

2.3 MMP/gelatin zymography

MMP-2 and MMP-9 activity in control and 500 nM SNOG-treated fibroblasts were assessed by gelatin zymography. Samples were separated under non-reducing conditions on 10%

SDS-PAGE mini-slab gels co-polymerized with 150 µg/ml type I gelatin, washed in 5% Triton X-100, and equilibrated with collagenase assay buffer (50 mM Tris, 200 mM NaCl, 5 mM $CaCl_2$, pH 7.2) at 37°C. Counterstaining with Coomassie brilliant blue revealed MMP-2 and -9 as cleared bands.

2.4 MMP and collagen gene expression

Total RNA was isolated from the non-diabetic and diabetic skin fibroblast cultures using TRIzol and then reverse transcribed using specific primers for MMP-2, -9 and -13, and Types I and III collagen. To determine the effects of NO donor on mRNA levels for each MMP, we performed real-time PCR analyses using 18S rRNA as the index gene, specific primers/probes for each MMP, and a Prism 7000 detection system (Applied Biosystems, Foster City, CA).

2.5 Determination of growth factor and cytokine levels

Release of cytokines and growth factors into the media of the cultures was quantified by use of Quantikine ELISA kits from R and D Systems. Colorimetric determination of interleukin-6 and PDGF-BB levels were done following manufacturer's specifications.

3. Results

3.1 Effects of NO donors on MMP expression

Expression of mouse MMP-2, MMP-9, and MMP-13 was measured using real time PCR. MMP-2 and MMP-9 were expressed in both normal and diabetic fibroblast cultures after 1 day of culture, but expression in the diabetic cells was 5-8 times higher than that found in normal (Figure 1). In contrast, MMP-13 was expressed by both cells at equivalent levels. When S-nitroso-N-acetylpenicillamine (SNAP), a NO donor with a half-life of 5 hours, was added to the cultures, a dose-dependent decrease in MMP-9 expression was observed (Figure 2). These results validate our previous findings in human skin fibroblasts (Burrow et al., 2007) and confirm that it is reasonable to expect mouse fibroblast MMP expression to be similar to that found with the human fibroblasts.

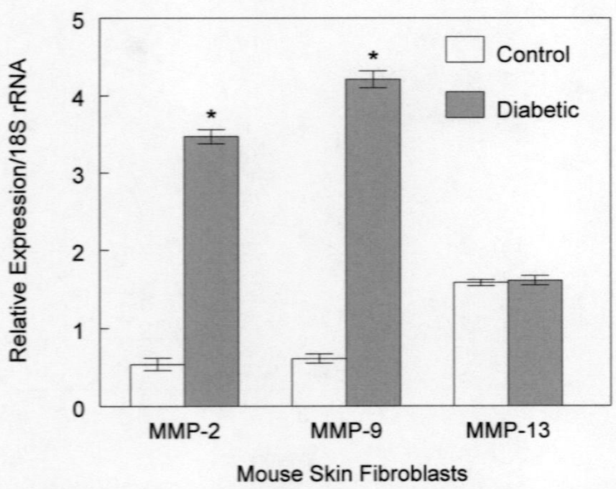

Fig. 1. Matrix metalloproteinase gene expression in control and diabetic mouse fibroblasts.

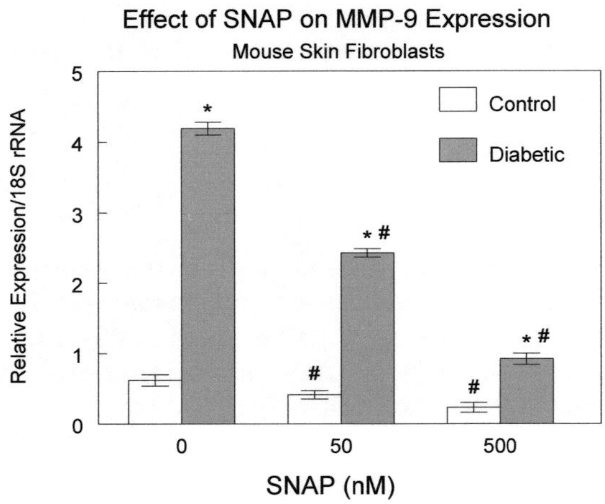

Fig. 2. Effect of NO donor SNAP on MMP-9 expression by control and diabetic mice fibroblast.

3.2 Effects of NO donors on skin wound healing

In the diabetic ulcer model, it can be clearly seen that wound area in the diabetic animals does not appreciably change over time. In contrast, normal mice mount a significant healing response and the wounds are virtually healed by 4 weeks. Treatment with 500 nM NO donor compound SNOG (Figure 3) or SNAP (data not shown) elicited a healing response in the diabetic animals that temporally approximated the normal healing process. Interestingly, normal animals treated with NO donors also displayed accelerated healing compared with normal controls. When 500 nM NOR-3, the fast acting donor was used, there was no effect on wound healing (Figure 4).

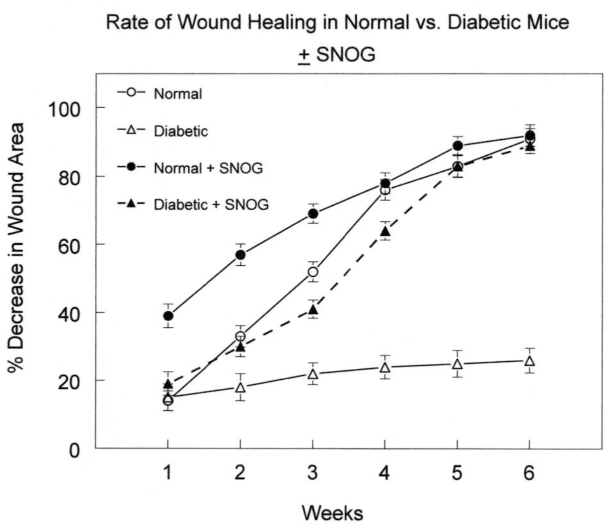

Fig. 3. Effect of NO donor SNOG on skin wound healing in normal and diabetic mice

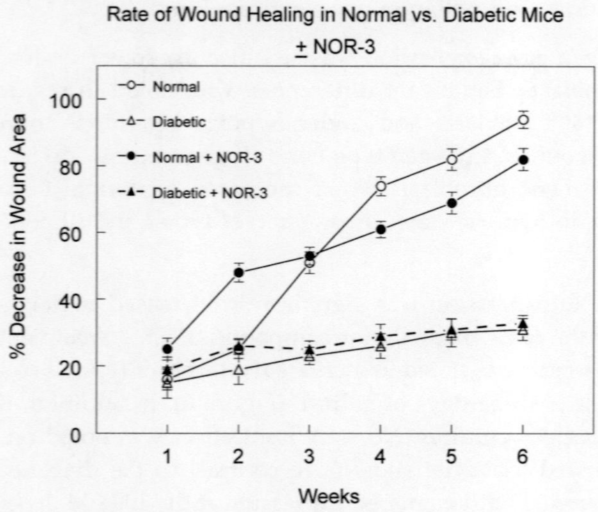

Fig. 4. Effect of NO donor NOR-3 on skin wound healing in normal and diabetic mice

3.3 Effects of NO donors on MMP activity determined by gelatin zymography

Cultured fibroblasts from the skin tissue of the normal and genetically-diabetic mice were examined for differences in MMP activity using gelatin zymography. Clear zones indicate MMP activity and the results demonstrate that equivalent cell numbers of diabetic fibroblasts show higher MMP-9 enzyme activity as compared to normal fibroblasts (Figure 5, compare MMP-9 signal in lane 3 versus lane 7). When treated for 24 hours with 500 nM SNOG, a significant reduction in MMP-9 activity was evident for both the non-diabetic and diabetic fibroblast cultures (see lanes 4 and 8). There was no such effect observed for MMP-2.

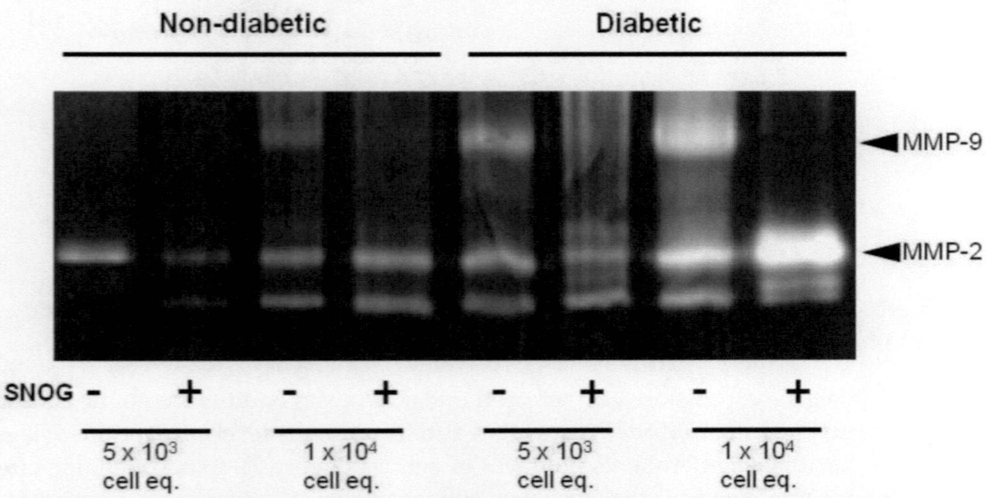

Fig. 5. Zymographic analysis of MMP enzyme activity before and after SNOG treatment of mouse fibroblast cultures.

3.4 Effects of NO donors on collagen gene expression

Type I and III collagen gene expression was significantly lower under hypoxic conditions and in diabetic fibroblasts. Significant differences were noted in regards to collagen gene expression in diabetic fibroblasts and under hypoxic conditions, mimicking the *in vivo* situation of chronic wounds. Collagen type I and III gene expression in our control samples was decreased in diabetic fibroblasts when compared to normal fibroblasts. Also, when comparing normoxic to hypoxic states, expression of type I and III collagen genes was less in the hypoxic group.

Type III collagen gene expression was significantly increased under normoxic conditions with the addition of the nitric oxide donor compound SNOG. Treatment with 1 nM SNOG, the long-acting NO donor, was noted to increase the levels of type III collagen expression by diabetic fibroblasts after three days of culture (Figure 6). In addition, the effect was dose-dependent for the diabetic cultures. No significant effect was noted on day 1 of culture at any concentration tested (data not shown). In contrast to the diabetic fibroblasts, normal fibroblasts only responded with increased expression at the 100 nM dose.

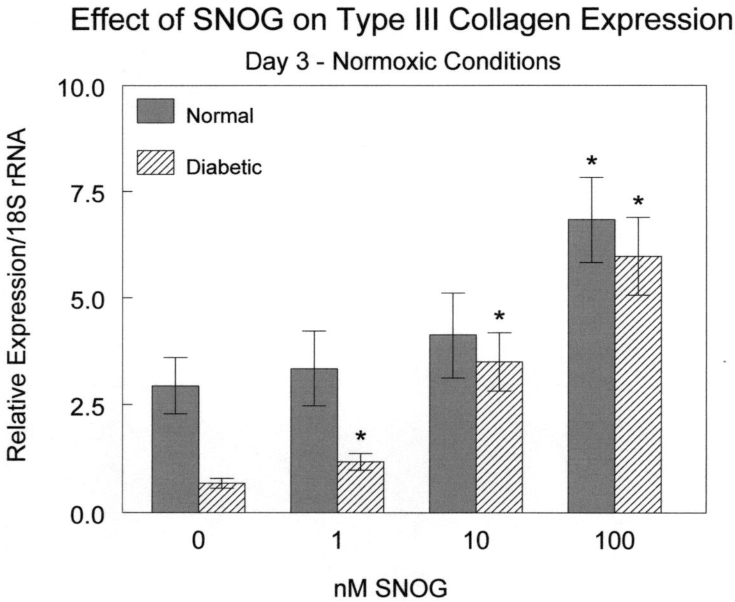

Fig. 6. Effect of NO donor SNOG on Type III collagen expression by normal and diabetic human fibroblasts cultured for three days under normoxic conditions.

Type III collagen gene expression was increased under hypoxic conditions with the addition of SNOG. Treatment with 1nM SNOG was noted to increase the levels of type III collagen expression by the diabetic fibroblasts on day 3 of culture (Figure 7). In addition, the effect was dose-dependent. However, the effect was only significant for the normal fibroblasts at 10 nM and 100 nM SNOG-treated cultures. No significant effect was noted on day 1 of culture at any concentration tested (data not shown).

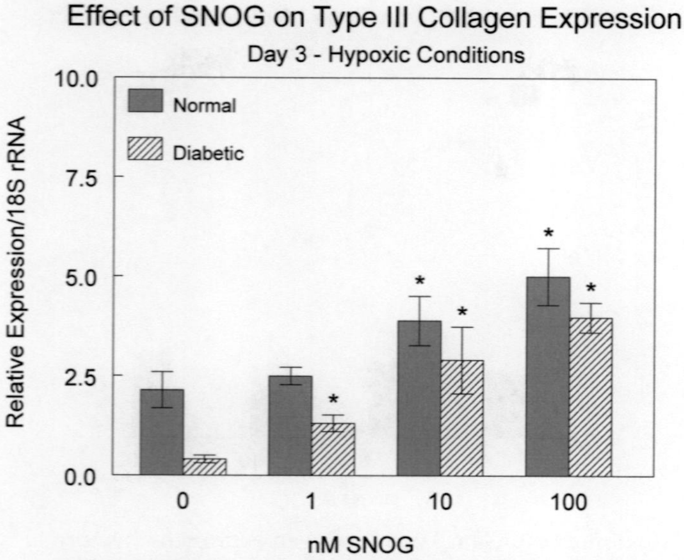

Fig. 7. Effect of NO donor SNOG on Type III collagen expression by normal and diabetic human fibroblasts cultured for three days under hypoxic conditions.

Type I collagen gene expression by normal fibroblasts at day 3 was not affected by SNOG treatment under normoxic conditions (Figure 8). A similar trend was noted with diabetic cells under normoxic conditions for type I collagen expression, except that a significant increase was observed with 100 nM SNOG treatment. No effect on type I collagen expression was noted for either normal or diabetic fibroblasts cultured for 3 days under hypoxic conditions (Figure 9).

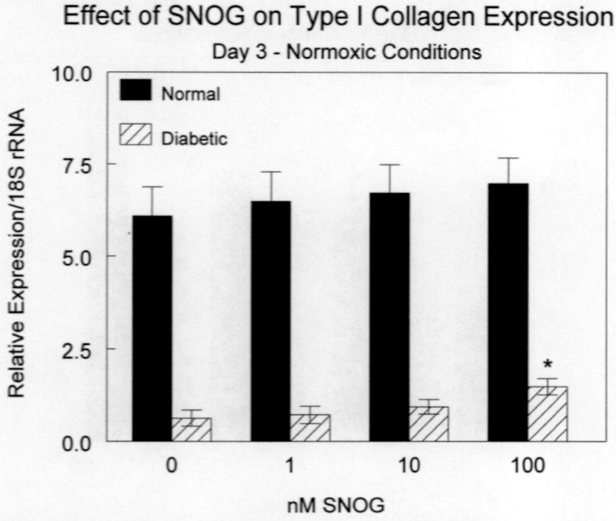

Fig. 8. Effect of NO donor SNOG on Type I collagen expression by normal and diabetic human fibroblasts cultured for three days under normoxic conditions.

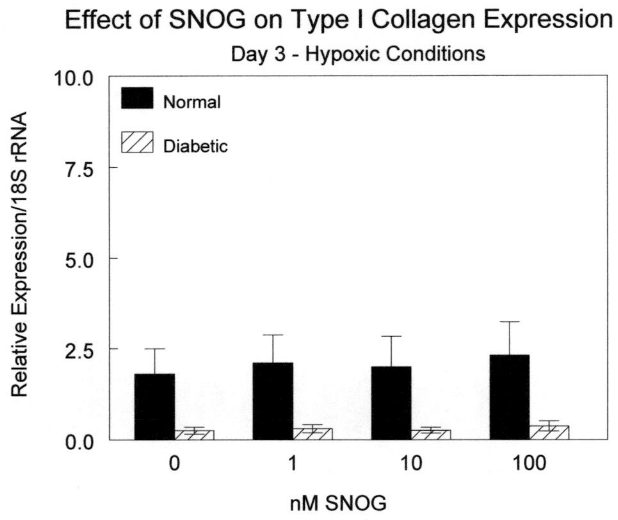

Fig. 9. Effect of NO donor SNOG on Type I collagen expression by normal and diabetic human fibroblasts cultured for three days under hypoxic conditions.

However, after seven days of culture under normoxic conditions following a single addition of SNOG, type I collagen expression by normal and diabetic fibroblasts was found to be increased (Figure 10). A significant increase was observed at 1nM SNOG for the normal fibroblasts and the effect was dose-dependent. Significant increases were also noted for the diabetic cultures, however only at the 10 and 100nM doses. Dose-dependent increases in type I collagen expression for normal and diabetic fibroblasts were also seen under hypoxic conditions (Figure 11).

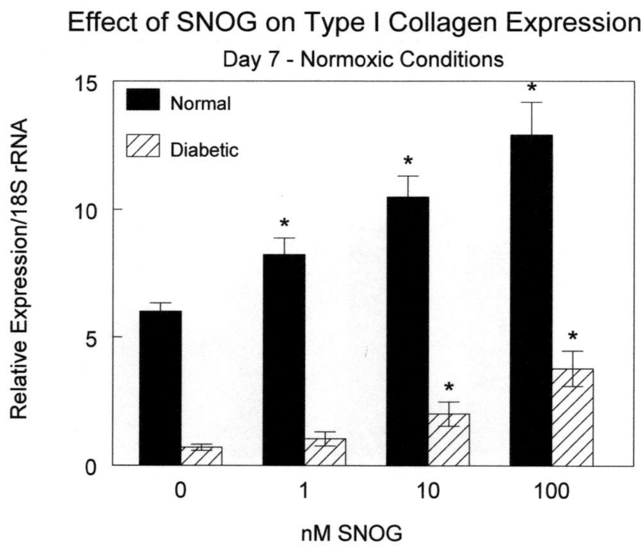

Fig. 10. Effect of NO donor SNOG on Type I collagen expression by normal and diabetic human fibroblasts cultured for seven days under normoxic conditions

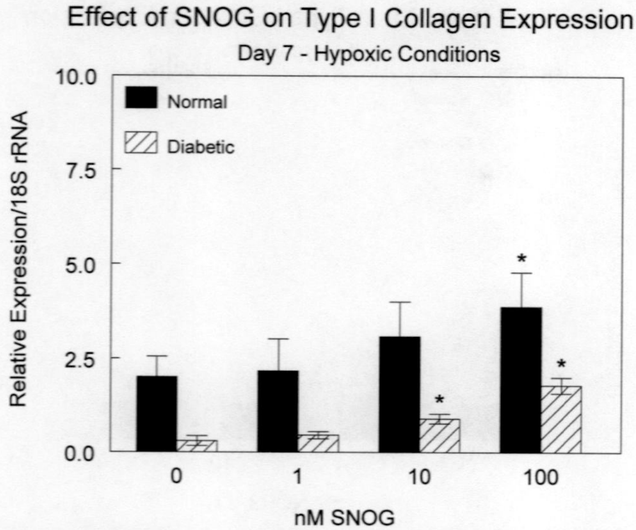

Fig. 11. Effect of NO donor SNOG on Type I collagen expression by normal and diabetic human fibroblasts cultured for seven days under hypoxic conditions.

In contrast, the short-acting NOR-3 NO donor had no significant effect upon collagen gene expression by either normal or diabetic fibroblasts cultured under either normoxic or hypoxic conditions. No effect was observed under normoxic (data not shown) or hypoxic conditions for type III collagen expression by normal or diabetic fibroblasts cultured for three days in the presence of NOR-3 (Figure 12). Similarly, there was no effect on type I collagen expression for cultures grown under hypoxic conditions for three days (Figure 13). Additonally, no effects were noted on days 1 or 7 of culture (data not shown).

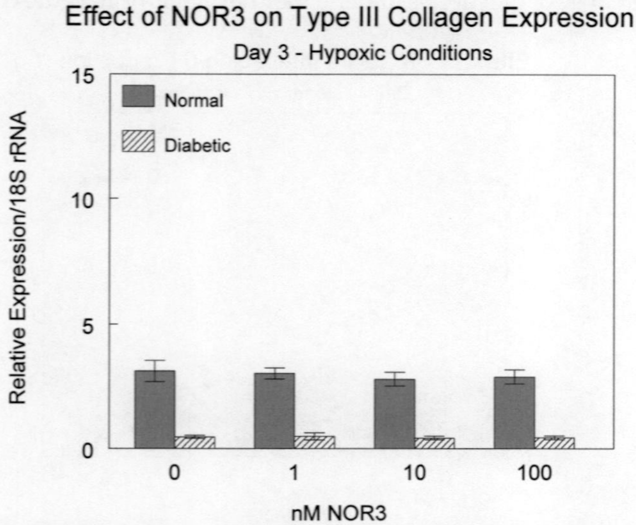

Fig. 12. Effect of NO donor NOR-3 on Type III collagen expression by normal and diabetic human fibroblasts cultured under hypoxic conditions.

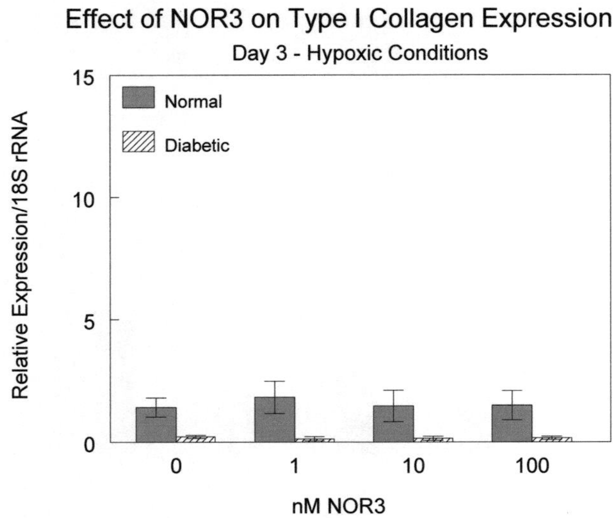

Fig. 13. Effect of NO donor NOR-3 on Type I collagen expression by normal and diabetic human fibroblasts cultured under hypoxic conditions.

3.5 Effects of NO donors on interleukin-6 production

The nitric oxide donor SNOG reduced IL-6 production by normal and diabetic skin fibroblasts grown under normoxic conditions and hypoxic conditions. At the control (0 nM) concentration, diabetic cells show significantly greater production of IL-6 than normal fibroblast cultures. The long-acting nitric oxide donor SNOG dose-dependently reduced IL-6 production for diabetic fibroblasts cultured either under normoxic conditions (Figure 14) or hypoxic conditions (Figure 15). In contrast, normal fibroblasts only demonstrated an effect at the highest dose of NO donor under either normoxic or hypoxic conditions.

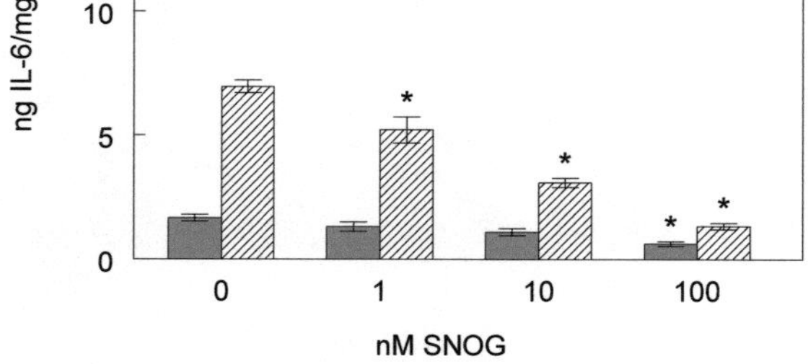

Fig. 14. Effect of NO donor SNOG on IL-6 production by normal and diabetic human fibroblasts cultured under normoxic conditions.

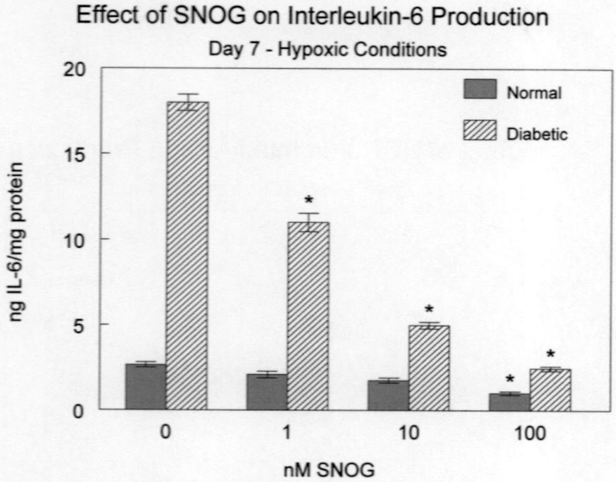

Fig. 15. Effect of NO donor SNOG on IL-6 production by normal and diabetic human fibroblasts cultured under hypoxic conditions.

The short-acting NO donor NOR-3 had no significant effect upon IL-6 production in either normal or diabetic fibroblasts cultures grown under either normoxic conditions (Figure 16) or hypoxic conditions (Figure 17).

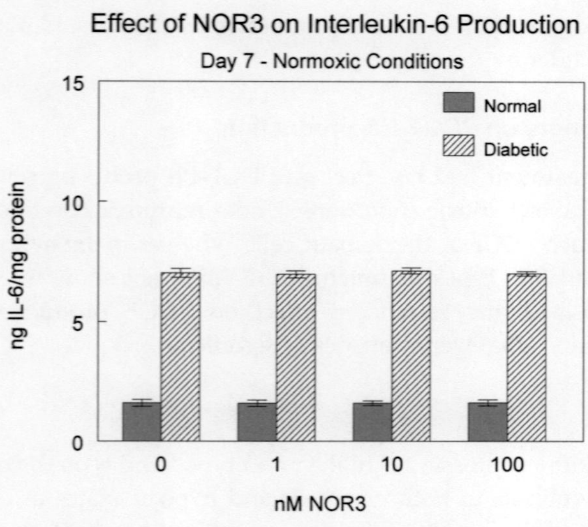

Fig. 16. Effect of NO donor NOR-3 on IL-6 production by normal and diabetic human fibroblasts cultured under normoxic conditions.

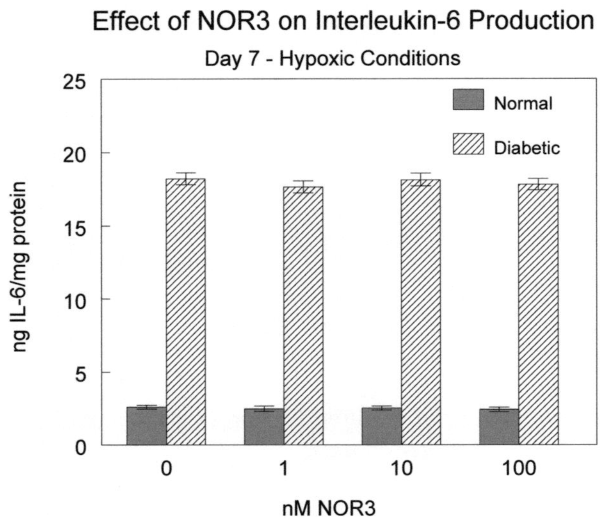

Fig. 17. Effect of NO donor NOR-3 on IL-6 production by normal and diabetic human fibroblasts cultured under hypoxic conditions.

3.6 Effects of NO donors on PDGF-BB production

Nitric oxide donor treatment had no effect on PDGF-BB production by normal fibroblasts grown under normoxic or hypoxic conditions. Under normoxic conditions, the normal cells produced twice as much PDGF as the diabetic cells, whereas in the hypoxic environment the normal cells produced five times as much PDGF (data not shown). Neither of the nitric oxide donors tested had any significant effect on PDGF production in either of the environmental conditions that were statistically significant.

3.7 Summary

MMP-9 and interleukin-6 expression is higher, and type I and type III collagen expression is lower, in diabetic fibroblasts in both normoxic and hypoxic states as compared to normal fibroblasts. With the addition of the NO donor with the relatively long half-life (SNOG), MMP-9 gene expression and enzyme activity were decreased. Additionally, production of the inflammatory cytokine interleukin-6 was decreased by increasing NO levels with SNOG. Concurrently, type I and type III collagen expression were increased. Treatment with SNOG resulted in a significant effect upon collagen type III production in a dose-dependent fashion in both normal and diabetic fibroblasts under both normoxic and hypoxic states. In diabetic fibroblasts, under a normoxic state, the effect did not become significant until the 1nM SNOG-treated cells on day 3, and continued at the 10nM and 100nM concentrations on days 3 and 7. The effect upon collagen type III production in diabetic fibroblasts, under a hypoxic state, was found to be significant at the 1nM, 10nM, and 100nM in SNOG-treated cells on days 3 and 7. The effect of the addition of SNOG to both normal and diabetic fibroblasts under both normoxic and hypoxic states also results in a significant increase in collagen type I production in a dose dependent fashion. The effect in diabetic fibroblasts, under a normoxic state, was noted to be significant at the 100nM concentration of the SNOG donor compound on day 3. The effect in diabetic fibroblasts, under a hypoxic state, was found to be significant at the 10nM and 100nM level on day 7. The addition of NOR-3 had no significant effect upon the production of type I or III collagen in normal or diabetic fibroblasts.

4. Conclusion

Chronic diabetic wounds present a significant challenge to healthcare providers and resources. Significant amounts of time, money and resources have gone into prevention and treatment of these wounds. However, despite these efforts, chronic wounds continue to pose a serious problem. This has led researchers to focus more on understanding the molecular organization and function of normal wound healing and how this process is altered in chronic diabetic wounds. This is a very complex process that occurs through a series of highly integrated interactions between a multitude of varying cell types, growth factors, and cytokines. In diabetics, these wound healing interactions are disrupted and the process of wound healing seems to be locked in a perpetual state of chronic inflammation.

In diabetic wound healing, a physiologic state consistent with decreased nitric oxide (NO) levels results, leading to an impaired inflammatory response, decreased collagen production, and decreased wound-breaking strength (Witte et al., 2002). Prior studies have also revealed the MMP levels are significantly elevated in chronic diabetic wounds, thus creating an imbalance in matrix breakdown and release of growth factors that are important for normal wound healing (Wysocki et al., 1993; Trengove et al., 1999; Lobmann et al., 2002). Chronic diabetic wounds appear to be physiologically trapped in the inflammatory stage of wound healing and nitric oxide may promote normal healing by selectively reversing dysregulated factors (e.g.: localized ischemia, cell proliferation, MMP/TIMP ratio, growth factors/ cytokines, matrix synthesis) which prevent progression to the reepithelialization phase of wound healing. Additionally, nitric oxide may play a larger role in diabetic foot problems as low levels of endothelial nitric oxide synthase, an enzyme responsible for nitric oxide production, is associated with bone fractures (Loveridge et al., 2002) and Charcot neuroarthropathy (La Fontaine et al., 2008).

Prior studies have shown that introduction of a NO donor can improve wound healing (Shabani et al., 1996; Bohl-Masters et al., 2002). The mechanism(s) responsible for NO-induced healing remains unclear. Our studies reveal significant differences in the levels of MMP-9, NO synthetases, PDGF-BB, interleukin-6 and types I and III collagen in normal and diabetic fibroblasts. With the addition of NO donor compounds, the levels of extracellular matrix-degrading MMP-9 and inflammatory mediator interleukin-6 were decrease in skin fibroblast cultures. NO donors stimulated type I and III collagen expression in both normal and diabetic fibroblasts and under both normoxic and hypoxic states. Thus, the results of this study combined with previous studies involving chronic diabetic wounds, the potential exists to develop a topical media to apply to chronic wounds that would introduce these NO donors to the wound site to improving the healing potential of these wounds.

Although it is known that diabetic patients display impaired wound healing, the mechanism for this impairment is not fully understood. Because fibroblasts are essential for dermal wound repair, the current study compared the *in vitro* behavior of human dermal fibroblasts. It has been reported that fibroblasts from diabetic wounds continue to display impaired proliferation even when taken out of their *in vivo* diabetic environment and cultured *in vitro* (Burrow et al., 2007; Loot et al., 1999; Hehenberger et al., 1998). Therefore, identical tissue culture conditions should not obscure differences between our experimental groups.

Diabetic cells when compared to normal cells demonstrated a decreased gene expression in types I & III collagen, eNOS and iNOS, and PDGF-BB, with an increased production of IL-6. Within the hypoxic condition the expression of types I & III collagen, eNOS and iNOS and PDGF-BB were further reduced in both the diabetic and normal cells, whereas the IL-6 production was only significantly increased within the diabetic fibroblasts. With the treatments of the NO donors, it was demonstrated that when evaluating the types I & III collagen and eNOS and iNOS only SNOG was seen to have an effect on either type, with its most profound effect on type III collagen in both environmental conditions. The IL-6 production was only decreased by the long-acting NO donor SNOG. Neither NO donor demonstrated a significant effect upon PDGF-BB production.

In 2005, we demonstrated that the addition of the NO donor SNAP to skin wounds in a diabetic mouse model significantly increased the rate and extent of wound healing (Stehly et al., 2005). The wound healing rates in the diabetic treatment groups approximated the normal mice. In a study by Bohl-Masters et al., 2002, a polyvinyl alcohol hydrogel impregnated with NO donor was used to increase the local NO concentration in a wound healing model in diabetic and normal mice. They found that wound healing in the NO donor-treated diabetic mice was either the same or slightly less than in the control group. However, the quality of granulation tissue was much improved in the presence of nitric oxide donor.

NO has been shown to be significantly reduced in chronic ulcers. Impaired healing of diabetic wounds is thought to be related to diminished NO production (Witte et al., 2002; Schaffer et al., 1997). Because the level of NO in chronic wounds is low, and elevation of NO enhances wound healing, a number of other approaches have been tried to deliver NO therapeutically. Studies using compounds such as L-arginine (Shi et al., 2003), vitamin B_{12} (Bauer et al., 1998), and multivitamin therapy using a combination of folic acid, vitamin B_6, and vitamin B_{12} (Boykin et al., 2005) have reported concomitant increases in wound tissue NO level and healing. The latter study demonstrated that serum homocysteine, an inhibitor of NOS, is elevated in patients with chronic wounds; with multivitamin therapy, this inhibitor is decreased and associated with enhanced healing. Both of these approaches employ systemic delivery of the compounds to raise NO, but do not involve a local targeted delivery of NO directly into the wound site. Very few investigations have sought to deliver NO directly into wounds. For example, one study using a NO-modified polyvinyl alcohol hydrogel effectively healed cutaneous wounds in diabetic mice (Bohl-Masters et al., 2002). Increased production of extracellular matrix molecules was noted in this study, but no attempt was made to measure changes in MMP activity. Other approaches used to deliver NO to the wound have used linear polyethyleneimine/NO adducts (Bauer et al., 1998) and delivery of iNOS naked DNA via a collagen sponge (Thornton et al., 1998). Both of these approaches reported toxic effects related to the delivery of excessive levels of NO to the wound, suggesting the need for a more finely controlled transient release of NO. The longer-acting NO donor compounds, SNAP and SNOG, used in the current study, and similar cell-permeable compounds which produce transient increases in tissue NO concentration, should provide a means of optimizing the therapeutic effect. NO donor compounds may ultimately provide a new therapeutic tool for the treatment of diabetic foot wounds.

The purpose of this study was to assess the effect that NO donor compounds would have upon the production of type I and type III collagen production in diabetic fibroblasts both in normoxic and hypoxic (representative of chronic diabetic wounds) states. Prior studies have mainly focused upon the effect in normal fibroblasts under normoxic conditions. This study demonstrated that collagen type I and type III production was decreased in diabetic fibroblasts under both normoxic and hypoxic states when compared to normal fibroblasts without the addition of NO donor compounds. Thus, providing a catalyst to increase the amount of type I and type III collagen could potentially improve wound healing in diabetic chronic wounds.

To examine the time dependence of NO action in wound healing, this study utilized a shorter acting NO donor compound (NOR-3) and a relatively long-acting NO donor, SNOG, to assess their effects upon collagen production. Through the introduction of these agents in this study, significant increases in collagen type I and type III production were observed. In fact, the effect of the SNOG NO donor compound upon type III collagen production in diabetic fibroblasts demonstrated a significantly greater dose dependent effect than that observed in normal fibroblasts. Type I collagen levels were also significantly increased with the addition of the SNOG NO donor compound in both diabetic and normal fibroblasts. However, the dose dependent relationship for collagen type I production was essentially the same for both normal and diabetic fibroblasts.

The short acting NO donor compound (NOR-3), was not found to have any significant effect upon collagen type I or III production in diabetic fibroblasts. This finding, along with previous findings with the use of NOR-3 potentially indicate that relatively longer-acting NO donor compounds are more effective at NO and collagen production in diabetic fibroblasts. Thus, using a relatively longer-acting NO donor compound could potentially expose the chronic wound to longer duration of NO further increasing the wound healing potential and being present throughout more of the wound healing stages.

The results observed in this study are very encouraging in regards to possible future treatment of chronic diabetic wounds. By studying the effects of these NO donor compounds in diabetic fibroblasts under normoxic and hypoxic states we have been able to create an environment more closely resembling a chronic wound state in human diabetic patients. From the results of this and other studies in our laboratory we now have the potential to develop a topical treatment for chronic diabetic wounds based upon optimal delivery of NO to assist with wound healing. Preliminary studies are currently being performed examining SNOG attachment and release from both collagen-based and hydroxyapatite-based scaffolds. The goals of these studies are to develop new types of synthetic graft materials for the treatment of diabetic skin and bone wounds respectively. Future research will be directed toward development and optimization of these and other NO delivery systems for the treatment of wounds and other diabetic complications.

5. Acknowledgments

The authors wish to thank Thomas L. Sanders, Hui-Hsiu Chuang and Weinan Zhong for their contributions to the work presented in this chapter. This research was supported by a grant from the Juvenile Diabetes Research Foundation (Grant 5-2005-179).

6. References

Bauer JA (1998). Hydroxocobalamins as biologically compatible donors of NO implicated in the acceleration of wound healing. *Medical Hypotheses* 51:65-67.

Bohl-Masters KS, Leibovich SJ, Belem P, West JL, Poole-Warren LA (2002). Effects of nitric oxide releasing poly(vinyl alcohol) hydrogel dressings on dermal wound healing in diabetic mice. *Wound Repair and Regeneration* 10:286-294.

Boykin JV, Baylis C, Allen SK, Humphries YM, Shawler LG, Sommer VL, Watkins MB, Young JK, Crossland MC (2005). Treatment of elevated homocysteine to restore normal wound healing: a possible relationship between homocysteine, NO, and wound repair. *Advances in Skin and Wound Care* 18:297-300.

Burrow JW, Koch JA, Chuang H-H, Zhong W, Dean DD, and Sylvia VL (2007). NO donors selectively reduce the expression of matrix metalloproteinases-8 and -9 by human diabetic skin fibroblasts. *Journal of Surgical Research* 140:90-98.

Chen C, Schultz G, Bloch M, Edwards P, Tebes S., Mast B (1999). Molecular and mechanistic validation of delayed healing rat wounds as a model for human chronic wounds. *Wound Repair and Regeneration.* 7:486-494.

Cook H, Davies KJ, Harding KG, Thomas DW (2000). Defective extracellular matrix reorganization by chronic wound fibroblasts is associated with alterations in TIMP-1, TIMP-2, and MMP-2 activity. *Journal of Investigative Dermatology.* 115:225-233.

Efron PA, Moldawer LL (2004). Cytokines and wound healing: the role of cytokine and anticytokine therapy in the repair response. *Journal of Burn Care & Rehabilitation.* 25(2):149-60.

Hehenberger K, Heilborn JD, Brismar K, Hansson A (1998). Inhibited proliferation of fibroblasts derived from diabetic wounds and normal dermal fibroblasts treated with high glucose is associated with increased formation of l-lactate. *Wound Repair & Regeneration* 6(2):135-141.

La Fontaine J, Harkless LB, Sylvia VL, Carnes D, Heim-Hall J, Jude E (2008). Levels of endothelial nitric oxide synthase and calcitonin gene-related peptide in the Charcot foot: A pilot study. *Journal of Foot and Ankle Surgery* 47(5):424-429.

Lobmann R, Ambrosch A, Schultz G, Waldmann K, Schieweck S, Lehnert H (2002). Expression of matrix-metalloproteinases and their inhibitors in the wounds of diabetic and non-diabetic patients. *Diabetologia* 45:1011-1016.

Loot MA, Lamme EN, Mekkes JR, Bos JD, Middelkoop E (1999). Cultured fibroblasts from chronic diabetic wounds on the lower extremity (non-insulin-dependent diabetes mellitus) show disturbed proliferation. *Archives of Dermatological Research* 291(2-3):93-99.

Loveridge N, Fletcher S, Power J, Caballero-Alias AM, Das-Gupta V, Rushton N, Parker M, Reeve J, Pitsillides AA (2002). Patterns of osteocytic endothelial nitric oxide synthase expression in the femoral neck cortex: Differences between cases of intracapsular hip fracture and controls.

Reiber GE. Epidemiology of foot ulcers and amputations in the diabetic foot. In: Bowker JH, Pfeifer MA, eds. *The Diabetic Foot*. 6th ed. St. Louis, MO: Mosby; 2001:13-32.

Schaffer MR, Tantry U, Efron PA, Ahrendt GM, Thornton FJ, Barbul A (1997b). Diabetes-impaired healing and reduced wound nitric oxide synthesis: a possible pathophysiologic correlation. *Surgery* 121(5):513-519.

Shabani M, Pulfer SK, Bulgrin JP (1996). Enhancement of wound repair with a topically applied nitric oxide-releasing polymer, *Wound Repair & Regeneration* 4: 353-362.

Shi HP, Most D, Efron DT, Witte MB, Barbul A (2003). Supplemental L-arginine enhances wound healing in diabetic rats. *Wound Repair and Regeneration* 11:198-203.

Singh N, Armstrong DG, Lipsky BA (2005) Preventing foot ulcers in patients with diabetes. *JAMA* 293:217-228.

Stehly EM, Sylvia VL, Dean DD, Bruggeman A (2005). Nitric oxide donor improves wound healing in diabetic mice. *Southern Medical Journal* 98(10): S75.

Thornton FJ, Schaffer MR, Witte MB, Moldawer LL, MacKay SL, Abouhamze A, Tannahill CL, Barbul A (1998). Enhanced collagen accumulation following direct transfection of the inducible nitric oxide synthase gene in cutaneous wounds. *Biochemical & Biophysical Research Communications* 246(3):654-659.

Trengove NJ, Stacey MC, MacAuley S, Bennett N, Gibson J, Burslem F, Murphy G, Schultz G (1999). Analysis of the acute and chronic wound environments: the role of proteases and their inhibitors. *Wound Repair & Regeneration*. 7(6):442-52.

Vandeberg JS, Rose MA, Haywood-Reid PL, Rudolph R, Payne, WG, Robson MC (2004). Cultured pressure ulcer fibroblasts show replicative senescence with elevated production of plasmin, plasminogen activator inhibitor-1, and transforming growth factor-β1. 2005. *Wound Repair and Regeneration*. 13:76-83.

Witte MB, Kiyama T, Barbul A (2002). Nitric oxide enhances experimental wound healing in diabetes. *British Journal of Surgery* 89:1594-1601.

Wysocki AB, Staiano-Coico L, Grinnell F (1993). Wound fluid from chronic leg ulcers contains elevated levels of metalloproteinases MMP-2 and MMP-9. *Journal of Investigative Dermatology*. 101(1):64-68.

11

Nutritional Treatment of Diabetic Foot Ulcers - A Key to Success

Patrizio Tatti[1] and Annabel Barber[2]
[1]*Diabetes and Endocrinology Unit – ASL RMH Roma*
[2]*University of Nevada, LV*
[1]*Italy*
[2]*USA*

1. Introduction

Diabetic Foot Ulcers (DFUs) represent a frequent occurrence in the diabetic population and up to 15% of these subjects may be expected to develop a foot ulcer at least one time in his/her life[1,2]. DFUs cause personal, social and economic problems and are a serious risk factor for death[3,4]. These ulcers can be broadly classified as neuropathic, vascular[5] or mixed, although the pathogenesis is much more complex. Biochemical[6], hygienic[7], structural deformity[8,9], dynamic, pressure, skeletal, nutritional, socioeconomic factors, reduced antibacterial activity[10,11,12], workplace influences, all concur to cause and maintain the lesion. A multicenter study attributed 63 percent of diabetic foot ulcers to the critical triad of peripheral sensory neuropathy, trauma, and deformity[13]. Most often healing requires the cooperation of many specialists, including surgeons, podiatrists, wound nurses and endocrinologists. In many cases, the definitive treatment demands minor or major surgery.

While the treatment of vascular ulcers is straightforward and requires a bypass or a radiologic procedure if the damage to the limb is to be limited or cured, the treatment of neuropathic ulcers is much more complex. Most often relief of the abnormal pressure does not lead to the healing of the ulcer, rather these wounds are characteristically chronic, with alternating periods of partial improvement and relapse. Sometimes a superimposing infection worsens the clinical condition. These ulcers in general do not lead to major amputation of the limb but frequently cause considerable economic, social and psychological burden on the patient and his relatives.

2. Etiology of the ulcer

The distinctive characteristic of the diabetic ulcer is the tendency to become chronic. There are many definitions of "chronic". The American Heritage Medical Dictionary and Stedman's Medical Dictionary define chronic ulcers as a "longstanding ulcer with fibrous scar at its base. A thorough search through the literature does not give an exact definition of this term. Sometimes one can read of "ulcers lasting more than six months" but this ignores the wide array of biological backgrounds and the phenotypic presentations of these ulcers. We propose an equally subjective but more realistic definition: "*an ulcer lasting more than one could expect on the basis of previous experience in nondiabetic subjects*". The characteristic chronicity of the DFU was one of the bases for the diagnosis of diabetes before the introduction of the blood glucose assay. This idea penetrated the lore, and it is still possible to hear sentences like "I do not have diabetes, my ulcers heal quickly".

Chronic neuropathic ulcers usually occur as a result of a repeated trauma in the most exposed areas of the foot and ankle. However, not infrequently, may be the result of an acute trauma that is not recognized at the time of injury due to the relative pain insensitivity. The acute pathologic process is probably different and the outcome more favorable in the acute events versus the chronic ones.

The neuropathic ulcers have many concurrent factors that come into play to initiate and sustain the ulcer process. Among the risk factors, the presence of peripheral neuropathy with the consequent reduced or absent pain sensation, of bone deformity that exposes the bone heads to an abnormal load, and of trauma are prevalent[13]. Some form of diabetic neuropathy is present in nearly 65 % of diabetic patients. Fifty percent of these have a peripheral[14] that causes the loss of protective sensation. The often associated autonomic nerve dysfunction decreases sweating and causes thin, dry, fissured skin[15,16] that breaks easily. This autonomic dysfunction is one of the main causes of the severely damaged "Charcot foot"[17,18]. Trauma of any kind almost always has an initiating role. Acute wounds often are inadvertently self-inflicted during nail care or minor inadvertent injuries. Due to concomitant nerve damage, patients may not recognize or remember the trauma. The use of heaters to warm the feet or of overheated water to wash may cause burns or blisters that later develop into chronic wounds. The initiating factor in chronic pressure wounds most often is the repeated impact of an ill-fitting shoe on one area of the foot. Furthermore, diabetic patients have a peculiar rigidity of the joints that do not allow the foot to mold to the shoe or the floor[19], thus creating an abnormal pressure and increasing the risk of injury. In many instances, calluses are an independent cause of injury, and is not uncommon to discover an ulcer beneath a callus.

Diabetic neuropathies appear with such wide array of different clinical presentations and in so many different places, sometimes symmetrically, less frequently as mononeuropathies, that finding a common cause has till now been impossible.[20,21] The most obvious culprit is hyperglycemia[22], and at least at the beginning of the disease the normalization of the blood glucose can frequently revert to normal symptoms and signs of neuropathy.[23,24] Chronic hyperglycemia plays an important role in the appearance of neuropathy. It is well known from the Diabetes Control and Complication Trial (DCCT) that strict control of blood glucose in newly diagnosed non complicated type 1 diabetics decreases the development of peripheral neuropathy in 60% of the cases over 5 years [25,26]. However, the exclusive role of hyperglycemia has been challenged on the basis of the failure in some cases to achieve improvement of neuropathy with blood glucose control[27,28] and other observations among which the increased incidence of this condition in prediabetes, [29,30,31] a state in which the blood glucose is still normal. Alternatively, a role of insulinopenia has been suggested.[32,33] Insulin receptors are present in the peripheral nervous system, and it is conceivable that any malfunction of insulin delivery[34] may damage the function of neurons. There is also proof that in an experimental model of diabetes, a modest reduction of insulin levels even without an increase of the blood glucose levels can reduce the pain threshold.[35,36] Thus it is possible that the insulin level required to regulate the nerve function is higher than that needed for glucose control. Further, neuropathy can appear early also in type 2 diabetes[37,38] where at least in the prediabetic stages, there is a compensatory hyperinsulinemia coupled with an increase in insulin resistance. This and the previous observation that a higher level of insulinemia is probably required for the regulation of the nervous than the glycemic system may point to a role of insulin resistance. In this case, the compensatory hyperinsulinemia could be present for many years and be effective to prevent the occurrence of overt diabetes, but not to prevent the nerve damage. Or, in turn, the insulin resistance could involve the nervous receptors to a higher degree than those involved in glucoregulation. It has also been shown that Insulin Growth Factor 1 (IGF1), a molecule that mimics many insulin effects,[39,40,41] induces recovery of the nerve function in rats[42]. Taken together, these hypotheses fail to explain the pathogenesis of diabetic peripheral neuropathy and do not confirm an exclusive role of hyperglycemia. On the other hand, there is no doubt that hyperglycemia causes the microvascular damage frequently associated with the DFU. In a recent study the Authors found a graded association between HbA1C and carotid Intima Media Thickness (IMT) that is currently considered the best marker of progression of atherosclerosis.[43] In this study LDL and HDL cholesterol, plasma triglycerides, and waist-to-hip ratio were significantly associated with HbA1c after multivariable adjustment. Among other factors interfering with healing at the cellular level, the prevalence of infections in diabetics should not be overlooked. Chemotaxis, phagocytosis and all the bactericidal actions of neutrophils are impaired in uncontrolled diabetes[4445]. Also the formation of Advanced Glycation Endo Products (AGE), that can bind to specific receptors on the leucocyte membrane (RAGE), may further impair the leucocyte antibacterial activity.[46] Thus, at present we have not identified a distinctive cause nor we have a definite role for the co-causal factors. One hypothesis put forward to explain the appearance and/or the progression of diabetic neuropathy is that impairment of synthesis of proteins may be the primary insult leading to the centripetal necrosis of the neuron [4748,49,50,51]. Because this aspect is strictly connected with the topic of nutrition we will deal with it later in this chapter. This and many other hypotheses and their support were recently discussed in depth[52] and are beyond the scope of his chapter

3. The body composition of the subjects with an ulcer

The body of a diabetic is different from the body of a person who has a normal blood glucose level. The well known changes at the molecular level, notably the accumulation of AGEs[53] cause in time morphological changes of the tissues, with diffuse damage to the vascular walls, reduction of the body cell mass and lean body mass[54], skin stiffness and prevalence of fat.

What we broadly define lean body mass is in reality a composite of what is mostly the structural - protein component of the body including muscle, parenchymal organs, red blood cells, enzymes, mitochondria and the like,[55] and has a critical role in maintaining the integrity of the body and permitting the survival. Although surprising there are very few studies of the body composition of type 2 diabetic subjects. To fill this gap we compared the body composition of 244 subjects with type 2 diabetes mellitus and demonstrated a reduction in the Body Cell Mass index (an index of the % mass of cells normalized for the actual height of the subject) in both sexes versus 266 non diabetic matched controls. Furthermore in 715 diabetics we also demonstrated that this reduction was proportional to both the prevailing level of HbA1c in the last year and the duration of disease, although with the multiple regression analysis the former appears to account for most of the actual reduction[52].

There are many possible explanations for the protein/lean body mass loss: (1) the body of the diabetic is in a continuous catabolic state due to insulin deficiency and to the phenomenon of neoglucogenesis continuously turning aminoacids and fat into harmful glucose. This process lasts throughout the day in uncompensated diabetes[56] without interruption at mealtime and is proportional to the blood glucose level[57], in accordance with our observations. (2) Most diabetics have a persistent microalbuminuria, which represents another source of protein loss[58] (3) the wound itself is a source of protein loss proportional to the size and depth of the lesion.[59] (4) Because of the concomitant kidney damage these patients are frequently put on a protein reduced diet, on unsupported grounds[60], thus aggravating their protein depletion.

Furthermore the presence of the wound tends to change the metabolic environment towards catabolism: the secretion of proinflammatory cytokines in proportion to the size and the condition of the lesion increases the insulin resistance deranging glucose metabolism, and drives the body into a catabolic state. This phenomenon is particularly dangerous in diabetics who already have high circulating levels of cytokines secreted by the excess abdominal fat. The increased cortisol secretion as part of the stress response to the wound adds to the catabolism: less energy is derived from the fat mass, and the protein catabolism is increased. In turn the release of aminoacids drives the neoglucogenesis in the liver.

To add further to this catabolic state, diabetic subjects have reduced levels of most anabolic hormones. Beyond the obvious absence or ineffectiveness of insulin on protein metabolism[61,62,63] these subjects have a subnormal level of testosterone (low testosterone syndrome)[64,65,66,67] with a characteristic hypogonadotropic hypogonadism[64] responsible for the decreases the lean body mass. In view of all these events occurring together it is not surprising that most of these subjects are in a protein depleted state. As suggested before, it is possible that the failure of proteins synthesis involved in nerve functioning may result in impaired nerve regeneration and death.[68,69,70,71]

Loss	Catabolism	Reduced supply
Kidney (microalbuminuria) Liver (neoglucogenesis) Ulcer (exudate)	Low testosterone Low GH Fat derived cytokines	Diet Protein losing enteropathy diarrhea

Table 1. Common causes of protein malnutrition in the diabetic

It is thus clear that decompensated diabetes is a catabolic condition further aggravated by the stress reaction and this creates a conflict with the ancestral mechanisms of survival of the body. A better comprehension of the wound healing process can be acquired through an analysis of these processes. The human body is programmed for survival and has a hierarchy of priorities for this aim[72]. The primary need is the conservation of the lean body mass defined as above as a composite of muscle, circulating enzymes, red blood cells, all the parenchymal organs, the immune organ and the water representing the metabolic and structural machinery of the body. Stated more simply the lean body mass is all that is not fat. Any reduction of this mass poses a risk to survival. This compartment is continuously refilled with the proteins derived from the diet. The average energy need of a healthy young 70 kg person is 2500 cal / die obtained from the diet. Usually 20% of these (125 gr) derive from protein. However in times of abundance, when the lean body mass is replete, the organism deals with the wound as a nutritional priority and any aminoacid and protein supply acquired through the diet are diverted to the wound to promote the closure[73]. This diversion to the skin is a damage to the lean body mass because subtracts the aminoacids from the diet in proportion to the size and the depth of the ulcer. If the lesion is exceedingly large and deep also the protein content of the lean body mass is catabolized to aminoacids to support the repair of the skin. When more than 15-20% [74,75,76] of the lean body mass is lost the survival mechanism changes radically its perspective and the true priority becomes the maintenance of this structure. Under these conditions the body uses all the hormonal and metabolic tools available to support the lean body mass, that includes antibodies and immune cells and almost nothing is left for the wound. The integrity of this lean mass is so critical that its reduction to $\leq$60% of the initial value usually leads to failure of the immune function and death due to pneumonitis[77].

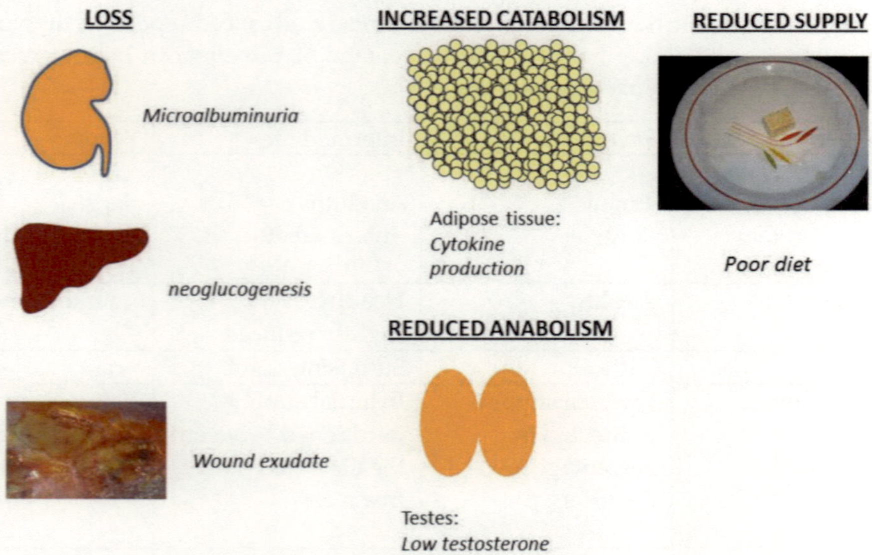

Fig. 1. Main causes of protein malnutrition in diabetes

We should envisage the body as a sophisticated system with a central compartment (Lean Body Mass, LBM) supplying the periphery on demand. If a peripheral lesion (the ulcer) supervenes the central compartment supplies protein until a danger level of depletion is reached. The human body does not have a reservoir of spare proteins, and these have a low energetic yield. Thus a critical level of depletion is reached soon. This phenomenon is even more prominent in the protein depleted diabetics. In these subjects the central compartment of LBM is frequently already in borderline-low conditions and subtracts all the alimentary supply of proteins. In these conditions an ulcer will never heal.

In summary, in the presence of a chronic ulcer in a longstanding diabetic subject, we must always assume the existence of a certain degree of lean body mass (LBM) loss. The Body Bioimpedance analysis (BIA) is a widely used method for estimating the body composition and the presence of this condition. The technology is relatively simple, quick and noninvasive and evaluates the electrical impedance of body tissues, which provides an estimate of total body water (TBW). This value can be used to calculate the fat-free mass (FFM) and body fat (adiposity).In addition this technology can be used to evaluate the body cell mass (BCM). When the BCM is corrected for the actual height of the subject (Body Cell Mass Index, BCMI) gives a very accurate estimate of the total cellular mass and is a useful tool to assess the nutritional state, more so if a previous report is available for comparison to estimate the degree of damage. [78]

Diabetic foot ulcers tend to occur in the advanced stages of the disease. The usual saying that a characteristic of early diabetes is the slow healing of wounds dates back to a period when the diagnosis of the disease was delayed. Today a diagnostic delay only occurs in the poor and the underprivileged. In these subjects the catabolic state is usually well advanced and the skin is thin with widespread loss of the subcutaneous tissue, and a chronic nonhealing ulcer can be a presenting sign of diabetes. We demonstrated in 700 diabetics that at this stage the loss of the lean body mass is already advanced, and that the use of re-feeding solutions containing an increased percentage of proteins can help to recreate the lean body mass[52] and the subcutaneous tissue[79]

Clinical scenario	Favorable	Intermediate	Worst
Wound: Size Caloric / protein requirement	 -Small -low	 -medium -intermediate	 -large -high
Lean body mass	-healthy	Healthy/ slightly reduced	-markedly reduced
Nutrition	Sufficient	Sufficient/scant	Scant
Pathophysiology	External supply redirected in percentage towards the ulcer	External supply partitioned between the ulcer and the fat free mass	External supply redirected towards the lean body mass
Ulcer	Heals rapidly	Ulcer healing delayed /absent	No ulcer healing

Current treatments

Since a single cause of the nonhealing diabetic foot ulcer has not been identified a variety of different products acting on, mimicking, or purportedly having magic qualities, have been introduced on the market without substantial proof of benefit, and often lacking rationale.

Although frequently emphasized, the general condition of the patient, the strict control of his blood glucose and the general nutritional status are too frequently overlooked, mostly in the general medical or surgical wards, where the attention is focused on the ulcer itself. The concern for the local factors and the commercial pressure of the pharmaceutical companies generated an incredible number of local treatments, including ointments, growth factors and the so called "advanced medications" containing a variety of metals and ions that should stimulate the reparative process. However the use of these substances did not demonstrate any substantial improvement in clinical studies. Although we do not think that these medications have a great role, we must acknowledge that proving the efficacy of these substances in healing ulcers with randomized controlled studies is a complicated and expensive task. It is evident that recruiting an adequate number of subjects with the same duration of disease, a similar degree of diabetic control, and an ulcer of the same characteristics for a randomized controlled trial is very difficult, and unless a substance has truly magical properties the statistical results will be open to discussion[80,81,82]

What starts the cascade of problems in the diabetic is an alteration of glucose metabolism that in turn causes a series of metabolic derangements, and the dire consequences that follow. In a recent study the Authors found a significant prevalence of HbA1c $\geq$7% (53 mmol/mol) and HDL $\leq$ 50 mg/dl in diabetic subjects with lower extremity disease versus those without.[83] But if things are so simple, why is the normalization of blood glucose alone not able to induce tissue regrowth and ulcer healing? The answer is that a diabetic foot ulcer only appears after a long period of decompensated diabetes, when the nerves, the skin and all the supporting tissues and structures are already severely damaged or impaired and the simple correction of the causal abnormality is not enough. In this respect is worthwhile to mention the results of the Accord study casting doubt on the feasibility of intensive blood glucose control in diabetic patients with complications. In this study after an average of 3.5 years, 257 people in the intensive blood glucose lowering strategy group died, compared to 203 participants in the standard strategy group. This difference of 54 deaths resulted in a 22 percent increased death rate in the intensive group. Since the presence of a DFU is a complication these results have an important bearing on the treatment of these subjects.[84]

Under normal circumstances the healing of an ulcer requires energy supplied by lipids and glucose. The role of glucose is probably the most complex because this molecule is part of the structural glycoproteins, of some enzymes[85,86] and fuels the inflammatory cells[87]. Lipids for the energetic needs of healing can be obtained from the diet or from fat deposits. As happens for glucose, lipids have multiple functions: the most well known is energy storage, but these molecules also have signaling capacity and are structural components of the cell membrane. Both glucose and lipids must be available for the normal healing processes of the ulcers, but diabetics have a characteristic difficulty disposing of glucose inside the cells that can be only partially reversed with the available treatments. Proteins are structural components of the skin, but these subjects almost always have a degree of preexistent protein deficiency that must be taken into account when planning a diet. Estimating the degree of deficiency is the difficult part because the body composition is an individual characteristic and no "normal values" exist. The available tools to evaluate the degree of LBM and indirectly the degree of protein loss, like Bioimpedance Analysis and Skin Fold Thickness, are only useful in the presence of previous records of the same subject. The body weight loss, another simple and sequentially available measurement does not give any information on the body compartments and is thus of limited utility. However the presence of a nonhealing ulcer implies the loss of at least 20% of the LBM. When estimating the calorie-protein need of a diabetic the most reasonable option is to err on the excessive side.

Although the role of nutrition is crucial and usually acknowledged, it is surprising how often is overlooked in practice. The most recent edition of the ADA book on the treatment of DFU[88] does not even mention the general condition and the nutritional status of the patient among the aspects to evaluate.

Our hypothesis is that the damage to the tissues is both preventable and at least partially reversible if the treatment is directed towards all the main causal factors. In other words, in our opinion if the vascular blood supply is normalized, the blood glucose level is kept under control, the abnormal pressure is reduced with adequate biophysical support and the texture of the skin is reconstituted there is absolutely no place for growth factors, colloids, metals or whatever else. The diabetic now has the same ability to heal as nondiabetics. The reconstitution of the skin requires the supply of proteins and other biological material that is usually reduced in the diabetic and must be supplied with adequate nutrition. The avoidance of relapses requires attention to postural and neurologic factors.

4. Treatment

The role of the nutritional condition of the patient with a DFU is crucial to the pathogenesis and treatment of the lesion, but infrequently recognized or treated. Accordingly, we think that the term "treatment of the DFU" is a misnomer and should be substituted with "treatment of the subject with a DFU". We suggest a series of steps[89]:

1. Whenever possible the nutritional condition should be assessed as accurately as possible, with Bio-Impedance Analysis, Skin Fold Thickness, Body Weight and Blood chemistry studies (protein electrophoresis, BUN, Hemogram). If previous values are available the change should be included as part of this assessment.
2. The resting caloric requirement should be calculated as 20-25 kcal/kg body weight. This value decreases in the elderly. The value so obtained should be multiplied by 1.2-1.5 according to the severity of the lesion.[90] This figure should be increased if there is evidence of malnutrition.
3. Add the caloric expenditure of activity. All these measurements can be obtained with the use of indirect calorimetry or with the recently introduced non-invasive tools worn at the arm that are worn over a longer period of time. The statistical elaboration of the Bio-Impedance Analysis can yield a reliable estimate of the Basal Metabolic Rate
4. The value so obtained should be multiplied by a "stress factor" that varies from 1.2 for clean wounds, to 1.5 in the case of infected wounds

All these calories should be replaced with an adequate diet, with no less that 20-22% protein given in at least three divided doses throughout the day. These values should be increased by 30-50% according to the co-morbidities of the subject. Paddon Jones suggests that non diabetic elders should have a minimum of 15 g of essential amino acids, equivalent to about

30 g of high-quality dietary protein at each meal.[91] Although there are no fast and hard rules this figure must be increased in the diabetic with a chronic wound.

Another critical component is hydration[92]. We suggest to drink at least 2-3 lt of water per day. In addition to the maintenance of the circulation and the tissue exchange of metabolites, the water induced diuresis helps the body to get rid of the excess glucose.

Some trace substances and vitamins are also absolutely needed for the healing process. In particular Vitamin C, E, Selenium and β-carotene with strong antioxidant properties that antagonize the harmful oxygen free radicals (ROS) present in excess in the chronic wound[93]. Vitamin C is also needed for collagen formation.[94]

The progression of the ulcer should be evaluated with inspection, with photographic records including a ruler close to the lesion, with the biochemical analytes useful to monitor the inflammation and the nutritional state (ESR, Hemogram, CRP, Albumin and Prealbumin levels), and the BIA.

5. The role of supplements

The body of the diabetic is in a general catabolic state and restituting the normal catabolism is a distinctive advantage for the treatment. According to this principle testosterone treatment has been instituted.[95] We use transdermal testosterone supplement in testosterone deficient subjects with apparent reduction in healing time, although we did not conduct a systematic study. Other anabolic hormones have been used with variable results.[96] We have a good experience with an oral nutritional supplement, a blend containing Argine, glutamine and β-hydroxy- β -methyl-butyrate (HMB). HMB is normally present in the muscle, is an active leucine metabolite and a potent stimulator of mTOR (Mammalian Target of Rapamycin), an intracellular protein controlling protein synthesis.[97,98] Due to this anabolic property, the substance is widely used by the athletes worldwide, and to reverse the effects of aging.[99] Glutamine also has a spectrum of positive effects[100], notably stimulation of protein synthesis and support of immune function.[101,102] and a positive effect on intestinal integrity.[103] Its effectiveness in collagen formation has also been consistently proven.[104] Arginine also has a positive effect on wound healing[105], and stimulates immune function.[106,107] Arginine also has a vasodilator action[108] that was exploited for male erectile dysfunction before the introduction of the phosphodiesterase inhibitors. In our experience the use of this blend reduced to 1/3 the time to healing in a group of 12 diabetic patients while improving the lean body mass.[109] We also found an unexpected reduction of microalbuminuria in 16 diabetic subjects under treatment with this blend, which might concur to explain the increase in lean body cell mass[110]

It should be emphasized that the use of anabolic substances or blends is no substitute for an adequate nutrition with enough protein, calories, minerals, vitamins and iron that can be found in the normal Western diet. Therefore, the best nutritional approach to the diabetic patient is: (1) the evaluation of the degree of wasting of the lean body mass and of the degree of current needs; (2) institution of a diet supplying what is missing and what is currently required, supplemented with enough protein, and distributed in at least three meals per day. This diet should be integrated with vitamins, minerals and iron; (3) use of anabolic agents or a blend of the three substances we used. Irrespective of which medical treatment will be used, the closure of a wound will be impossible unless these steps are followed.

6. References

[1] McNeely MJ, et Al: The independent contributions of diabetic neuropathy and vasculopathy in foot ulceration. *Diabetes Care* 18:216–219, 1995

[2] National Diabetes Data Group: *Diabetes in America*. Vol. 2. Bethesda, MD, National Institutes of Health, 1995 (NIH publ. no.95–1468)

[3] Van Baal J, MSC et Al. Mortality Associated With Acute Charcot Foot and Neuropathic Foot Ulceration. *Diabetes Care* 33:1086–1089, 2010

[4] Leese GP, et Al A: Predicting foot ulceration in diabetes: validation of a clinical tool in a population-based study. Int J Clin Prac 60:541–545, 2006

[5] Tan PL, Teh J. MRI of the diabetic foot: differentiation of infection from neuropathic change. *Br J Radiol. Nov 2007;80(959):939-48.*

[6] Christian Weigelt, MD et Al. Immune Mediators in Patients With Acute Diabetic Foot Syndrome. *Diabetes* Care 32(2009):1491–1496,

[7] Calle-Pascual A. et Al, Reduction in Foot Ulcer Incidence (letter). *Diabetes Care, Volume 24, N 2, (2001):405-7*

[8] Van Schie C. H.M., PHD et Al. Muscle Weakness and Foot Deformities in Diabetes. *Diabetes Care, Vol 27, N 7, (2004):1668-73*

[9] Sicco A. Intrinsic Muscle Atrophy and Toe Deformity in the Diabetic Neuropathic Foot. *Diabetes Care 25 (2002):1444–1450*

[10] Boulton AJ, Vileikyte L: The diabetic foot: the scope of the problem. *J Fam Pract 49 (Suppl. 11):S3–S8, 2000*

[11] Levin M: Pathophysiology of diabetic foot lesions. In Clinical Diabetes Mellitus: A Problem-Oriented Approach. *Davidson JK, Ed. New York, Theme Medical, 1991, p. 504 –510*

[12] Lawrence A. L . et Al Risk Factors for Foot Infections in Individuals With Diabetes. *Diabetes Care 29 (2002):1288 –1293*

[13] Reiber GE et Al Causal pathways for incident lower-extremity ulcers in patients with diabetes from two settings. *Diabetes Care.1999;22:157–62.*

[14] Vinik A. et Al. Diabetic Autonomic neuropathy. *Diabetes Care, Vol 26, N 5, (2003):1553-79*

[15] Vinik, AI. Et Al. Diabetic neuropathies: an overview of clinical aspects. In: LeRoith, D.; Taylor, SI.; Olefsky, JM., editors. *Diabetes Mellitus. Philadelphia, New-York: Lippincott-Raven Publishers; 1996. p. 737-751.*

[16] Boulton AJM. The diabetic foot: from art to science. The 18th Camillo Golgi lecture. *Diabetologia (2004);47:1343–1353*

[17] Armstrong DG, et Al. The natural history of acute Charcot's arthropathy in a diabetic foot specialty clinic. *Diabet Med (1997);14:357-63*

[18] Brower AC, Allman RM. The neuropathic joint: a neurovascular bone disorder. *Radiol Clin North Am (1981);19:571-80*

[19] Zimn S et Al. The Role of Limited Joint Mobility in Diabetic Patients With an At-Risk Foot. *Diabetes Care 27(2004):942–946*

[20] Dyck PJ. Detection, characterization, and staging of polyneuropathy: assessed in diabetics. *Muscle Nerve (1988);11:21–32. [PubMed: 3277049]*

[21] Boulton AJ,et Al . Diabetic neuropathies: a statement by the American Diabetes Association. *Diabetes Care (2005);28:956–962. [PubMed: 15793206]*

[22] Adler AI et Al. Association between glycated haemoglobin and the risk of lower extremity amputation in patients with diabetes mellitus – review and meta-analysis. *Diabetologia (2010) 53:840–849*

[23] Thomas PK. Diabetic neuropathy: mechanisms and future treatment options. *J Neurol Neurosurg Psychiatry (1999);67:277–279. [PubMed: 10449543]*

[24] Thomas PK. Classification, differential diagnosis, and staging of diabetic peripheral neuropathy. *Diabetes (1997);46 (Suppl 2):S54–S57. [PubMed: 9285500]*

[25] Lasker RD. The diabetes control and complications trial. Implications for policy and practice. *NE J Med (1993);329:1035–1036. [PubMed: 8366905]*

[26] The Diabetes Control and Complications Trial Research Group (DCCT). The effect of intensive treatment of diabetes on the development and progression of long term complications in insulin-dependent diabetes mellitus. *N Engl J Med (1993);329:977–986. [PubMed: 8366922]*

[27] Sugimoto K, Murakawa Y, Sima AA. Diabetic neuropathy--a continuing enigma. *Diabetes Metab Res Rev (2000);16:408–433. [PubMed: 11114101]*

[28] Young RJ et Al. A controlled trial of sorbinil, an aldose reductase inhibitor, in chronic painful diabetic neuropathy. *Diabetes (1983);32:938–942. [PubMed: 6225686]*

[29] Argoff CE, et Al. Diabetic peripheral neuropathic pain: clinical and quality-of-life issues. *Mayo Clin Proc (2006);81:S3–11. [PubMed: 16608048]*

[30] Singleton JR, et Al. Increased prevalence of impaired glucose tolerance in patients with painful sensory neuropathy. *Diabetes Care (2001);24:1448–1453. [PubMed: 11473085]*

[31] Novella SP, et Al. The frequency of undiagnosed diabetes and impaired glucose tolerance in patients with idiopathic sensory neuropathy. *Muscle Nerve (2001);24:1229–1231. [PubMed: 11494278]*

[32] Brussee V, et Al. Direct insulin signaling of neurons reverses diabetic neuropathy. *Diabetes (2004);53:1824–1830. [PubMed: 15220207]*

[33] Huang TJ, et Al. Insulin prevents depolarization of the mitochondrial inner membrane in sensory neurons of type 1 diabetic rats in the presence of sustained hyperglycemia. *Diabetes (2003);52:2129–2136. [PubMed: 12882932]*

[34] Sugimoto K, et Al. Insulin receptor in rat peripheral nerve: its localization and alternatively spliced isoforms. *Diabetes Metab Res Rev (2000);16:354–363. [PubMed: 11025559]*

[35] Singhal A et Al. Near nerve local insulin prevents conduction slowing in experimental diabetes. *Brain Res (1997);763:209–214. [PubMed: 9296561]*

[36] Brussee V, et Al. Direct insulin signaling of neurons reverses diabetic neuropathy. *Diabetes (2004);53:1824–1830. [PubMed: 15220207]*

[37] Singleton JR, et Al . Polyneuropathy with Impaired Glucose Tolerance: Implications for Diagnosis and Therapy. *Curr Treat Options Neurol (2005);7:33–42. [PubMed: 15610705]*

[38] Russell JW, Feldman EL. Impaired glucose tolerance--does it cause neuropathy? *Muscle Nerve (2001);24:1109–1112. [PubMed: 11494263]*

[39] Frasca F, et Al. Insulin receptor isoform A, a newly recognized, high-affinity insulin-like growth factor II receptor in fetal and cancer cells. *Mol Cell Biol (1999);19:3278–3288. [PubMed: 10207053]*

[40] Rajkumar K, et Al. Impaired glucose homeostasis in insulin-like growth factor binding protein-1 transgenic mice. *J Clin Invest (1996);98:1818–1825. [PubMed: 8878433]*

[41] Meier C, et Al . Developing Schwann cells acquire the ability to survive without axons by establishing an autocrine circuit involving insulin-like growth factor, neurotrophin-3, and platelet-derived growth factor-BB. *J Neurosci (1999);19:3847–3859. [PubMed: 10234017]*

[42] Zhuang HX et Al. Insulin-like growth factor (IGF) gene expression is reduced in neural tissues and liver from rats with non-insulin-dependent diabetes mellitus, and IGF treatment ameliorates diabetic neuropathy. *J Pharmacol Exp Ther (1997);283:366–374. [PubMed: 9336345]*

[43] Selvin E et Al. Glycemic control, atherosclerosis and risk factors for cardiovascular disease in individuals with diabetes. *Diabetes Care 28:1965–1973, 2005*

[44] Delamaire, M et Al. Impaired leucocyte functions in diabetic patients *Diabet. Med. (1997), 14, 29-34*

[45] Davidson, N.J. et Al Defective phagocytosis in insulin controlled diabetics: evidence for a reaction between glucose and opsonising proteins. *J. Clin. Pathol., (1984),37, 783-6.*

[46] Collison, K.S et Al. RAGE-mediated neutrophil dysfunction is evoked by advanced glycation end products (AGEs), *J. Leukoc. Biol. (2002), 71, 433-44*

[47] Thomas PK. Diabetic neuropathy: mechanisms and future treatment options. *J Neurol Neurosurg Psychiatry (1999);67:277–279. [PubMed: 10449543]*

[48] Zochodne DW. Neurotrophins and other growth factors in diabetic neuropathy. *Semin Neurol (1996);16:153–161. [PubMed: 8987129]*

[49] Britland ST et Al. Association of painful and painless diabetic polyneuropathy with different patterns of nerve fiber degeneration and regeneration. *Diabetes (1990);39:898–908. [PubMed: 2373262]*

[50] Sima AA. Peripheral neuropathy in the spontaneously diabetic BB-Wistar-rat. *An ultrastructural study. Acta Neuropathol (Berl) (1980);51:223–227. [PubMed: 7445976]*

[51] Liuzzi FJ, Bufton SM, Vinik AI. Streptozotocin-induced diabetes mellitus causes changes in primary sensory neuronal cytoskeletal mRNA levels that mimic those caused by axotomy. *Exp Neurol (1998);154:381–388. [PubMed: 9878176]*

[52] Dobretsov M et Al. Early diabetic neuropathy: Triggers and mechanisms. *World J Gastroenterol. (2007) January 14; 13(2): 175–191.*

[53] Peppa M et Al. Glucose, Advanced Glycation End Products, and Diabetes Complications: What Is New and What Works. *Clinical Diabetes, Volume 21, Number 4, (2003):186-7*

[54] Tatti P et Al. Reduced body cell mass in type 2 diabetes mellitus: reversal with a diabetes specific nutritional Formula. *Mediterr J Nutr Metab (2010) 3:133–136*

[55] *Webster's Medical Dictionary*

[56] Monnier L, Colette C. Contributions of fasting and postprandial glucose to hemoglobin A1c._*Endocr Pract (2006) Jan-Feb;12 Suppl 1:42-6*

[57] DeFronzo RA, Banting Lecture. *Diabetes, Vol. 58, April 2009:773-95*

[58] Guerrero-Romero F, Rodriguez-Mòran M. Relationship of microalbuminuria with the diabetic foot ulcers in type II diabetes. *J Diabetes Complications, (1998) Jul-Aug;12(4):193-6.*

[59] M. Lehnhardt et Al. A qualitative and quantitative analysis of protein loss in human burn wounds. *Burns Vol 31, issue 2, (March 2005); 159-67*

[60] Koya D et Al. Long term effect of modification of dietary protein intake on the progression of diabetic nephropathy: a randomized controlled trial. *Diabetologia (2009)52:2037-45*

[61] Biolo G, et Al. Physiological hyperinsulinemia stimulates protein synthesis and enhances transport of selected amino acids in human skeletal muscle. *J Clin Invest 95 (1995): 811–819*

[62] Fryburg DA, et Al. Insulin and insulin-like growth factor-1 enhance human skeletal muscle protein anabolism during hyperaminoacidemia by different mechanisms. *J Clin Invest 96 (1995): 1722–1729,.*

[63] Mo¨ller-Loswick AC, et Al. Insulin selectively attenuates breakdown of nonmyofibrillar proteins in peripheral tissues of normal men. *Am J Physiol Endocrinol Metab 266 (1994): E645–E652,.*

[64] Grossmann M, et AL. Low testosterone levels are common and associated with insulin resistance in men with diabetes. *J Clin Endocrinol Metab 93 (2008):1834-40.*

[65] Sandeep Dhindsa, et Al. Testosterone Concentrations in Diabetic and Nondiabetic Obese Men. *Diabetes Care 33 (2010):1186–1192,*

[66] Dhindsa S, et Al. Frequent occurrence of hypogonadotropic hypogonadism in type 2 diabetes.*J Clin Endocrinol Metab (2004);89:5462–5468*

[67] Dhindsa S, et Al. The effects of hypogonadism on body composition and bone mineral density in type 2 diabetic patients. *Diabetes Care (2007);30:1860–1861*

[68] Zochodne DW. Neurotrophins and other growth factors in diabetic neuropathy. *Semin Neurol (1996);16:153–161. [PubMed: 8987129]*

[69] Britland ST et Al. Association of painful and painless diabetic polyneuropathy with different patterns of nerve fiber degeneration and regeneration. *Diabetes 39 (1990);898–908. [PubMed: 2373262]*

[70] Sima AA. Peripheral neuropathy in the spontaneously diabetic BB-Wistar-rat. An ultrastructural study. *Acta Neuropathol (Berl) (1980);51:223–227. [PubMed: 7445976]*

[71] Liuzzi FJ, et AI. Streptozotocin-induced diabetes mellitus causes changes in primary sensory neuronal cytoskeletal mRNA levels that mimic those caused by axotomy. *Exp Neurol (1998);154:381–388. [PubMed: 9878176]*

[72] Moore FD, Brennan M. Surgical injury, body composition, protein metabolism and neuron-endocrinology. In: *Ballinger W, Collins J, eds. Manual of Surgical Nutrition. Philadelphia, Pa: W. B. Saunders; (1975);169–202.*

[73] Wernerman J, et Al. The effect of stress hormones on the interorgan flux of amino acids and concentration of free amino acids in skeletal muscle. *Clin Nutr. (1985);4:207–16*

[74] Say J. The metabolic changes associated with trauma and sepsis [review]. *Nurs Crit Care. (1997);2:83–7.*

[75] Chiolíro R, et Al. Energy metabolism in sepsis and injury [review]. *Nutrition. (1997);13, suppl 9:45S–51S.*

[76] Cartwright M. The metabolic response to stress: a case of complex nutrition support management [review]. *Crit Care Nurs Clin North Am. (2004);16:467–87.*

[77] Moran L, et Al. Nutritional assessment of lean body mass. *J Pen. (1980);4:595.*

[78] A. Talluri. The application of body cell mass index for studying muscle mass changes in health and disease conditions. Acta Diabetologica. Volume 40, Supplement 1, s286-s289, DOI: 10.1007/s00592-003-0088-9

[79] Tatti P et Al. Extremely accelerated healing of diabetic foot ulcers with medical nutrition therapy: *Int J Diabetes & Metabolism (2009) 17:115-116*

[80] Ritu Jones et Al. The external validity of published randomized controlled trials in primary care BMC Family Practice *(2009), 10:5 doi:10.1186/1471-2296-10-5*

[81] Tones K. Evaluating health promotion—beyond the RCT. In: *Norheim L, Waller M, eds. Best Practices, Quality and Effectiveness of Health Promotion. Helsinki, Finland: Finnish Centre for Health Promotion; 2000: 86–101*

[82] Sibbald B, Roland M. Understanding controlled trials: Why are randomised controlled trials important? *BMJ 316 : 201 (Published 17 January 1998)*

[83] Dorsey RR, et Al. Control of risk factors among people with diagnosed diabetes, by lower extremity disease status. Prev Chronic Dis 2009;6(4). http://www.cdc.gov/pcd/issues/2009/oct/08_0224.htm

[84] The Action to Control Cardiovascular Risk in Diabetes Study Group. Effects of Intensive Glucose Lowering in Type 2 Diabetes. N Engl J Med 2008; 358:2545-2559 June 12, 2008

[85] Irelton-Jones C, Liepa R. Carbohydrates and wound healing in nutrition. In: *Molner J, ed. Nutrition and Wound Healing. Boca Raton, Fla: CRC press; (2006):5.*

[86] Patel G. The role of nutrition in managing lower extremity wounds. *Int J Low Extrem Wounds. (2005);4:12–22*

[87] Hart D, Wolf S, Zhang X, et al. Efficacy of a high energy carbohydrate diet in catabolic illness. *Crit Care Med. (2001);29:1318*

[88] American Diabetes Association. Clinical Care of the diabetic Foot, *2nd Edition (2010)*

[89] Demling RH. Nutrition, Anabolism, and the Wound Healing Process: *An Overview. ePlasty, published Feb 3, Vol 9(2009):65-94*

[90] Dorner B et al. The role of nutrition in pressure ulcer prevention and treatment: National Pressure Ulcer Advisory Panel White Paper. *Adv Skin Wound Care 2009;22:212-221.*

[91] Paddon-Jones D et al. Dietary protein recommendations and the prevention of sarcopenia.*Curr Opin Clin Nutr Metabolic Care 2009;12:86-90.*

[92] Institute of Medicine. National Academy of Sciences: Dietary Reference Intakes for Water, Potassium,Sodium, Chloride, and Sulfate. *Washington, DC, 2004. Http://www.iom.edu/?id=54343 "http://www.iom.edu/?id=54343*

[93] Clark RAF. Oxidative stress and "senescent" fibroblasts in nonhealing wounds as potential therapeutic targets. *J Invest Dermatol (2008);128:2361-2364.*

[94] Morris SM. Recent advances in arginine metabolism: roles and regulation of the arginases. *Br J Pharmacol (2009);157:922-930*

[95] Demling R, DeSanti L. The anabolic steroid oxandrolone reverses the wound healing impairment in corticosteroid dependent burn and wound patients. *Wounds. (2001):203–8.*

[96] Lang C, Frost R. Role of growth hormone, insulin-like growth factor-1 and insulin-like growth factor binding proteins in the catabolic response to injury and infection. *Curr Opin Clin Nutr Metab Care.* 2002:271–9.

[97] Manzano M, et Al. Is β-hydroxy-β-methylbutyrate (HMB) the bioactive metabolite of L-leucine (LEU) in muscle? Molecular evidence and potential implications. *Abstract presented at: European Society for Clinical Nutrition and Metabolism 31st Congress; Vienna, Austria; August 29-September 1, (2009). Abstract P267.*

[98] Baxter J et Al. *4th cachexia conference 2007, Abstract 1.18*

[99] Wilson GJ et Al. Effects of beta-hydroxy-beta-methylbutyrate (HMB) on exercise performance and body composition across varying levels of age, sex, and training experience: *A review. Nutrition & Metabolism 2008, 5:1 doi:10.1186/1743-7075-5-1*

[100] Peng Xi et Al. Clinical and protein metabolic efficacy of glutamine granules-supplemented enteral nutrition in severely burned patients. *Burns, Vol 31, issue 3 (2005):342-6*

[101] Wilmore DW. The Effect of Glutamine Supplementation in Patients Following Elective Surgery and Accidental Injury. *J Nutr. (2001);131, Suppl 9:2543S-9S*

[102] Moccheggiani E et Al. Effect of L-arginine on thymic function. Possible role of L-arginine: Nitric oxide (no) pathway. *Archives of Gerontology and Geriatrics. Volume 19, Supplement 1,*(1994): 163-170

[103] Van del Hulst et Al. Glutamine and the preservation of gut integrity. *Lancet., 1993 May 29;341(8857):1363-5.*

[104] Williams JZ. Effect of a Specialized Amino Acid Mixture on Human Collagen Deposition. *Ann Surg. (2002) September; 236(3): 369–375.*

[105] Curran JN et Al. Biological fate and clinical implications of arginine metabolism in tissue healing. *Wound Repair and Regeneration, Volume 14, Issue 4 July–August (2006): 376–386, 2006*

[106] Barbul A et Al. Arginine enhances wound healing and lymphocyte immune responses in humans. *Surgery. (1990) Aug;108(2):331-6*

[107] Witte MB, Barbul A. Arginine physiology and its implication for wound healing. *Wound Repair and Regeneration, Volume 11, Issue 6, November (2003):419–423,*

[108] Rhodes P et Al. Arginine, lysine and ornithine as vasodilators in the forearm of man. *European Journal of Clinical Investigation, Volume 26, Issue 4, April (1996) pages 325–331*

[109] Tatti P, Barber AB. Nutritional supplement is associated with a reduction in healing time and improvement of fat-free body mass in patients with diabetic foot ulcers. *EWMA Journal vol 10 no 3(2010): 13-17*

[110] Tatti P et Al. Effect of a nutritional supplement used for diabetic foot ulcers on microalbuminuria. DOI 10.1007/s12349-011-0072-9

12

Intralesional Human Recombinant Epidermal Growth Factor for the Treatment of Advanced Diabetic Foot Ulcer: From Proof of Concept to Confirmation of the Efficacy and Safety of the Procedure

Pedro A. López-Saura et al.*
Center for Genetic Engineering and Biotechnology, Havana, Cuba

1. Introduction

Foot ulceration is among the most significant complications of diabetes. It is estimated that 15% of the diabetic patients develop ulcers at some point in their lives (Reiber, 1996). The therapeutic management of a diabetic patient carrying a diabetic foot ulcer (DFU) is currently based on: metabolic control, debridement (Brem et al., 2004), moist cures, wound dressing, local pressure off-loading, antimicrobial treatment of infections, and revascularization procedures, when indicated. More recent therapies such as topical growth factors (Tsang et al., 2003; Brem et al., 2004; Eldor et al., 2004; Hong et al., 2006; Viswanathan et al., 2006), skin substitutes (Marston et al., 2003; Veves et al., 2001), and others have shown efficacy in pure neuropathic, non-complicated ulcers. However, these products would still have to be tested in advanced lesions including those with an ischemic etiopathogenic component. Still 10 to 30% of the cases progress to amputation, frequently preceded by gangrene and infection (Lipsky, 2004). After amputation of a lower limb, the five year mortality rate reaches 50-60% (Reiber, 1996). Therefore, despite progress in the diagnosis and treatment of infection and other complications (Lipsky, 2004; Williams et al., 2004), the advanced DFU is still an unmet medical need.

The local (intralesional) instillation of recombinant human epidermal growth factor (rhEGF) to promote granulation and healing of chronic, advanced DFU has been recently introduced in medical practice in some countries. This chapter will review the rationale, experimental background, and clinical development of such procedure.

---

* Jorge Berlanga-Acosta[1], José I. Fernández-Montequín[2], Carmen Valenzuela-Silva[1], Odalys González-Díaz[1], William Savigne[2], Lourdes Morejon-Vega[2], Amaurys del Río-Martín[1], Luis Herrera-Martínez[1], Ernesto López-Mola[1] and Boris Acevedo-Castro[1]
[1]*Center for Genetic Engineering and Biotechnology, Havana, Cuba*
[2]*National Institute for Angiology and Vascular Surgery, Havana, Cuba*

2. Why can Epidermal Growth Factor (EGF) be used for the treatment of Diabetic Foot Ulcers (DFU)?

Epidermal growth factor (EGF) is a 53 aminoacid polypeptide that was isolated for the first time by Cohen from mice submaxillary glands (Cohen, 1962). It stimulates the proliferation of fibroblasts, keratinocytes and vascular endothelial cells, which contribute to its scar tissue formation property. Its action is launched by the interaction with specific receptors located on the cellular membrane. The EGF receptor is a glycoprotein with an extracellular binding domain, a transmembrane region and a cytoplasmic portion with tyrosine kinase activity (Bazley & Gullick, 2005). This receptor is expressed on most human cell types including those which play critical roles for wound repair such as fibroblasts, endothelial cells and keratinocytes (undifferentiated, marginal, leading edge, hair follicles, sweat ducts and sebaceous glands). Only hematopoietic cell lineages lack the EGF receptor (Werner & Grose, 2003). The rationale of the use of Epidermal Growth Factor (EGF) for the treatment of (DFU) is based on:

2.1 Impairment of healing in diabetic patients, partially due to a relative deficit of growth factors (EGF among them) in the wound area

Wound healing is an ancestral mechanism evolutionarily designed to ensure the structural and functional restoration of an injured area. The mechanism involves cellular responses from two major classes: (i) repair-committed cells such as fibroblasts, other mesenchymal-derived cells, endothelial / angiogenic precursor cells and epithelial keratinocytes and (ii) inflammatory cells that are transiently recruited and temporarily infiltrate the wound (Eming et al., 2007). Under physiological conditions this process is ensued by inflammatory cells' progressive apoptosis and inflammation cessation. Although in diabetic wounds the cells and the pro-inflammatory cytokines are the same than in non-diabetic, acute counterparts; inflammation is more a condition than a reaction. The perpetuation of neutrophils, macrophages and their related pro-inflammatory cytokines in diabetic wounds contribute to the onset of a pro-degradative microenvironment which results from the imbalance between matrix synthesis and degradation (Berlanga et al., 2008).

Under these circumstances the local pool of growth factors (GFs) and their corresponding receptors turn detrimental due to a reduced transcriptional expression by the wound bed committed cells and/or to increased enzymatic degradation (Clark, 2008). The role of GFs turns more important in the context of a diabetic wound since high glucose levels and other associated metabolic by-products are toxic for endothelial and fibroblastic cells, which become arrested and senescent. In this environment the granulation tissue promoting cells launch a pro-apoptogenic program which eventually hinders the granulation process (Goren et al., 2006). The observation that diabetic wounds are enriched in proteases supports the premise that impaired GFs availability may act as a rate limiting factor in diabetic wound healing (Burrow et al., 2007), which justifies an appropriate wound bed preparation and a GFs replacement therapy.

2.2 The growth stimulating, healing promoting, and cytoprotective actions of EGF, including angiogenesis

The EGF family of ligands exhibit mitogenic activity upon binding to four different high-affinity receptors: EGFR/ErbB1, HER2/ErbB2, HER3/ErbB3, and HER4/ErbB4. Upon ligand binding, the formation of a functionally active EGFR-EGFR homodimer or EGFR-HER2, EGFR-HER3, or EGFR-HER4 heterodimers causes the ATP-dependent phosphorylation of specific tyrosine residues in the EGFR intracellular domain, which triggers a complex program of intracellular signals to the cytoplasm and then to the nucleus (Citri & Yarden, 2006).

Another biological action unleashed by the EGF-EGFR binomium is the locomotion stimulation of epithelial and fibroblastic cells (Barrandon & Green, 1987). This pro-motogenic impulse induced by the EGF-EGFR complex on keratinocytes is important for re-epithelialization. EGF can also control fibroblasts extension, attachment or detachment directly or indirectly via modifications of the injured tissue extracellular matrix composition (Maheshwari et al., 1999).

The EGF-induced mitogenic, motogenic, and cyto-protective actions are instrumental for healing events that may be summarized as: (a) stimulation of productive cells migration toward the injured area, (b) stimulation of granulation tissue outgrowth - including extracellular matrix accumulation, maturation and de novo angiogenesis, (c) stimulation of wound contraction by myofibroblast activation and proliferation, (d) stimulation of the damaged area resurfacing by epithelial cells migration and proliferation (Werner & Grose, 2003).

EGF is also endowed with angiogenic activity thus promoting the growth of a vascular mesh within the wound bed. The mechanisms behind this angiogenic effect appears to be related to chemotaxis of endothelial cells and the enhancement of other angiogenic factors expression (van Cruijsen et al., 2005). This EGF-mediated neoangiogenic action is significant for ischemic wounds (Grazul-Bilska et al., 2003).

2.3 The nerve restoration action of EGF in sciatic nerve section experiments, where it prevented distal limb ulcers and toe loss

Several experiments demonstrated that single or repeated EGF systemic injections exerted cyto-protective and proliferative responses, supporting the intrinsic ability of EGF at supra-physiological concentrations to unleash biological events required for an effective tissue repair (Berlanga et al., 1998a, 1999, 2001, 2002a, 2002b).

The effect of an EGF local injection was evaluated for the first time in tissues unrelated to the digestive system (which at the moment was the most common experimental substrate - Curling's ulcers prevention) through the perilesional injection of EGF in rats that had been subjected to a complete sciatic nerve section. Two independent studies demonstrated that the intralesional injection of EGF produced: (i) recovery of the motor nerve impulse conduction; (ii) axonal recovery and remyelination, and (iii) prevented or delayed the onset of trophic changes of the hind limb soft tissues (plantar ulcers and toe necrosis). These sciatic nerve experiments suggested the possibility for a pharmacological management of trophic ulcers derived from a neurogenic ischemia (Prats et al., 1998). This animal model somewhat mirrored the condition of a neurogenic diabetic lower extremity in which both neuropathy and angiopathy concertedly predispose to ulceration (Dyck & Giannini, 1996).

3. Why EGF has to be injected intralesionally?

3.1 The availability of the growth factor on the surface of the wound is limited as it can be degraded by proteases from the biofilm that covers the lesion and/or from its fluid

The need for a prolonged interaction between EGF and its receptor to achieve a significant granulation tissue response in controlled wounds in mice had been reported (Buckley et al., 1985). Proteolysis exerted by the wound-derived exudate was observed incubating the ulcers´ material at neutral pH with a fluorescent-synthetic peptide at room temperature. Pre-incubation with a protease inhibitor prevented substrate's degradation. These observations suggested a possible reduction of EGF bioavailability by proteases derived from controlled wounds (Berlanga et al., 1998b). Other studies had already established proteolysis of growth factors and their receptors in chronic circumstances (Mast & Schultz, 1996; Saarialho-Kere, 1998; Trengove et al., 1999;, Medina et al., 2005).

Furthermore, profiles of ^{125}I-EGF in a rat full-thickness wound model, demonstrated tissue-bound radioactivity 2 h after the administration. Within this period, ^{125}I-EGF degraded subspecies with no diffusion of the peptide to the surrounding skin were identified. The receptor expression was increased 2 h after wounding, followed by a slow decline up to 12 h below baseline. These results point out that ^{125}I-EGF is rapidly cleared from the application site probably by protease-driven cleavage and receptor-mediated endocytosis. The mean residence time (MRT) values suggested that more than 60% of the amount administered could have disappeared as early as 2 hour post-administration (Prats et al., 2002). Previous clinical evidences of topically applied EGF had already rendered disappointing results possibly due to local bioavailability limitations (Falanga et al., 1992;, Falanga, 1992).

3.2 Responding granulation tissue develops from the deep layers of the wound

An immuno-histochemical characterization of biopsy cylinders from diabetic wound beds shed more light on the biological sustentation for the infiltrative modality. Granulation tissue biopsy cylinders (approximately 7 millimeters length) from neuropathic patients were collected and paraffin-processed for different histochemical techniques and for incubation with anti-EGF receptor and anti-prohibitin (PHB) antibodies. The monoclonal antibody against EGF receptor EGFR-pY1197 (1:250, DAKO) binds to tyrosine residue 1197 when it is phosphorylated, indicating downstream signaling activation. Prohibitin rabbit monoclonal (Abcam. EP2804Y) was diluted at 1:200. EnVision + Dual Link System-HRP was used to develop the reaction. Slides were hematoxylin counterstained. Pictures were obtained at X 40 constant magnification. The figure shows three strata along the longitudinal axis of the biopsy material were defined: upper, middle, and bottom. Fibroblasts populating the more superficial stratum expressed more prohibitin and less EGF-receptor. Prohibitin is an inhibitor of cell cycle progression and may therefore contribute to the onset of wound's chronic phenotype. (Mishra et al., 2010; Lee et al., 2010; Dong et al. 2010). This expression profile became progressively inverted going through deeper cells layers (Fig. 1). Advanced glycation end products and elastase also appeared more intensely labeled next to the wound surface than in deeper cells strata (not shown).

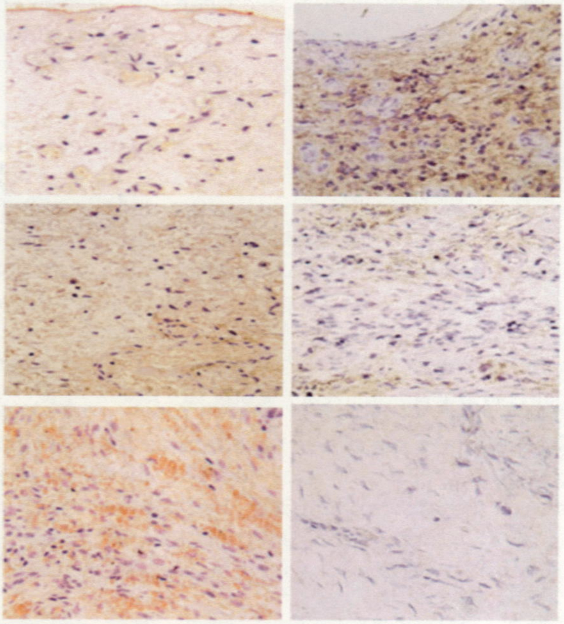

Fig. 1. EGF receptor (left) and prohibitin (right) expressions along the biopsy longitudinal axis.

4. Clinical development of intralesional recombinant human EGF in advanced DFU. Efficacy results

A formulation of recombinant human Epidermal Growth Factor (rhEGF) for intralesional administration in DFU has been developed. The growth factor is purified from a transformed *Saccharomyces cerevisiae* strain and presented as a lyophilized preparation containing 25 or 75 µg of rhEGF per vial. The efficacy and safety of the intervention has been tested in five exploratory and one confirmatory randomized, double-blind, placebo control clinical trials (Berlanga et al., 2006; Fernandez-Montequin et al., 2007, 2009a, 2009b). A total of 344 patients took part in these studies (Table 1).

This clinical development has dealt with a type of patient not usually recruited in DFU clinical trials. The characteristics of the patients included have been quite homogeneous across the trials, given essentially by (i) long-lasting Diabetes Mellitus, mostly type 2; (ii) median age >60 years; (iii) chronic ulcers (more than one month of evolution); (iv) deep ulcers (exposes cellular subcutaneous tissue or tendons, or joint capsule); (v) advanced, given by large size (median area always > 20 cm^2), baseline infection (that had to treated before the use of rhEGF), necrotic tissue (that had to be removed surgically); (vi) approximately one half of the patients with deficient irrigation of the corresponding leg (ischemia). The three latter features are usually exclusion criteria in DFU clinical trials. Such ulcers corresponded to grades 3 or 4 of the Wagner´s classification (Armstrong et al., 1998).These patients, which can represent 50% of the whole DFU population, lead to most of the amputations.

Patients with hemoglobin <100 g/l, uncontrolled chronic diseases, psychiatric disorders, malignancies, pregnant or breastfeeding, were excluded. Signed, informed consent was an inclusion requisite in all trials, which were approved by the corresponding Ethics Committees and by the National Regulatory Authority.

Intralesional rhEGF was administered adjuvant to the conventional good wound care measures: metabolic control, thorough debridement of necrotic and infected tissue, pressure off-loading, and antimicrobials if needed. The product was dissolved in 5 ml of water for injection or saline and distributed evenly throughout the lesion in 5 to 10 punctures, starting from the cleanest zones. The needle was changed between injections in order to prevent infection dissemination. Treatment was given three times per week on alternate days, until complete granulation response or a maximum of 8 weeks. Only in trial No. 0705 treatment was continued until wound closure. Subjects were hospitalized during treatment in all trials and then followed-up, generally for one year, as outpatients.

The main outcome variable in most of the studies was the development of granulation tissue, classified, according to the lesion area covered, in: (i) no response: less than 25% granulation; (ii) minimal response: 25 to 50%; partial response: 50 to 75%; complete response: more than 75% of the lesion area, that could support a skin graft to complete ulcer closure. A 100% granulation response was nonetheless achieved in most complete responders.

In these, more advanced ulcers, granulation is a valid outcome since it is part of the healing process and should necessarily precede the final healing. Besides, granulation over the ulcer area permits skin grafting to attain final healing, so a group of patients does not reach complete spontaneous healing to be evaluated. Additionally, a significant correlation was found between granulation and healing in the confirmatory study No. 0503 (Fernandez-Montequin et al., 2009b). Previous studies had identified partial wound closure as predictive of complete healing for Wagner's grade 1 or 2 DFU (Sheehan et al., 2006), and other ulcers (van Rijswijk & Polansky, 1994; Kantor & Margolis, 2000), but this was the first report of an early surrogate endpoint in Wagner's grade 3 or 4 DFU.

4.1 Pilot, exploratory trial in 29 patients who were bound to amputation

Patients bore advanced DFU, Wagner´s grade 3 (10 cases) or 4 (19 cases); 23 of them were ischemic and had no other therapeutic alternative. Some granulation response was obtained in 25 cases (86%) and the complete response and lesion closure in 17 (59%; one of them through skin graft), thus preventing amputation. Recurrence appeared in only one patient after a one-year follow-up (Berlanga et al., 2006). An immuno-histochemical study suggested that TGF β could be the main effector mediating the EGF-stimulated granulation process. Biopsies taken from neuropathic and ischemic patients showed the stimulation of granulation tissue growth and organization as well as the formation of new blood vessels after the treatment with rhEGF, illustrating its angiogenic effect (Figure 2 in Berlanga et al., 2006).

4.2 Dose exploratory trial

A controlled, double-blinded, randomized and multicenter clinical trial was later carried out in five institutions to explore a possible dose-dependent response (Fernandez-Montequín et al., 2007).

Forty-one patients bearing Wagner's grade 3 and 4 lesions were included. They were randomly distributed in two groups receiving rhEGF at 75 µg or 25 µg. A tendency to better results with the higher dose was observed: higher granulation response rate and faster, but groups behaved similar concerning wound closure during follow-up. Only one patient relapsed in the follow-up. In some of the cases wound contraction could be evidenced as part of the healing process (Figure 2). This property is usually abolished in diabetic patients.

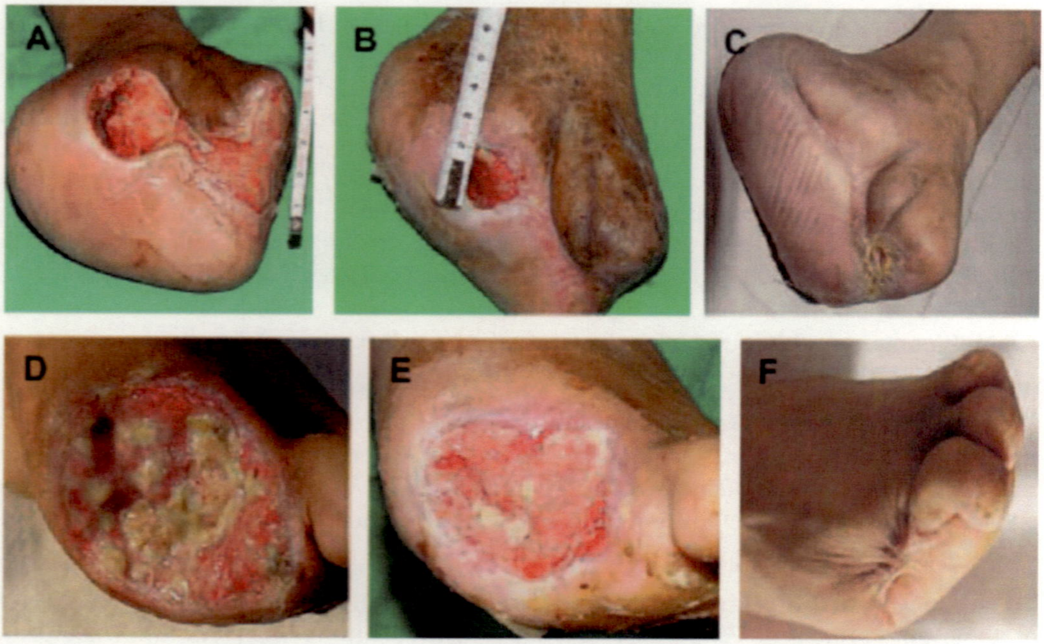

Fig. 2. Evidence of granulation and healing in two patients from study No. 0202. Upper line: 65 years-old female. An ischemic 38 cm^2 transmetatarsal amputation base was treated with rhEGF. A: before the beginning of treatment; B: after 5 weeks (15 infiltrations) complete granulation was achieved; C: healing occurred at 29 weeks. Lower line: 46 years-old female with ischemic and infected DFU. After toe disarticulation and antibiotics, she was treated with rhEGF. D: before treatment; E: after 4 weeks (12 infiltrations) complete granulation was achieved; F: Healing was reported at 17 weeks. Wound contraction is evident as part of the healing mechanism. (Picture taken from Fernandez-Montequin et al. 2007)

4.3 Series of 12 patients treated with the 75 µg dose (not published)

The results obtained agree with those obtained in previous trials. Most of the patients responded satisfactorily. The observed total response rate was 75%. Major amputations were carried out in 3 patients (25%), all ischemic, associated to the occurrence of local infection in two of them.

4.4 Monitoring of patients treated after initial conditional marketing approval of the product (not published)

A multicenter, non-controlled, phase IV-type study was based on the reports of all treated cases after an initial conditional marketing approval in Cuba. The rhEGF began to be used throughout the country and was administered at 25 µg, three times per week until complete granulation or up to 8 weeks. Results were consistent with the previous ones. Relapse was present in only one patient after one year follow-up.

4.5 Series of patients treated with 75 µg up to wound closure

Twenty patients were included and treated with intralesional rhEGF, three times per week, until the lesion closure was attained (Fernandez-Montequín et al, 2009a). According to Wagner's classification, 16 patients (80%) were grade 3 and 4 (20%) were grade 4. The mean initial area of the lesions was 16.3 ± 21.3 cm^2. There was evidence of ischemia in 5 patients (25%), whose limb occlusion pattern was at a distal level. A complete granulation response was obtained in all cases, complete lesion closure in 17 (85%) and none of them required amputation. The mean healing time was only 6 weeks. There was one wound recurrence 6 months after healing. This study indicated that rhEGF can be used after total granulation until the lesion is completely closed or until its area is significantly reduced (≤ 1 cm^2).

4.6 Multicenter, double-blind, placebo-controlled confirmatory trial

A confirmatory, multicenter, randomized, double-blind trial was carried out (Fernandez-Montequín et al, 2009b). Besides, it was compared to placebo. The latter was required to provide unquestionable evidence on the efficacy of intralesional rhEGF administration; to rule out that the results obtained were explained by good wound care that improves under clinical trial settings or due to the endogenous local production of growth factors induced by the debridement and injection procedures.

The study was carried out at 20 institutions in all Cuban provinces. The treatment consisted of three applications of 75 µg EGF, 25 µg, or placebo for 8 weeks or until complete granulation, adjuvant to general good wound care.

Due to ethical reasons, to avoid giving placebo to a non-responder, if less than 25% of the ulcer area was covered by granulation tissue after two weeks of treatment, the patient´s code was opened and the patient switched to 25 µg rhEGF, when on the placebo, or 75 µg, when on 25 µg. The main evaluation variable was the existence of at least a partial response (50% of the lesion area covered by granulation tissue) after two weeks of treatment, since this was the period when all patients were randomized and double-blinded in their original treatment groups. The hypothesis of the trial was to obtain at least 30% advantage in the proportion of individuals with an objective response at that moment in the groups treated with rhEGF as compared to the placebo. The secondary variables taken into account were the existence of a complete granulation response at the end of treatment, the time to complete response, lesion closure during the 12 months follow-up, time to closure, the occurrence of relapses and the need for amputation. Safety was evaluated by adverse events monitoring and laboratory variables. All the analyses were made under the principle of "intention to treat".

One hundred and forty-nine patients were included. Groups were equivalent in regard to demographic and baseline variables. Both dosage groups fulfilled the study hypothesis of more than 30% advantage over the placebo group, in the proportion of patients with more than 50% of the lesion area covered by granulation tissue. Differences (and their 95% CI) with respect to the placebo are shown in Table 1. Superiority in relative terms (OR) was 7.5 (2.9 – 18.9) and 3.7 (1.6 – 8.7) for the high and the low doses, respectively.

After eight weeks, the proportion of patients with complete granulation response was significantly higher only for the 75 µg treatment compared to placebo. The benefits of the treatment were more evident for the neuroinfectious origin cases than in those with an ischemic component. The time required for a complete response was 3 weeks for each group receiving EGF and 5 weeks for the placebo. This difference was statistically significant for both dosage levels.

The evaluation of the complete closure of the ulcers was performed during the 12-month follow-up. The statistical multivariate analysis of lesion healing showed that the factors that favored ulcer closure were rhEGF 75 µg vs. control (OR: 3.6; 95% CI: 1.4 – 9.5), the "pure" neuropathic vs. ischemic character (5.5; 2.3 – 13.5), and an initial smaller ulcer size (0.98; 0.96 – 0.99). Relapses only occurred in the placebo group. Although amputations were too few to support any statistical analysis, it is remarkable that there was only one amputation among the neuropathic patients treated with rhEGF at any of the dosages, while 15% of the neuropathic cases required amputation in the placebo group. There was only one failure after two weeks in the group receiving rhEGF at 75 µg.

This trial confirmed the efficacy of intralesional rhEGF in advanced DFUs. The results were better in the group using the high dose, although both dosage levels fulfilled the efficacy hypothesis for the main variable (partial granulation response after two weeks). Besides, only the high dose showed significant differences compared to the control group for some secondary variables, suggesting a dose-dependent effect. This is particularly important for patients with ischemia, which is an adverse condition for granulation and healing

Study details	Variables evaluated	Treatment		
		75 µg rhEGF	25 µg rhEGF	Placebo
Code: 0102	N		29	
Pilot; exploratory; grades 3 and 4 ulcers, ischemic and	Complete granulation at the end of treatment		17 (59%)	
neuropathic; high risk of amputation	Wound closure during follow-up		17 (59%)	
Treatment: 25 µg, 3 times per week until complete granulation or 8 weeks	Time to complete granulation in weeks (mean ± SD)		4.7 ± 1.5	
maximum. Follow-up for one year.	Time to wound closure in weeks (95% CI)		7 (1; 13)	
Ref: Berlanga et al. 2006	Amputations		12 (41%)	
Code: 0202	N	23	18	
Dose exploratory study; grades 3 and 4 ulcers,	Complete granulation at the end of treatment	19 (83%)	11 (61%)	

Study details	Variables evaluated	Treatment		
		75 µg rhEGF	25 µg rhEGF	Placebo
ischemic and neuropathic; Design: multicenter, randomized, double blind. Treatment: 25 µg or 75 µg, 3 times per week until complete granulation or 8 weeks maximum. Follow-up for one year Ref.: Fernandez et al., 2007	Wound closure during follow-up	13 (57%)	9 (50%)	
	Time to complete granulation in weeks (mean ± SD)	3.8 ± 2.2	4.9 ± 2.2	
	Time to wound closure in weeks (95% CI)	21 (17; 24)	20 (16; 23)	
	Amputations	8 (35%)	6 (33%)	
Code: 0504 Lineal, patient series. Ulcers: grade 4, ischemic and neuropathic; Treatment: 75 µg, 3 times per week until granulation or 8 weeks maximum Not published	N	12		
	Complete granulation at the end of treatment	9 (75%)		
	Amputations	3 (25%)		
Code: 0604; Lineal, phase IV – type study after conditional approval; Ulcers: grade 3 and 4, ischemic and neuropathic. Treatment: 25 µg, 3 times per week until granulation or 8 weeks maximum. 3- year follow-up. Not published	N		93	
	Complete granulation at the end of treatment		78 (84%)	
	Wound closure during follow-up (16 patients lost)		46 (49%)	
	Time to wound closure in weeks (95% CI)		10 (9; 11)	
	Amputations		26 (28%)	
Code: 0705; Lineal, patient series. Ulcers: grade 3 and 4, ischemic and neuropathic; Treatment: 75 µg, 3 times per week until healing or 12 weeks maximum Ref.: Fernandez et al., 2009a	N	20		
	Complete granulation at the end of treatment	20 (100%)		
	Wound closure	17 (85%)		
	Time to complete granulation in weeks (mean ± SD)	3.4 ± 0.5		
	Time to wound closure in weeks (95% CI)	6.3 (4; 9)		
	Amputations	0		
Code: 0503 Confirmatory multicenter, randomized, double blind, placebo-controlled trial; 20 sites; Ulcers: grade 3 and 4,	N	53	48	48
	No response at 2 weeks; code opened	1 (2%)	5 (10%)	8 (17%)
	≥50% granulation at 2 weeks (95% CI of the difference with placebo)	44 (83%) (24; 63)	34 (71%) (10; 52)	19 (40%)

Study details	Variables evaluated	Treatment		
		75 µg rhEGF	25 µg rhEGF	Placebo
ischemic and neuropathic; Treatment: 25 µg, 75 µg, or placebo 3 times per week	Complete granulation at the end of treatment (95% CI of the difference with placebo)	46 (87%) (6; 39)	35 (73%) (-8; 29)	28 (58%)
until complete granulation or 8 weeks maximum. Follow-up for one year.	Time to complete granulation in weeks (95% CI)	3 (2.6; 3.4)	3 (2.2; 3.8)	5 (3.4; 6.6)
If no response at 2 weeks, code opened and if placebo, switched to 25 µg; if 25 µg, switched to 75 µg.	Wound closure during follow-up (95% CI of the difference with placebo)	41 (77%) (1; 41)	25 (52%)	27 (56%)
Ref.: Fernandez et al., 2009b	Time to wound closure in weeks (95% CI)	15.7 (10; 22)	17.3 (11; 24)	21.4 (8; 35)
	Amputations	7 (13%)	10 (21%)	12 (25%)
Pooled analysis	N	108	188	48
	Complete granulation at the end of treatment	94 (87%)	141 (75%)	28 (58%)
	Wound closure during follow-up	71/96 (74%)	97 (52%)	27 (56%)
	Time to wound closure in weeks (95% CI)	14 (12; 16)	12 (10; 14)	21.4 (8; 35)
	Amputations	18 (17%)	54 (29%)	12 (25%)

Table 1. Summary of characteristics and results of clinical trials with rhEGF in DFU. SD: standard deviation; CI: confidence interval

4.7 Long-term follow-up of the patients included in all clinical trials

Overall, 323 individuals were enrolled in clinical trials since 2001 (one patient took part in studies 0604 and 0503). They were visited in 2010 looking for information on survival, recurrences, new foot ulcers, amputations, adverse events and co-morbidities, including neoplasia. The median follow-up period was 3 years (maximum, 8 years). The results are summarized in Table 2. Patients from study No. 0705 were not followed-up since they live abroad. Patients from study No. 0503 were considered "per protocol" for this evaluation, since some had switched treatment at 2 weeks.

No evidence was gathered indicating that intralesional rhEGF administration could stimulate cancer growth. Two patients had developed malignancies: one who had received rhEGF at 25 µg; the other was from the placebo group of the phase III trial.

Thirty nine percent of the patients had deceased. The more frequent causes of death were heart infarct, chronic renal failure, and stroke. Median survival was longer in patients that had attained ulcer-healing: 5.7 ± 0.8 years vs. 4.2 ± 0.7 years in those who did not heal ($p=0.004$).

The frequency of relapses at any moment was significantly lower ($p<0.001$) in patients that received rhEGF (10% and 4% for the 75 µg and 25 µg doses, respectively) as compared to the control group of the confirmatory, No. 0503, trial (23%). This effect was obtained for both neuropathic and ischemic patients. On the contrary, no effect was seen on the appearance of DFU on other locations (mainly on the contralateral limb). The rates were 26%, 24%, and 32% for patients treated with 75 µg rhEGF, 25 µg, and placebo, respectively. It seems as if the tissue keeps a sort of "memory" of the treatment received, which is not transferable to non-treated zones. Molecular and immunohistochemistry studies are in course to elucidate these mechanisms.

Trial	Dose	Enrolled	Followed-up	Recurrences	New ulcers	Amputations	Cancer
0102	25 µg	29	29	1	7	13	
0202	25 µg	18	18	0	6	9	
	75 µg	23	22	1	11	12	
0504	75 µg	12	11	1	0	4	
0604	25 µg	93	66	3	20	29	1
0503	25 µg	49	43	1	12	15	
	75 µg	57	51	5	11	16	
	Placebo	43	42	8	13	15	1

Table 2. Long term follow-up of patients from all clinical trials with rhEGF in DFU

Amputations were necessary in 114 patients at some moment after rhEGF treatment. The amputation rates were 35% for both rhEGF dose levels, the same as for the control group of the confirmatory trial. However, if only neuropathic and mild ischemic patients are taken into account amputations were less among patients treated with rhEGF 75 µg (14%) or 25 µg (20%) than among those who only received the good standard care (33%). Thus, severe and critic ischemia is still an adverse condition, difficult to overcome. Probably rhEGF should be used in those cases after appropriate revascularization procedures that improve tissue blood supply.

4.8 Consistency of the efficacy results from the different trials

Efficacy measurements across the different studies, summarized in Table 1, are consistent. More than 80% granulation was obtained globally for both dose levels used. They are much better than what was obtained for a group of patients that received only standard care (the placebo group of study No. 0503). The fact than only one study had a control group is a limitation to this comparison, but there is homogeneity among the different studies with respect to the results obtained and the 95% confidence interval of the result in the placebo group falls below those of the treated groups. There seems to be a dose-dependent effect, since results were always better for the higher dose. Subgroup analyses, limited by the fact that they were not previewed in the protocols, suggest that the difference between doses is given by patients with more complicated ulcers (larger, with more severe ischemia).

Results on healing are clinically relevant as well, for the 75 µg dose. Treatment-dependency was also found for complete closure, despite being reached during follow-up, as outpatients, only under general wound care measures (except for study No. 0705, where treatment was continued until healing). This apparent "EGF-memory" effect on wound closure can be explained by the granulation tissue stimulation, which was predictive of closure. Granulation can also reduce the probability of infection progression, since the fresh tissue is better prepared to "fight" against invading micro-organisms and better irrigation can increase the local bioavailability of systemic antibiotic treatment. As mentioned above, some persistent action of rhEGF treatment should take place, leading to less relapses as well. Time-to-closure was also shortened in approximately 4 weeks, which is a clinically significant feature.

With respect to amputations, the number of events has been very small in each study in order to make a proper statistical analysis. For that reason this outcome has been secondary in all trials. The pooled analysis after long-term follow-up, mentioned above is interesting for the 75 µg dose.

5. Overview of safety

Since all trials included very similar populations and the same therapeutic schedule (only the dose varied), a pooled analysis was done. Intralesional rhEGF was well tolerated. About half of the included patients (58.5%) reported some adverse event. Those occurring in more than 1% of the patients are summarized in Table 3. Pain and burning sensation at the administration site were the most frequent. A dose-effect relation associated to the appearance of shivering and chills was systematically obtained in all trials that used both doses and in the pooled analysis.

Concerning intensity, the adverse events reported were 65.6 % mild, 28.6% moderate, and only 3.7% severe. Serious adverse events were reported in 13% of the patients from the clinical studies. Local infection was the more frequent serious adverse event. It caused hospitalization and/or amputation. It was the adverse event that most frequently lead to treatment interruption. It is difficult to establish a causal relationship between its appearance and rhEGF administration since this event is also a frequent complication of Wagner´s grade 3 and 4 DFU and a significant risk factor for amputation. It has been reported that lower extremities infection is the most frequent reason for the hospitalization of patients with diabetes (Edmonds & Foster, 2004). Likewise, it appeared in the placebo group of the controlled study 0503. Some of the factors that leave patients predisposed to the progress of local infection include the presence of an entryway for bacteria and the fact that the immune response of diabetic patients is often compromised.

The analysis of the relationship of adverse events with demographic or baseline characteristics only yielded significant results for the age and ulcer etiopathogeny. A multivariate logistic regression model yield a significant more frequent appearance of any adverse event in patients ≥ 65 years old vs. younger (OR: 1.86; 95% CI: 1.09 – 3.15), and less frequent if the ulcer was neuropathic (OR: 0.25; 95% CI: 0.14 – 0.45). Local infection appeared significantly more frequently in patients with Diabetes type II than in type I: 45/222 (16.9%) vs. 2/62 (3.1%).

Three of the patients in the clinical trials died: one with placebo and one with each of the doses. Other 8 deaths occurred during follow-up (up to one year). None of the deaths can be considered as related to treatment but to the underlying diabetes and/or the age of the patients. The death causes were: acute myocardial infarct (4), bronchopneumonia (2), mesenteric thrombosis, acute renal failure, acute pulmonary edema, and infection. At the time of follow-up, 12 months after the conclusion of the treatment, no long term adverse effects related to the product were reported.

Adverse events	75 µg N=116		25 µg N=181		Placebo N=48	
	N	%	N	%	N	%
Pain at the administration site	21	18.1%	52	28.7%	20	41.7%
Burning sensation at the administration site	26	22.4%	25	13.8%	14	29.2%
Shivering	34	29.3%	18	9.9%	2	4.2%
Local infection	20	17.2%	18	9.9%	8	16.7%
Chills	30	25.9%	15	8.3%	1	2.1%
Fever	9	7.8%	18	9.9%	6	12.5%
Anemia	5	4.3%	5	2.8%	5	10.4%
Vomiting	7	6.0%	4	2.2%	1	2.1%
Pain on the lesion	9	7.8%	2	1.1%	0	
Nauseas	5	4.3%	3	1.7%	2	4.2%
Chest pain	3	2.6%	4	2.2%	0	

Table 3. Frequency of patients with each adverse event in Clinical Trials. Events that appeared in more than 1% of the patients (pooled).

The presence of anti-EGF autoantibodies has not been considered detrimental for adult animals (Raaberg et al., 1995a, 1995b) or in the healing process (Casaco et al., 2004). Nevertheless, immunogenicity of rhEGF was evaluated in three studies since, as a recombinant protein, it could exert antibody production and this is an important safety issue for all agencies. Anti-EGF antibodies were detected in some patients (4 in study 0202 and 5 in study 0503). Some other patients had these antibodies naturally, before treatment. All the titers found were very low and there was no clear relationship with efficacy or safety results.

The adverse event profile from the first report of the postmarketing pharmacovigilance in Cuba (from 1851 patients) is very similar to that from clinical trials. The most frequent events are shivering, pain and burning sensation at the administration site, and chills. Local infection is less frequent, but the most frequent among the serious events found (manuscript in preparation).

A particular concern on the therapeutic use of growth factors is the possibility of development or stimulation of a pre-existing malignancy in the patients. The concern is justified by the growth stimulating property of these active principles. Practically, anti-growth factor therapy is approved or extensively experimented for several neoplasia (Gonzalez et al., 2011; Caraglia et al., 2006; Geva et al., 2010). Additionally an increase in any-site cancer incidence was observed in DFU patients treated with platelet-derived-growth factor (PDGF; becaplermin), which generated a warning from regulatory agencies (FDA-USA, 2008).

EGF is not an exception to this concern. In fact, the presence or history of neoplasia has been an exclusion criteria in all clinical trials with intralesional rhEGF and is a precaution for the use of the procedure in medical practice. However, there are several theoretical and experimental considerations that do not support the idea that EGF treatment, at the doses and schedules used, could stimulate any tumor growth. These aspects are thoroughly discussed by Berlanga et al., 2009. Briefly:

EGF, although growth stimulating and thus a possible tumor promoter, does not induce malignant transformation.

EGF stimulation of cell lines and tumor grafts growth is not a consistent result. There are cases of growth inhibition by exogenously administered EGF. (Knowles et al., 1985; Barnes, 1982)

EGF overexpression in transgenic animals not always lead to increase in tumor development (Chan & Wing-Chuen, 2000).

No increase in tumors in patients treated with topical EGF for burns, in a controlled trial done in Cuba in 1993-94. These patients were visited in 2008 – 2009 and their incidence of cancer was not above that expected for that age group in Cuba for that long period of time (not published result, reported by Berlanga et al., 2009)

The pharmacokinetics study in DFU patients showed short residence in blood of intralesionally administered rhEGF. After 2 hours all EGF was cleared and no accumulation was detected after repeated injections (not published result; manuscript in preparation). These data are inconsistent with long-term systemic actions.

Treatments with rhEGF are short-term: not more than 8-12 weeks, contrary to a tumor promoting action that would require a longer exposure.

Lack of treatment-related cancer development in the long-term follow up of patients from clinical trials with rhEGF (mentioned above). This argument is nonetheless still weak since the result comes from few individuals.

6. Benefit-risk analysis

The clinical studies in patients with advanced DFU (Wagner´s grade 3 or 4, median size >20 cm^2, ischemic not excluded) have shown that intralesionally injected rhEGF, adjuvant to standard good wound care, has the potential to promote granulation, complete wound healing, even in subjects unresponsive to other treatments, faster than subjects treated with standard good wound care alone. The relapse rate is reduced as well. The procedure has the potential to reduce amputation rates, particularly in neuropathic or mild ischemic patients, with a considerable personal and public health improvement.

Potential risks of the use of intralesional rhEGF in DFU can be evaluated by the safety profile obtained from the clinical trials and the possibility of cancer stimulation, discussed above. No particular treatment-related serious adverse event was observed. All can be explained by the underlying disease. No increase in cardiovascular, respiratory or renal complications was reported. Adverse events attributed to treatment have been generally limited to shivering, chills, and injection site pain. These have been mild and self-limiting. No increase in cancer development in treated patients has been observed. Local infection progression is the more frequent serious adverse event. Since the injection procedure can potentially contribute to infection spreading, caution is recommended in this sense. Clinical signs of infection should be cleared before treatment with rhEGF.

This benefit-risk balance seems quite favorable. This was also suggested by the analysis done using a Bayesian approach (Spiegelhalter et al., 2004) comparing the probability of benefit (given by complete healing) with the probability of risk (given by the occurrence of serious adverse events, including amputation), taking into account data from all clinical trials. These results are shown in Fig. 3.

Assuming that there are two hypotheses H_1 (benefit, given by ulcer healing) and H_2 (risk, given by the occurrence of serious adverse events or amputation) proposed for the patients outcome data set and under H_k the data are related to the parameter vector ψ_k by a distribution with probability density $p(X \mid \psi_{k,} H_k)$. Given the prior probabilities p(*benefit*) and p(*risk*) = 1 - p(*benefit*), the data produce the posterior probabilities $p(benefit \mid X)$ and $p(risk|X) = 1 - p(benefit|X)$.

The Bayes Factor (B_{br}) is then:

$$B_{br} = \frac{p(x|benefit)}{p(x|risk)}$$

representing a summary of the evidence provided by the data in favor of benefit, as opposed to risk. A value larger than 1 means a favorable benefit-risk ratio.

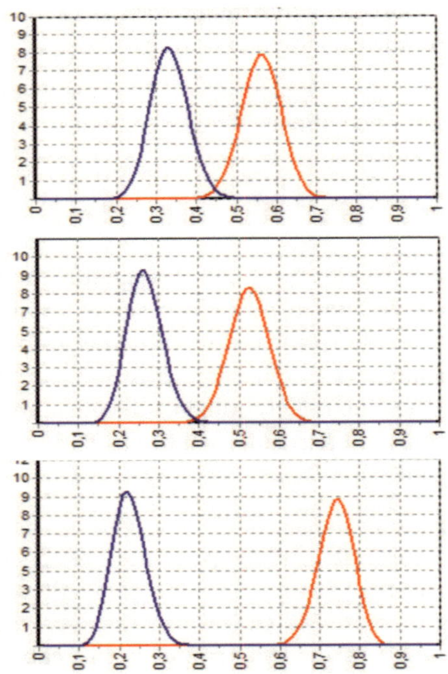

Fig. 3. Benefit and risk probability distributions of the outcome of DFU patients treated with intralesional rhEGF.

The results shown are:

Upper graph: placebo (study No. 0503): B_{br}= 1.69; difference between the probabilities: 23% (95% CI: 11% – 36%).

Middle graph: treatment with 25 µg rhEGF; B_{br}= 1.92; difference between probabilities: 26% (95% CI: 13% – 40%).

Lower graph: treatment with 75 µg rhEGF. B_{br}= 3.36; difference between probabilities: 51% (95% CI: 40% – 63%).

In all cases the differences between benefit and risk probabilities favor the former; the Bayes factors and differences are larger for the rhEGF treated groups than for the controls. The balance of the higher dose is much favorable.

7. Conclusion

The intralesional administration of rhEGF offers a new alternative for the treatment of advanced DFU, reluctant to other treatments, which frequently lead to a lower limb amputation. Further extension of the procedure should yield impact data (pharmacoeconomic, limb salvage).

8. References

Armstrong, DG., Lavry, LA. & Harkless, LB. (1998) Validation of a Diabetic Wound Classification System: The contribution of depth, infection, and ischemia to risk of amputation. *Diabetes Care*, Vol. 21, No. 5 (May, 1998) pp. (855-859), ISSN: 0149-5992

Barnes DW. (1982) Epidermal growth factor inhibits growth of A431 human epidermoid carcinoma in serum-free culture. *Journal of Cell Biology*, Vol. 93, No. 1 (April, 1982), pp. (1–4), ISSN :0021-9525

Barrandon, Y. & Green H. (1987) Cell migration is essential for sustained growth of keratinocyte colonies, pp. (the roles of transforming growth factor-alpha and epidermal growth factor. *Cell*, Vol. 50, No. 7 (September, 1987), pp. (1131–1137), ISSN: 0092-8674

Bazley, LA. & Gullick WJ. (2005) The epidermal growth factor receptor family. *Endocrine Related Cancer*, Vol. 12, Suppl. 1 (July, 2005), pp. (S17–S27), ISSN: 1351-0088

Berlanga, J., Caballero, ME., Ramirez, D., Torres, A., Valenzuela, C., Lodos, J. & Playford, R. (1998a) Epidermal growenth factor protects against carbon tetrachloride-induced hepatic injury. *Clinical Science (London)*, Vol. 94, No. 3 (March, 1998) pp. (219-223), ISSN: 0143-5221.

Berlanga, J., Lodos, J., Reyes, O., Infante, JF., Caballero, E. & López-Saura, P. (1998b) Epidermal growth factor stimulated re-epithelialization in pigs. The possible role of acute-wound proteases. *Biotecnología Aplicada*, Vol. 15, No. 1 (April, 1998), pp. (83-87), ISSN: 0684-4551

Berlanga, J., Caballero, E., Prats, P., Lopez-Saura, P. & Playford, RJ. (1999) The role of the epidermal growth factor in cell and tissue protection. *Medicina Clinica (Barcelona)*, Vol. 113, No. 6 (September, 1999), pp. (222-229), 0025-7753

Berlanga-Acosta, J., Playford, RJ., Mandir, N. & Goodlad RA. (2001) Gastrointestinal cell proliferation and crypt fission are separate but complementary means of increasing tissue mass following infusion of epidermal growth factor in rats. *Gut*, Vol. 48, No. 6 (January, 2001), pp. (803-807), ISSN: 0017-5749

Berlanga, J., Lodos, J. & Lopez-Saura, P. (2002a) Attenuation of internal organ damages by exogenously administered epidermal growth factor (EGF) in burned rodents. *Burns*, Vol. 28, No. 5 (August, 2002), pp. (435-42), ISSN: 0305-4179

Berlanga, J., Prats, P., Remirez, D., Gonzalez, R., Lopez-Saura, P., Aguiar, J., Ojeda, M., Boyle, JJ., Fitzgerald, AJ. & Playford RJ. (2002b) Prophylactic use of epidermal growth factor reduces ischemia/reperfusion intestinal damage. *American Journal of Pathology*, Vol. 161, No. 2 (August, 2002), pp. (373-379), ISSN: 0002-9440

Berlanga, J., Savigne, W., Valdez, C., Franco, N., Alba, JS., del Rio, A., López-Saura, P., Guillén, G., Lopez E., Herrera, L. & Férnandez-Montequín, J. (2006) Epidermal Growth Factor Intra-lesional can prevent amputation in diabetic patients with advanced foot wounds. *International Wound Journal*, Vol. 3, No. 3 (September, 2006), pp. (232-239), ISSN: 1742-4801

Berlanga-Acosta, J., del Barco, DG., Vera, DC., Savigne, W., Lopez-Saura, P., Guillen, NG. & Schultz, GS. (2008) The pro-inflammatory environment in recalcitrant diabetic foot wounds. *International Wound Journal*, Vol. 5, No. 4 (October, 2008), pp. (530-539), ISSN: 1742-4801

Berlanga-Acosta, J., Gavilondo-Cowley, J., López-Saura, P., González-López, T., Castro-Santana, MD., López-Mola, E., Guillén-Nieto, G. & Herrera-Martinez, L. (2009) Epidermal Growth Factor (EGF) in clinical practice- A review of its biological actions, clinical indications and safety implications. *International Wound Journal*, Vol. 6, No. 5 (October, 2009) pp. (331–346), ISSN: 1742-4801

Brem, H., Sheehan, P. & Boulton, AJ. (2004) Protocol for treatment of diabetic foot ulcers. *American Journal of Surgery*, Vol. 187, No. 5A (May, 2004), pp. (1S-10S), ISSN: 0002-9610

Buckley, A., Davidson, JM., Kamerath, CD., Wolt, TB. & Woodward, SC. (1985), Sustained release of epidermal growth factor accelerates wound repair. *Proceedings of the National Academy of Sciences USA*, Vol. 82, No. 21 (November, 2005), pp. (7340-7344), ISSN: 0027-8424

Burrow, JW., Koch, JA., Chuang, HH., Zhong, W., Dean, DD. & Sylvia, VL. (2007) Nitric oxide donors selectively reduce the expression of matrix metalloproteinases-8 and -9 by human diabetic skin fibroblasts. *The Journal of Surgical Research*, Vol. 140, No. 1 (June, 2007), pp. (90-98), ISSN: 0022-4804

Caraglia, M., Marra, M., Meo, G., Addeo, SR., Tagliaferri, P., & Budillon, A. (2006) EGF-R small inhibitors and anti-EGF-R antibodies: advantages and limits of a new avenue in anticancer therapy. *Recent Patents on Anticancer Drug Discovery.*, Vol. 1, No. 2 (June, 2006), pp. (209-222), ISSN: 1574-8928

Casaco, A., Diaz, Y., Ledon, N., Merino, N., Valdes, O., Garcia, G., Garcia, B., Gonzalez, G. & Perez, R. (2004) Effect of an EGF-cancer vaccine on wound healing and inflammation models. *The Journal of Surgical Research*, Vol. 122, No. 1 (November, 2004), pp. (130-134), ISSN: 0022-4804

Chan, SY. & Wing-Chuen, RW. (2000) Expression of epidermal growth factor in transgenic mice causes growth retardation. *Journal of Biological Chemistry*, Vol. 275, No. 49 (December, 2000), pp. (38693–38698), ISSN: 0021-9258

Citri, A. & Yarden, Y. (2006) EGF-ERBB signaling: towards the systems level. *Nature reviews. Molecular cell biology*, Vol. 7, No. 7 (July, 2006), pp. (505-516), ISSN: 1471-0072

Clark, RA. (2008) Synergistic signaling from extracellular matrix-growth factor complexes. *The Journal of investigative dermatology*, Vol. 128, No. 6 (June, 2008), pp. (1354-1355), ISSN: 0022-202X

Cohen S. (1962) Isolation of a mouse submaxillary gland protein accelerating incisor eruption and eyelid opening in the new-born animal. *Journal of Biological Chemistry*, Vol. 237, No. 5 (May, 1962), pp. (1555-1562), ISSN: 0021-9258

Dong, P., Flores, J., Pelton, K. & Solomon, KR. (2010), Prohibitin is a cholesterol-sensitive regulator of cell cycle transit. *Journal of Cell Biochemistry*, Vol. 111, No. 5 (December, 2010), pp. (1367-1374), ISSN:0730-2312

Dyck, PJ. & Giannini, C. (1996) Pathologic alterations in the diabetic neuropathies of humans: a review. *Journal of Neuropathology and Experimental Neurology*, Vol. 55, No. 12 (December, 1996), pp. (1181–1193), ISSN:0022-3069

Edmonds, M. & Foster, A. (2004), The use of antibiotics in the diabetic foot. *American Journal of Surgery.*, Vol. 187 No. 5A (May, 2004), pp. (25S-28S), ISSN:0002-9610

Eldor, R., Raz, I., Ben Yehuda, A. & Boulton, AJ. (2004) New and experimental approaches to treatment of diabetic foot ulcers: a comprehensive review of emerging treatment strategies. *Diabetic Medicine*, Vol. 21, No. 11 (November, 2004), pp. (1161-1173), ISSN:0742-3071

Eming, SA., Krieg, T. & Davidson, JM. (2007) Inflammation in wound repair: molecular and cellular mechanisms. *The Journal of Investigative Dermatology*, Vol. 127, No. 3 (March, 2007), pp. (514-525), ISSN:0022-202X

Falanga, V. (1992) Growth factors and chronic wounds: the need to understand the microenvironment. *The Journal of Dermatology*, Vol. 19, No. 11 (November, 1992), pp. (667-672), ISSN: 0385-2407

Falanga, V., Eaglstein, WH., Bucalo, B., Katz, MH., Harris, B. & Carson, P. (1992) Topical use of human recombinant epidermal growth factor (h-EGF) in venous ulcers. *The Journal of Dermatologic Surgery and Oncology*, Vol. 18 No. 7 (July, 1992), pp. (604-606), ISSN: 0148-0812

Fernández-Montequín, JI., Infante-Cristiá, E., Valenzuela-Silva, C., Franco-Pérez, N., Savigne-Gutierrez, W., Artaza-Sanz, H., Morejón-Vega, L., González-Benavides, C., Eliseo-Musenden, O., García-Iglesias, E., Berlanga-Acosta, J., Silva-Rodríguez, R., Betancourt, BY. & López-Saura, PA. Cuban Citoprot-P Study Group. (2007) Intralesional Injections of Citoprot P® (Recombinant Human Epidermal Growth Factor) in Advanced Diabetic Foot Ulcers with Risk of Amputation. *International Wound Journal*, Vol. 4, No. 4, December, 2007), pp. (333-343), ISSN: 1742-4801

Fernández-Montequín, JI., Betancourt, BY., Leyva-Gonzalez, G., López Mola, E., Galán-Naranjo, K., Ramírez-Navas, M., Bermúdez-Rojas, S., Rosales, F., García-Iglesias, E., Berlanga-Acosta, J., Silva-Rodriguez, S., Garcia-Siverio, M. & Herrera Martinez, L. (2009a) Intralesional administration of epidermal growth factor-based formulation (Heberprot-P) in advanced diabetic foot ulcer: Treatment up to complete wound closure. *International Wound Journal*, Vol. 6, No. 1 (February, 2009), pp. (67-72), ISSN: 1742-4801

Fernández-Montequín, JI., Valenzuela-Silva, CM., González-Díaz, O., Savigne, W., Sancho-Soutelo, N., Rivero-Fernández, F., Sánchez-Penton, P., Morejón-Vega, L., Artaza-

Sanz, H., García-Herrera, A., González-Benavides, C., Hernández-Cañete, CM., Vázquez-Proenza, A., Berlanga-Acosta, J. & López-Saura, PA., for the Cuban Diabetic Foot Study Group. (2009b) Intralesional injections of recombinant human Epidermal Growth Factor promote granulation and healing in advanced diabetic foot ulcers. Multicenter, randomized, placebo-controlled, double blind study. *International Wound Journal*, Vol. 6, No. 6 (December, 2009), pp. (432–443), ISSN: 1742-4801

Food and Drug Administration (USA). (2008) Update of Safety Review: Follow-up to the March 27 Communication about the Ongoing Safety Review of Regranex (becaplermin). *http://www.fda.gov/Drugs/DrugSafety/PostmarketDrugSafetyInformationforPatientsandProviders/DrugSafetyInformationforHeathcareProfessionals/ucm072148.htm*

Geva, R., Prenen, H., Topal, B., Aerts, R., Vannoote, J. & Van Cutsem, E. (2010) Biologic modulation of chemotherapy in patients with hepatic colorectal metastases: the role of anti-VEGF and anti-EGFR antibodies. *The Journal of Surgical Oncology,* Vol. 102, No. 8 (December, 2010), pp. (937-945), ISSN:0022-4804

Gonzalez, G., Crombet, T., & Lage, A. (2011) Chronic vaccination with a therapeutic EGF-based cancer vaccine: a review of patients receiving long lasting treatment. *Current Cancer Drug Targets.*, Vol. 11, No. 1, (January, 2011), pp. (103-110), ISSN:1568-0096

Goren, I., Muller, E., Pfeilschifter, J. & Frank, S. (2006) Severely impaired insulin signaling in chronic wounds of diabetic ob/ob mice: a potential role of tumor necrosis factor-alpha. *American Journal of Pathology,* Vol. 168, No. 3 (March, 2006), pp. (765-777), ISSN: 0002-9440

Grazul-Bilska, AT., Johnson, ML., Bilski, JJ., Redmer, DA., Reynolds, LP., Abdullah, A. & Abdullah, KM. (2003) Wound healing: the role of growth factors. *Drugs of Today (Barcelona).*, Vol. 39, No. 10 (October, 2003), pp. (787-800), ISSN:1699-3993

Hong, JP., Jung, HD. & Kim, YW. (2006) Recombinant human epidermal growth factor (EGF) to enhance healing for diabetic foot ulcers. *Annals of Plastic Surgery,* Vol. 56, No. 4 (April, 2006), pp. (394-398), ISSN:0148-7043

Kantor, J. & Margolis, DJ. (2000) A multicentre study of percentage change in venous leg ulcer area as a prognostic index of healing at 24 weeks. *The British Journal of Dermatology,* Vol. 142, No. 5 (May 2000), pp. (960–964), ISSN:0007-0963.

Knowles, AF., Salas Prato, M. & Villela, J. (1985) Epidermal growth factor inhibits growth while increasing the expression of an ecto-calcium-ATPase of a human hepatoma cell line. *Biochemical and Biophysical Research Communications,* Vol. 126, No. 1 (January, 1985) pp. (8–14), ISSN:0006-291X

Lee, H., Arnouk, H., Sripathi, S., Chen, P., Zhang, R., Bartoli, M., Hunt, RC., Hrushesky, WJ., Chung, H., Lee, SH. & Jahng, WJ. (2010) Prohibitin as an oxidative stress biomarker in the eye. *International Journal of Biological Macromolecules,* Vol. 47, No. 5 (December, 2010), pp. (685-690), ISSN: 0141-8130

Lipsky, BA. (2004) Medical treatment of diabetic foot infections. *Clinical Infectious Diseases,* Vol. 39, Suppl 2 (August, 2004), pp. (S104-114), ISSN:1058-4838

Maheshwari, G., Wells, A., Griffith, LG. & Lauffenburger, DA. (1999) Biophysical integration of effects of epidermal growth factor and fibronectin on fibroblast migration. *Biophysical Journal,* Vol. 76, No .5 (May, 1999), pp. (2817-2823), ISSN:1058-4838

Marston, WA., Hanft, J., Norwood, P. & Pollak, R. Dermagraft Diabetic Foot Ulcer Study Group. (2003) The efficacy and safety of Dermagraft in improving the healing of chronic diabetic foot ulcers: results of a prospective randomized trial. *Diabetes Care*, Vol. 26, No. 6 (June, 2003), pp. (1701–1705), ISSN: 0149-5992

Mast, BA. & Schultz, GS. (1996) Interactions of cytokines, growth factors, and proteases in acute and chronic wounds. *Wound Repair and Regeneration*, Vol. 4, No. 4 (October, 1996), pp. (411-420), ISSN:1067-1927

Medina, A., Scott, PG., Ghahary, A. & Tredget, EE. (2005) Pathophysiology of chronic nonhealing wounds. *The Journal of Burn Care and Rehabilitation*, Vol. 26, No. 4 (July-August, 2005), pp. (306-319), ISSN: 0273-8481

Mishra, S., Ande, SR. & Nyomba, BL. (2010) The role of prohibitin in cell signaling. *The FEBS Journal*, Vol. 277, No. 19 (October, 2010), pp. (3937-3946), ISSN:1742-464X

Prats, PA., Castañeda, LO., Falcón, V., de la Rosa, MC., Menéndez, I., Labarta, V. & Ortega, V. (1998) Effect of Epidermal Growth Factor on the regeneration of transected sciatic nerve in rats. *Biotecnología Aplicada*, Vol. 15, No. 4, December, 1998), pp. (237-241), ISSN: 0684-4551

Prats, PA., Duconge, J., Valenzuela, C., Berlanga, J., Edrosa, CR. & Fernandez-Sanchez, E. (2002) Disposition and receptor-site binding of (125)I-EGF after topical administration to skin wounds. *Biopharmaceutics & Drug Disposition*, Vol. 23, No. 2 (March, 2002), pp. (67-76), ISSN: 0142-2782

Raaberg, L., Nexo, E., Poulsen, SS. & Jorgensen, PE. (1995a) An immunologic approach to induction of epidermal growth factor deficiency: induction and characterization of auto-antibodies to epidermal growth factor in rats. *Pediatric Research*, Vol. 37, No. 2 (Februray, 1995), pp. (169-174), ISSN: 0031-3998

Raaberg, L., Nexo, E., Jorgensen, PE., Poulsen, SS. & Jakab, M. (1995b) Fetal effects of epidermal growth factor deficiency induced in rats by auto-antibodies against epidermal growth factor. *Pediatric Research*, Vol. 37, No. 2 (Februray, 1995), pp. (175-181), ISSN: 0031-3998

Reiber GE. (1996) The epidemiology of diabetic foot problems. *Diabetic Medicine*, Vol. 13 Suppl 1 (February, 1996), pp. (S6-S11), ISSN: 0742-3071

Saarialho-Kere, UK. (1998) Patterns of matrix metalloproteinase and TIMP expression in chronic ulcers. *Archives of Dermatological Research*, Vol. 290, Suppl (July, 1998), pp. (S47-S54), ISSN:0340-3696

Sheehan, P., Jones, P., Giurini, JM., Caselli, A. & Veves. A. (2006) Percent change in wound area of diabetic foot ulcers over a 4-week period is a robust predictor of complete healing in a 12-week prospective trial. *Plastic and Reconstructive Surgery*, Vol. 117, Suppl. 7 (June, 2006), pp. (239S–244S), ISSN: 0032-1052

Spiegelhalter, DJ., Abrams, KR. & Myles, JP. (2004). *Bayesian Approaches to Clinical Trials and Health-Care Evaluation*, John Wiley & Sons, Ltd, ISBN: 0-471-49975-7, West Sussex, UK

Trengove, NJ., Stacey, MC., MacAuley, S., Bennett, N., Gibson, J., Burslem, F., Murphy, G. & Schultz, G. (1999) Analysis of the acute and chronic wound environments: the role of proteases and their inhibitors. *Wound Repair and Regeneration*, Vol. 7, No. 6 (November-December, 1999), pp. (442-452), ISSN:1067-1927

Tsang, MW., Wong, WK., Hung, CS., Lai, KM., Tang, W., Cheung, EY., Kam, G., Leung, L., Chan, CW., Chu, CM. & Lam EK. (2003) Human epidermal growth factor enhances healing of diabetic foot ulcers. *Diabetes Care*, Vol. 26, No. 6, (June, 2003), pp. (1856-1861), ISSN: 0149-5992

van Cruijsen, H., Giaccone, G. & Hoekman, K. (2005) Epidermal growth factor receptor and angiogenesis: Opportunities for combined anticancer strategies. *International Journal of Cancer*, Vol. 117, No. 6 (December, 2005), pp. (883–888), ISSN:0020-7136

van Rijswijk, L. & Polansky, M. (1994) Predictors of time to healing deep pressure ulcers. *Ostomy/Wound Management*, Vol. 40, No. 8 (October, 1994), pp. (40–48), ISSN: 0889-5899.

Veves, A., Falanga, V., Armstrong, DG., Sabolinski, ML. and the Apligraf Diabetic Foot Ulcer Study. (2001) Graftskin, a human skin equivalent, is effective in the management of noninfected neuropathic diabetic foot ulcers: a prospective randomized multicenter clinical trial. *Diabetes Care*, Vol. 24, No. 2 (February, 2001), pp. (290–295), ISSN:0149-5992

Viswanathan, V., Pendsey, S., Sekar, N. & Murthy, GSR. (2006) A phase III study to evaluate the safety and efficacy of recombinant human Epidermal Growth Factor (REGEN-D™ 150) in Healing Diabetic Foot Ulcers. *Wounds*, Vol. 18, No. 7 (July, 2006), pp. (186-196), ISSN:1746-6814

Werner, S. & Grose, R. (2003) Regulation of wound healing by growth factors and cytokines. *Physiological Reviews*, Vol. 83, No. 3 (July, 2003), pp. (835-870), ISSN: 0031-9333

Williams, DT., Hilton, JR. & Harding, KG. (2004) Diagnosing foot infection in diabetes. *Clinical Infectious Diseases*, Vol. 39, Suppl 2 (August 2004), pp. (S83-S86), ISSN:1058-4838

13

Lactoferrin as an Adjunctive Agent in the Treatment of Bacterial Infections Associated with Diabetic Foot Ulcers

Maria Elisa Drago-Serrano[1], Mireya De la Garza[2] and Rafael Campos-Rodríguez[3]
[1]*Departamento de Sistemas Biológicos, Universidad Autónoma Metropolitana Unidad Xochimilco,*
[2]*Departamento de Biología Celular, Centro de Investigación y de Estudios Avanzados del IPN,*
[3]*Laboratorio de Inmunidad en Mucosas, Escuela Superior de Medicina del IPN, México*

1. Introduction

Lactoferrin is a protein of mammalian origin secreted in the milk of several animals, including human beings, cows, horses, pigs, goats and mice (Masson & Heremans, 1971). From the moment that bovine (Tomita et al., 2009) and human lactoferrin (Weinberg, 2001) were isolated from the milk of their respective species, they began to receive great attention due to their multifunctional properties that are distinctive from lactoferrin from other mammals. In general, lactoferrin is regarded as a modulator of humoral and cellular components involved in inflammatory and immune responses (Actor et al., 2009; Legrand et al., 2004), which has broad implications. For instance, lactoferrin displays antimicrobial activity against a wide range of pathogens, including virus, bacteria, fungi and parasites (Jenssen & Hancock, 2009). It is also able to promote skin integrity by regulating the generation of humoral components of the inflammatory and immune responses, including such cytokines as the tumor necrosis factor (TNF) alpha and interleukin (IL) 1beta, as well as the migration of Langerhans cells (Kimber et al., 2002). Moreover, lactoferrin enhances collagen gel contractile activity of fibroblasts, leading to skin wound healing (Takayama & Takezawa, 2006).

The broad scope of activities of lactoferrin with potential clinical applications, depicted in the Table 1, has led to large scale production of native and recombinant preparations of this glycoprotein for commercial and/or clinical applications (Drago-Serrano, 2007). Among these products are Talactoferrin alfa ®, a recombinant human lactoferrin (Agennix, Houston TX, USA), and Bioferrin®, a native lactoferrin from bovine origin (Glanbia, Nutritionals Inc, Monroe, WI, USA). Through the modulation of inflammation, Talactoferrin alfa has proven effective as a wound healing factor in the experimental model of diabetic mice (Engelmayer et al., 2008). Indeed, the promising healing properties of Talactoferrin alfa have been tested in a phase 1/2 clinical study for the treatment of ulcers in patients with diabetic

ORIGIN	ACTIVITY	REFERENCE
	Antibacterial effect	
Bovine Lf	↓ *Pseudomonas aeruginosa* anti-biofilm formation in combination with xilitol (a sugar derivative alcohol) (*in vitro* test)	Ammons et al., 2011A Ammons et al, 2009
	Phagocytic cell function	
Neutrophil human Lf	↑ Bacterial killing by enhancing reactive oxygen species (ROS) generation (*in vitro* test)	Ambruso & Johnston, 1981
Neutrophil human Lf	↓ oxidative effect of ROS released by degranulated neutrophils (*in vitro* test)	Britigan et al, 1991
	Anti-Inflammatory effect	
Bovine Lf	↓ Tumor necrosis factor (TNF) production induced during bacteremia in mice	Zimecki et al., 2004
Human Lf	↓ Lipopolysaccharide (LPS)-induced expression of endothelial adhesion molecules (E-selectin, ICAM) (*in vitro* test)	Baveye et al., 2000A
	Pro-inflammatory effect	
bLf/hLf	↑ human neutrophil derived interleukin (IL)-8 production (*in vitro* test)	Shinoda et al., 1996
recombinant human Lf (rHLf)	↑ human dendritic cell derived IL-8 production (*in vitro* test)	Spadaro et al., 2008
	Granulopoiesis	
Bovine Lf	↑ output of neutrophil precursors in human volunteers	Zimecki et al., 1999B
Mouse Lf	↑ colony stimulating factor (CSF) in mice	Sawatzki & Rich, 1989
Human Lf	↓ output of granulocyte macrophage progenitor cells from spleen and femur of mice	Gentile & Broxmeyer, 1983
	Effects on skin	
Human Lf	anti-allergen effect by decreasing Langerhans cell migration induced by allergens in humans	Griffiths et al., 2001
rHLf	↑ re-epithelialization (*in vitro* test)	Tang et al., 2010A Tang et al., 2010B
Bovine Lf	↑ gel contractile activity in human fibroblasts (*in vitro* test)	Takayama et al., 2003
Bovine Lf	↑ nerve growth factor synthesis/secretion in mouse fibroblasts (*in vitro* test)	Shinoda et al., 1994
Bovine Lf	↑ hyaluronan synthesis in human dermal fibroblast (*in vitro* test)	Saito et al., 2011
	Wound healing	
(rHLf)	Healing enhancement of foot ulcers in diabetic mouse model	Engelmayer et al., 2008
(rHLf)	Healing enhancement of diabetic foot ulcers in human patients	Lyons et al., 2007

Table 1. Overview of multifunctional properties of lactoferrin

foot (Lyons et al., 2007). Bioferrin, on the other hand, has been found to have antibacterial activity, for which reason it has been used in the control of bacterial infections associated with diabetic foot ulcers (Ammons et al., 2011A; Ammons et al., 2009). Such infections represent a serious challenge, since they can lead to devastating consequences and possibly to limb amputations (Powlson & Coll, 2010). Hence, this glycoprotein is endowed with natural antibacterial and wound healing properties that can be beneficial in the treatment of either infected or uninfected diabetic foot ulcers. However, given the complex convergence of pathologies which encompass diabetic foot syndrome, lactoferrin should not be considered as a *panacea* able by itself to cure this disorder.

The aim of this chapter is to describe the applications of lactoferrin as an antibacterial and wound healing agent. We explore its use as an adjunctive agent to enhance the antibacterial activity of antibiotics and/or improve the efficacy of other adjunctive methods of antibiotic treatment, the latter of which include growth factors, dressings and other topical applications, debridement, and hyperbaric oxygen therapy (O´Meara et al., 2000). In parallel we give an overview of the biological and modulating properties of lactoferrin in relation to the inflammatory and immune responses, as these properties underlie the reestablishment of homeostasis at the dermal level and thus contribute to ulcer skin healing. Finally, we discuss the precautions that should be taken into account for the clinical applications of this glycoprotein.

2. Lactoferrin: An overview

2.1 Structural features

Lactoferrin is a member of transferrins, a family of proteins with iron chelating properties. This monomeric glycoprotein has a molecular weight of 80 kDa, and is highly cationic with an isoelectric point of 9.6 (Baker & Baker, 2009). Its tertiary structure consists of two main N and C lobes, within which are found the N1/N2 and C1/C2 domains, respectively. The N and C lobes are linked at the N1 and C1 domains by a three turn alpha chain (Baker & Baker, 2009). Human milk lactoferrin contains two sites of glycosylation (Anderson et al., 1987) with N-acetylneuraminic acid, N-acetylglucosamine, galactose and mannose (Spik et al., 1982). In spite of the fact that bovine milk lactoferrin has five glycosylation sites, only four of them are actually glycosylated (Moore et al., 1997) with N-acetylneuraminic acid, galactose, manose, fucose, N-acetylglucosamine and N-acetylgalactosamine (Coddeville et al., 1992). Between the N1/N2 and C1/C2 regions, a cleft is formed by R amino acid groups of an aspartic, a histidine and two tyrosine residues. At this cleft, iron in ferric form (Fe^{3+}) along with the bicarbonate (HCO_3^{1-}) ion can be bound reversibly to lactoferrin (Anderson et al., 1987; Moore et al., 1997). The iron loaded state of lactoferrin is called hololactoferrin, while its iron free form is known as apolactoferrin. On the other hand, the N1 domain, devoid of any iron chelating activity, has a region known as lactoferricin, which is characterized by its strong cationic charge. Lactoferricin can be obtained as a free peptide by the enzymatic proteolysis of parental lactoferrin with pepsine. The iron independent properties of lactoferrin, such as some forms of antibacterial activity as well as various modulating properties of the immune and inflammatory responses, arise from this lactoferricin domain (Gifford et al., 2005).

2.2 Biological properties

2.2.1 Distribution

Lactoferrin is secreted in the milk of several mammals and is regarded as an essential component of innate mechanisms of host defense. Evidence of this role is the strategic location of lactoferrin at mucosal surfaces, which are frequently colonized and/or invaded by pathogenic micro-organisms (Russell et al., 2005). Lactoferrin is also stored in secondary (specific) granules of neutrophils, which upon degranulation normally release this glycoprotein in serum (Levay &Viljoen, 1995). The extent of neutrophil degranulation and the level of lactoferrin in serum increase during an inflammatory response from infectious origin (Legrand et al., 2004).

2.2.2 Effects on cellular components of the adaptive immune response

As aforementioned, lactoferrin is a modulator of humoral and cellular components involved in inflammatory and immune responses. Among its effects on the cellular components of the adaptive host defense, lactoferrin positive or negatively modifies the activity of B lymphocytes, T cells, macrophages, dendritic cells, neutrophils, and Langerhans cells involved in specific immune responses (Actor et al., 2009). For instance, it is a factor in B lymphocyte maturation, a process that defines the phenotype and function of these cells (Zimecki et al., 1995). On the other hand, T cell proliferation (Bi et al., 1997) and maturation (Zimecki et al., 1991) are enhanced by lactoferrin, evidenced by an increased expression of CD4 antigen in the presence of this glycoprotein (Bi et al., 1997; Zimecki et al., 1991; Dhennin-Duthille et al., 2000). Other studies show that lactoferrin abrogates the inhibitory effect of the iron saturated transferrin on T cell proliferation (Djeha & Brock, 1992), and inhibits the proliferative response and cytokine production of Th1 but not Th2, which logically affects the activity of Th1/Th2 subpopulations (Zimecki et al., 1996).

Lactoferrin is also able to modulate macrophages, as antigen presenting cells, to induce a Th1 response. That is, in the presence of this glycoprotein, there is an increase of IL 12, which in turn is required to combat intracellular pathogens (Wilk et al., 2007). It has been reported that lactoferrin expressed on the surface of neutrophils of healthy patients interacts with TCD4+ cells to up-regulate the production of IL 10 and down-regulate the production of interferon (IFN) gamma. In contrast, in patients with systemic lupus erythematosis, lactoferrin expressed on the surface of neutrophils negatively modulated the production of IL 10 and IFN gamma by TCD4+ cells. These results suggest that endogenous lactoferrin is able to regulate the expression of interleukins by interacting with TCD4+ lymphocytes (Li et al., 2006). Moreover, Lactoferrin acts as a maturation factor of antigen presenting cells, such as dendritic cells (De la Rosa et al., 2008; Spadaro et al., 2008) and macrophages (Sorimachi et al., 1997), evidenced by an up-regulated expression of CD80/86, the increased priming of T cells, and the enhanced secretion of pro-inflammatory mediators such TNF and IL 8.

The modulatory effects of lactoferrin on cellular components (neutrophils, keratinocytes and Langerhans cells) as well as humoral components (cytokines) of the inflammatory response involved in the innate mechanisms of bacterial control or dermal homeostasis are addressed in section 4 of this chapter.

3. Anti-bacterial activity of lactoferrin

3.1 Importance of iron in infections

Human beings as well as microorganisms that infect them require iron for living, since this metal is necessary for all redox reactions. This transition element is part of the heme group in hemoglobin and is a cofactor of enzymes such as ribonucleotide-reductase, indispensable for DNA synthesis (Andrews et al., 2003).

In the body, iron is usually bound to proteins. It is important for the body to maintain a low free-iron concentration, as otherwise free iron would lead to the overproduction of reactive oxygen species by the Fenton reaction, and these molecules are toxic for proteins, DNA and lipids. Moreover, an excessive free-iron concentration would easily be employed by invading pathogens for their survival and proliferation. The extracellular iron concentration in humans is approximately 10^{-18} M, a level too low to sustain the growth of microbes trying to colonize and invade a host (Bullen et al., 2005; Nairz et al., 2010; Weinberg, 2009).

Mammals have evolved a general strategy of decreasing the free-iron concentration in order to protect themselves against invading microbes. Complex iron-withholding systems are based on iron-binding proteins that chelate this ion, such as transferrin that transports and delivers iron to all cells, ferritin that stores iron inside the cells in order to avoid its toxicity and to maintain cell iron homeostasis (Chiancone et al., 2004), and lactoferrin that, as a cationic glycoprotein of the innate immune system, sequesters iron in mucosae and infection sites, precisely to avoid the accessibility of iron to all intruders (Bullen et al., 1972, 2005; Arnold et al., 1977; Jenssen & Hancock, 2009). Indeed, this was one of the first properties of this glycoprotein to be discovered.

3.2 Bacterial species that infect the diabetic foot

One major problem caused by pathogenic bacteria to a human host is the constant infection suffered by diabetic patients in their inferior extremities. Infected foot ulcers are complex interactions of microorganisms that often progress to deeper spaces and tissues. These infections can become chronic and incurable, and may even degenerate into septic gangrene, which could require foot amputation. Although chronic infections are frequently polymicrobial, it has been reported that acute infections in patients not previously treated with antibiotics are mainly caused by a single pathogen, usually a Gram-positive coccus (Edmonds, 2006; Armstrong & Lipsky, 2004; Powlson & Coll, 2010). Accordingly, early surface infections of skin ulcers on the feet of untreated diabetic patients are associated with aerobic Gram positive cocci, including *Staphylococcus aureus* and beta haemolytic streptococci group A and B. On the other hand, for diabetic patients with chronic lesions, infections are characterized by a polymicrobial mixture of aerobic Gram positive and Gram negative bacteria (*Escherichia coli, Proteus spp., Klebsiella spp.*), anaerobic bacteria (*Bacteroides spp, Clostridium spp, Peptococcus spp* and *Peptostreptococcus spp*) and *Pseudomonas aeruginosa* (Citron et al., 2007; Dowd et al., 2008).

Staphylococcus aureus methicillin-resistance strains (MRSA) and *Pseudomonas aeruginosa* are the most prominent components of biofilms, and bacterial biofilm is a major contributor to non-healing chronic lesions of diabetic patients. For instance, *Pseudomonas aeruginosa* is an opportunistic pathogen in chronic lesions that is refractory to the killing activity of phagocytic cells (e.g., neutrophils), and it is an underlying factor promoting bacterial resistance to antibiotics (Guo & DiPietro, 2010).

Some anaerobes are also responsible for infection in foot ulcers, and even skin commensal bacteria may cause damage to tissue (Edmonds, 2006). For mild and severe infections, some antibacterials have been shown to be effective in clinical trials, but have numerous side effects for patients. Both specific antibiotics as well as those of a wide spectrum have been reported to produce distinct side effects, such as nephro- and hepato-toxicity, blood dysplasias, diarrhea, and disorders in the commensal flora equilibrium that lead to other syndromes by opportunistic microbes (López-Novoa et al., 2011). A very serious problem with antibiotic treatments is the emergence of multiresistant strains, generally in long-standing infections, a result of the fact that the rate of development of new antimicrobial drugs is slower than the evolution of resistance. In the case of anaerobes, metronidazole is the drug of choice, used together with antibiotics. However, metronidazole is toxic, causing nausea, vomiting, abdominal pain and other effects. In addition, it might be carcinogenic to patients when used at high doses and/or as a long-term treatment, evidenced by DNA breakages and chromosome aberrations caused by this drug in cultured cells, and by its carcinogenic effects in animal tests (Roe, 1983; Dobias et al, 1994; El-Nahas & El-Ashmawy, 2004; Kapoor et al., 1999; Mudry *et al.*, 1994).

3.3 Lactoferrin as an option in therapy against microbial infections

Due to the aforementioned problems with antibiotics and other drugs, alternative therapies against microbial pathogenic populations have been explored in the last few years. One such alternative is lactoferrin, mainly prescribed when infections are chronic and when bacteria are found to be resistant to all treatments. Lactoferrin is abundant in colostrum and milk as a defense mechanism in newborns. Its iron-free form (apolactoferrin) is secreted by the acinar glands to mucosae or by neutrophils in infection sites. This form can be microbiostatic, depriving pathogens of iron and thus leaving them in a latent state, or microbicidal, leading to the death of pathogens (Jenssen & Hancock, 2009; Ling & Schryvers, 2006; Yamauchi et al., 2006).

3.4 Lactoferrin is able to synergize with other proteins and antimicrobials

3.4.1 Natural synergy of lactoferrin with innate immune-system proteins to combat pathogenic microorganisms

It has been demonstrated that lactoferrin synergizes with other proteins of the innate immune system, such as lysozyme and IgA, in order to eliminate microbial infections. Indeed, these three proteins are secreted together to mucosae (Leitch & Willcox, 1998; Vaerman, 1984). Lactoferrin has large cationic patches on its surface, facilitating direct interaction with anionic lipid A from the lipopolysaccharide (LPS) in Gram-negative bacteria. This interaction leads to a greater permeability of the outer membrane of such bacteria (Jenssen & Hancock, 2009). In the case of *Staphylococcus epidermidis*, a Gram-positive bacterium, it has been proposed that lactoferrin interacts with lipoteicoic acid on the bacterial surface, leading to a decrease of the negative charge on the membrane, which in turn allows lysozyme to reach the cell wall-associated peptidoglycan where this enzyme acts (Leitch & Willcox, 1999A).

3.4.2 Lactoferrin also synergizes with drugs and antibiotics, enhancing their microbicidal action

Lactoferrin has the great advantage of synergizing with antiviral and antiparasitic drugs as well as with antibiotics, intensifying the antimicrobial activity. In some cases an antibiotic dose can be decreased if administered with lactoferrin, which diminishes the side effects to patients (Jenssen & Hancock, 2009; Bullen et al., 1972; Arnold et al., 1977; Farnaud & Evans, 2003; Leon-Sicairos *et al.*, 2006; Sanchez & Watts, 1999; Diarra et al., 2002; Viani et al., 1999). Another adjunctive effect of lactoferrin is that biofilms of *Staphylococcus epidermidis* become more susceptible to lysozyme and vancomycin treatment when used in combination with this glycoprotein (Leitch & Willcox, 1999B). Interestingly, it was found that lactoferrin synergized with bacteriophages (bacterial viruses) in a patient suffering a prolonged antibiotic-resistant post-influenza otitis media infection due to *Staphylococcus epidermidis,* and the infection was resolved (Weber-Dabrowsca et al., 2006).

3.5 Lactoferrin and lactoferricins are able to prevent the formation of biofilms

Biofilms are a matrix-encased colonial organization of cells that more readily become resistant to drugs, antibiotics and antibodies than their free-living, planktonic counterparts. This matrix is composed of exopolysaccharide, and its formation is under the control of quorum sensing, a bacterial mechanism for assessing population density and altering gene expression in order to carry out processes that require the cooperation of a large number of cells (Miller & Bassler, 2001). Lactoferrin and its derivative peptides have been used against bacteria in biofilms. Furthermore, the synthetic peptides derived from the N-terminal of bovine lactoferrin, lactoferricin and lactoferrampin, and a fusion peptide of both, lactoferrin chimera, have been assayed against a wide range of pathogens, showing a very high probability of success against multiresistant bacteria as well as those accustomed to organizing and forming biofilms (Bolscher et al., 2009; Xu et al., 2010; Flores-Villaseñor et al., 2010). Furthermore, synergistic activity of bovine lactoferricin (11 amino acids) with antibiotics was demonstrated against multiresistant clinical isolates of *Staphylococcus aureus* and *Pseudomonas aeruginosa in vitro* and in a model of corneal infection in mice. Lactoferricin also had an anti-inflammatory effect in cornea, suggesting that it leads to a decrease of cytokines and mediators involved in inflammation (Oo et al., 2010). Hence, lactoferrin as well as its derived peptides could be potential adjuncts to conventional antibiotics in combating these pathogens, which also infect diabetic foot ulcers.

Singh et al. (2002) evaluated the effect of lactoferrin on biofilm development by *Pseudomonas aeruginosa*. In this study, the use of a green fluorescent protein, GFP, as a marker of the bacterial cells in continuous-culture allowed for the tracking of biofilm development over time. Interestingly, they demonstrated that lactoferrin disrupted biofilm pattern development, even at concentrations lower than those needed to kill bacteria or prevent their regular growth. By chelating iron, lactoferrin stimulated bacterial twitching, which is a specialized surface motility in which bacteria wander across the surface instead of forming cell clusters and biofilm. As was hypothesized, this lactoferrin effect was iron-dependent and only the iron-free form, apolactoferrin, showed this antimicrobial action. However, bacteria in an established biofilm were resistant to lactoferrin.

Neutrophil derived lactoferrin also was able to prevent bacteria biofilm development of *Pseudomonas aeruginosa* (Leid et al., 2009). Other assays show that lactoferrin in combination with xylitol (a sugar derived penta-hidroxy alcohol) decreases the viability of established *Pseudomonas aeruginosa*, a consequence of both the disruption of the biofilm structure and the permeabilization of the bacterial membrane (Ammons et al., 2009).

3.5.1 Lactoferrin and lactoferricins in the battle against infections associated with diabetic foot

Reproducing diabetic foot in animal models with the aim of studying ulcer infections has not proved easy. Nevertheless, an *in vitro* model of chronic lesion biofilms used to evaluate antimicrobial susceptibilities was recently reported. This model imitates the lesion environment and allows researchers to study various aspects of the physiology of biofilms, as well as the effect of drugs and antibiotics on the same. In this model, pretreatment with lactoferrin was employed to test for the inhibition of biofilm development by clinical isolates of diverse bacteria species. Results showed that this pretreatment did not affect biofilm formation or the number of bacteria, leading the authors to conclude that a continuous exposure of biofilm to lactoferrin is necessary in order to achieve this effect, as has been suggested in reports by other researchers (Hill et al., 2010).

In relation to foot ulcers of diabetic patients, there are scant reports about the use of lactoferrin. The anti-biofilm efficacy of adjunctive methods, such as silver wound dressings, for the therapy of infections associated with chronic ulcers is significantly increased when combined with lactoferrin-xylitol. The mechanisms underlying this cooperative antimicrobial effect are the iron chelating property of lactoferrin, which destabilizes the bacterial membrane, and the inhibitory effect of xylitol on the ability of the bacteria to produce siderophores under conditions of iron restriction (Ammons et al., 2011A, 2011B). As is well-known, iron deprivation promotes siderophore secretion for acquisition of iron essential for bacterial growth (Skaar, 2010). These studies point to the great potential of lactoferrin and lactoferricins as an adjunct in the treatment of diabetic foot infections. Further studies are needed to explore this potential.

4. Modulatory activities of lactoferrin on inflammation

The pleitropic property of lactoferrin spans a wide array of regulatory activities on cellular and humoral components of the inflammatory response. The capacity of lactoferrin to modulate the inflammatory response has been explored *in vitro* and *in vivo*. The animal models include the use of exogenous lactoferrin from bovine and human origin (Legrand et al., 2004), as well as the observation of untreated animals in order to explore the role of endogenous lactoferrin (Legrand & Mazurier, 2010). Here we focus on the regulatory effects of lactoferrin on mielopoiesis, the production of cytokines and the generation of reactive oxygen species (ROS), and in particular on the inflammatory response in skin allergy and skin healing in non-infected lesions.

4.1 Modulatory effects on ROS generation

4.1.1 Up-regulation

Lactoferrin is a key component of immune homeostasis, able to positively or negatively regulate the function of cellular components of innate mechanisms of defense involved in inflammation, such as mononuclear cells (monocytes and macrophages) and neutrophils. According to *in vitro* assays with neutrophils treated with bovine lactoferrin, the ability of this glycoprotein to enhance phagocytosis may be a result of its direct contact along with an opsonin-like action on phagocytic cells (Miyauchi et al., 1998). However, the role of lactoferrin in phagocytosis has been linked with its ability to positively regulate the generation of ROS with bactericidal activity. Evidence of this up-regulating action is the fact that lactoferrin in secondary granules of neutrophils enhances the intracellular killing of *Pseudomonas aeruginosa* by promoting the generation of ROS during phagocytosis (Bullen & Armstrong, 1979). It has been reported that exogenous lactoferrin enhances the activity of ROS production in neutrophils (Ambruso & Johnston, 1981; Gahr et al., 1991) and macrophages (Lima & Kierszenbaum, 1987), and that the presence of iron is necessary for this effect to take place (Gahr et al., 1991; Lima & Kierszenbaum, 1987). Hololactoferrin (the iron- loaded form) seems to deliver the iron that can act as an enzymatic catalyst of Haber-Weiss reactions, which in turn generate various types of ROS, including hydrogen peroxide (H_2O_2), superoxide anion (O^{2-}) and the hydroxyl radical ($OH\cdot$) (Actor et al., 2009). Reactive oxygen species are substrates for the enzymatic generation of antibacterial molecules. For instance, H_2O_2 is a precursor of hypochlorous (HClO). The latter is a strong bactericidal molecule generated enzymatically by mieloperoxidase (MPO) (Hampton et al., 1998), a prominent component of azurophil granules in neutrophils (Leffell & Spitznagel, 1974).

4.1.2 Down-regulation

Lactoferrin can also have a down-regulatory effect on ROS production, such as is the case with phagocytes. The mechanism of this effect is the reduction of oxidative stress and the control of an excessive inflammatory response (Actor et al., 2009). During the oxidative burst, intracellular generation of ROS is essential for the control of bacterial growth (Hampton et al, 1998). However, under conditions of oxidative stress the excessive release of ROS to the extracellular milieu has devastating effects on the structure of macromolecules and cell functions (Actor et al., 2009). Unlike azurophil granules that store MPO, usually associated with phagosomes during bacteria phagocytosis, secondary (specific) granules that contain lactoferrin usually become degranulated (Leffell & Spitznagel, 1974). Evidence from in *vitro* assays shows that lactoferrin released during neutrophil degranulation decreases the overproduction of ROS (Britigan el al., 1989). Moreover, the uptake of exogenous lactoferrin by mononuclear phagocytes that do not contain endogenous lactoferrin inhibits their ability to form the hydroxyl radical and protects them from membrane auto-peroxidation (Britigan et al., 1991). This effect may be linked to the property of lactoferrin to inhibit lipid peroxidation (Gutteridge et al., 1981). In the mouse model of pollen induced allergic airway, lactoferrin has been effective in inhibiting the generation of the superoxide anion. Pollen grains contain reduced nicotinamide adenine dinucleotide phosphate (NADH) oxidases. Their product, O^{2-}, is a precursor of H_2O_2 and $OH\cdot$, which increase pollen induced airway inflammation (Kruzel et al., 2006).

Apart from its role in inhibiting the overproduction of ROS by phagocytes, lactoferrin can also down-regulate ROS production by neutrophils that are stimulated by LPS. Lipopolysaccharide interacts with the soluble receptor lipopolysaccharide binding protein (LPB), which in turn enables the binding of LPS to CD14, a membrane receptor of phagocytes (Van Amersfoort et al., 2003). After binding to the surface membrane via the

LBP/CD14 receptor complex, LPS released by dead or growing bacteria causes neutrophil activation, as evidenced by the oxidative burst accompanied with ROS generation. Moreover, when LPS is massively released, such as in septic shock, it binds to L-selectin, an integral glycoprotein of membrane leukocytes, and this complex also results in the production of ROS (Malhotra et al., 1996). Both of these mechanisms of ROS production are impeded by the capacity of lactoferrin to bind to LPS (Wang et al., 1995). Additionally, lactoferrin blocks the interaction of LPS with the L-selectin of neutrophils, which also avoids the production of ROS (Baveye et al., 2000B). It has been shown that either endogenous lactoferrin secreted by neutrophils (Wang et al., 1995) or exogenous lactoferrin (Cohen et al., 1992) can inhibit the ability of LPS to prime neutrophils for enhanced superoxide production.

Interestingly, the IL 10 receptor (IL-10R), a component of secondary granules, also has an anti-inflammatory effect, like lactoferrin, in the presence of LPS. This receptor is exported from secondary granules to the membrane of neutrophils primed with LPS. When interacting with its respective ligand, these IL 10 receptors reduce the production of ROS stimulated by LPS (Elbim et al., 2001).

4.2 Modulatory effects of lactoferrin on pro-inflammatory cytokines

Lactoferrin is a modulatory agent whose positive or negative effects on cytokine production and phagocytes involved in the inflammatory response is highly dependent on the type of inductor recognized by the immune system and also on environmental conditions (Actor et al., 2009). The modulatory activity of lactoferrin in inflammation has been addressed in animal models, such as that of colitis induced by dextran sulfate (Håversen et al., 2003A; Togawa et al., 2002) and that of hind-foot inflammation by carrageenan (Zimecki et al., 1998). This modulatory activity has also been assessed under *in vitro* and *in vivo* conditions by using LPS as an inducer (Puddu et al., 2010). The proven substantive regulatory effects of lactoferrin on inflammation induced by LPS are not fully understood. However, it is known that the intrinsic binding properties of lactoferrin to LPS and/or LPS receptors results in an interaction with toll like receptor (TLR)-4 and possibly with other unknown receptors, leading to the increase (Na et al., 2004) or decrease (Håversen et al., 2002) of cytokine production.

4.2.1 Down-regulation

The effects of lactoferrin on inflammation have been correlated with a decrease in three pro-inflammatory mediators: TNF (Håversen et al., 2003A; Togawa et al., 2002; Zimecki et al., 1998), IL 6 (Togawa et al., 2002; Zimecki et al., 1998) and IL 1 (Togawa et al., 2002). These effects have also been associated, in some cases, with an increase in two anti-inflammatory interleukins: IL 4 and IL 10 (Togawa et al., 2002). In animal models of infection with *Shigella flexneri* (Gómez et al., 2002), *Salmonella typhimurium* (Mosquito et al., 2010) and *Lysteria monocytogenes* (Lee et al., 2005), lactoferrin from bovine or human origin has been effective in reducing inflammatory necrosis in liver (Lee et al., 2005) and intestine (Mosquito et al., 2010), as well as in intestinal edema (Gomez et al., 2002). Owing to its anti-inflammatory effect, as evidenced by the reduced levels of TNF (Lee et al., 2005; Komine, et al., 2006; Zimecki et al., 2004) and IL 6 (Håversen et al., 2003B), lactoferrin contributes to a decrease in tissue damage caused by the inflammation induced by bacterial pathogens. Other assays also have shown that lactoferrin released by phagocytes acts as a negative feedback factor by decreasing the TNF released from these cells, which in turn prevents their excessive recruitment and activation of phagocytes. In this way, lactoferrin modulates the recruitment to sites of inflammation (Crouch et al., 1992).

There is also evidence that lactoferrin increases the expression of LFA-1, an adhesion molecule of blood mononuclear cells (Zimecki et al., 1999A). This is another molecule involved in the migration of phagocytes to inflammatory sites. On the other hand, lactoferrin inhibits LPS-induced expression of two adhesion molecules, E-selectin and ICAM-1, by endothelial cells (Baveye et al., 2000A). Furthermore, it decreases the IL 8 production induced by LPS and competes with this chemokine for its binding to proteoglycans of endothelial cells (Elass et al., 2002).

4.2.2 Up-regulation

In addition to its role as a down-regulator of some pro-inflammatory cytokines, lactoferrin has also been found to stimulate the production of other pro-inflammatory cytokines associated with resistance to bacteria. For instance, the activation by lactoferrin of mononuclear cells and polymorphonuclear leukocytes has been correlated with its ability to stimulate the release of IL 8 (Spadaro et al., 2008; Sorimachi et al., 1997; Shinoda et al., 1996). Up-regulatory properties of lactoferrin on TNF levels increase the efficacy of the BCG vaccine by inducing the increase of pro-inflammatory cytokines like IL 6 and IFN gamma, involved in the resistance against *Mycobacterium tuberculosis* (Hwang et al., 2007). In transgenic mice carrying a functional human *Lf* gene and infected with *Staphylococcus aureus*, causing septic arthritis, the increase of a pro-inflammatory Th1 response due to greater TNF and IFN gamma levels (and a decreased Th2 response of anti-inflammatory mediators IL 5 and IL 10) was associated with a reduced incidence of arthritis and mortality (Guillén et al., 2002). Thus, the pro-inflammatory effects of lactoferrin contribute to resistance to infections caused by the aforementioned pathogens.

4.3 Modulatory effects on mielopoiesis

Another protective effect of bovine lactoferrin in the protection against *Escherichia coli* bacteremia in mice has been associated with an increased turnover of neutrophils (Zimecki et al., 2004). In this regard, the demand for neutrophils greatly increases in the inflammatory response caused by infections. Thus, the effect of lactoferrin on bacterial resistance may be linked to its regulatory properties on cytokines involved in mielopoiesis, including IL 1,IL 6, IL 8 and TNF, as well as on mielopoietic growth factors, such as granulocyte macrophage colony stimulating factor (GM-CSF), G-CSF and M-CSF (Artym & Zimecki, 2007). These soluble factors favor mielopoiesis, i.e., the process of the generation of granulocyte and monocyte leukocytes from a bone marrow pluripotent cell.

The modulatory activity on mielopoiesis has been described in relation to lactoferrin released by human neutrophils and exogenous lactoferrin tested with culture cells or administered to animals or human volunteers (Artym & Zimecki, 2007). The modulatory role of lactoferrin upon progenitor cells of the granulocyte/macrophage lineage has been controversial (Artym & Zimecki, 2007). In healthy humans orally treated with bovine lactoferrin, the up-regulatory action of lactoferrin on granulopoiesis was linked to the increased output of neutrophil precursors along with an attenuated release of TNF and IL-6 (Zimecki et al., 1999B). The effect of lactoferrin in promoting granulopoiesis apparently results from its ability to stimulate the increase in CSF production, as was shown under *in vitro* and *in vivo* conditions (Sawatzki & Rich, 1989). With assays of mouse bone marrow and peritoneal cells, both cultured with or without indomethacin (a non-steroidal anti-inflammatory drug used as an inhibitor of prostaglandin synthesis), mouse or human lactoferrin promoted an increase in CSF. On the other hand, injection of mice with endotoxin free mouse lactoferrin stimulated an early increase in CSF production, and a more delayed increase in bone marrow granulocyte macrophage progenitor cells (GM-CFC) (Sawatzki & Rich, 1989).

Lactoferrin also can have a negative effect on mielopoiesis, as evidenced by the iron dependent capacity of human lactoferrin to suppress the number of granulocyte macrophage progenitor cells from femur and spleen of mice (Gentile & Broxmeyer, 1983). This iron dependent suppressor effect of human lactoferrin, when tested in human bone marrow derived cells and blood monocytes, was linked to the decrease of GM-CSF (Broxmeyer et al., 1980). However, the role of lactoferrin as a modulating agent on granulopoiesis was not at all confirmed by some other studies (DelForge et al., 1985; Winton et al., 1981).

These divergent results in regard to the modulatory effects of lactoferrin on leukocyte generation have probably arisen from variations in experimental design. After all, the inflammatory response is a very complex spatio-temporal process of multiple steps. The effect of lactoferrin on mielopoiesis must therefore be dependent on the stage of the inflammatory response. Lactoferrin as an immunoregulatory protein should presumable act first by enhancing the inflammatory response, and later by suppressing the same (Artym & Zimecki, 2007).

4.4 Modulatory effects of lactoferrin on inflammation in models of skin allergy and skin wound healing

The skin is the largest organ of the human body, made up of three main layers: epidermis, dermis and the hypodermis (Kanitakis, 2002). The epidermis layer contains no blood vessels and is made up of 90-95 % keratinocytes and 5% Langerhans cells, melanocytes and Merkel cells. Keratinocytes, upon dying due to a lack of blood supply, are responsible for skin keratinization by releasing keratin to extracellular surroundings. Langerhans cells are mobile dendritic presenting cells derived from CD34+ bone marrow precursor cells. Melanocytes produce melanin, a natural dye to protect skin from ultraviolet radiation. Merkel cells display neuroendocrine and epithelial features and function as mechanoreceptors by their contact through synaptic junctions with dermal sensory axons.

The dermis, the second layer of the skin, is tightly connected to epidermis by a basement membrane which protects the latter layer from stress. The dermis is a vascularized layer formed by an elastic and compressible connective tissue that contains fibroblasts, dermal dendrocytes (mesenchymal dendritic cells), mast cells and a dense network of collagen fibers.

The hypodermis represents the inner layer of skin and is made up of loose connective tissue and elastin. The main types of cells present in this layer are fibroblasts, macrophages and adipocytes. This layer contains 50% body fat and plays a relevant role in thermoregulation, insulation and supply of energy. It also acts as a shield against mechanical injuries (Kanitakis, 2002).

Lactoferrin displays a role in skin homeostasis by its ability to positively or negatively modulate the generation cytokines derived from keratinocytes and Langerhans cells, with an essential role in immune and inflammatory responses (Wang et al., 1999).

4.4.1 Modulation of the inflammatory response associated with skin allergy

Trials with human volunteers and assays on mice have addressed down-regulatory properties of bovine or human lactoferrin on pro-inflammatory cytokines generated during dermal allergic responses induced by diphenylcyclopropenone (DPC) (Griffiths et al., 2001; Kimber et al., 2002) and oxazolone (Cumberbatch et al., 2000).

In models of skin allergy induced by DPC or oxazolone, epidermal Langerhans cells migrate to skin-draining lymph nodes. As a consequence, there is an accumulation and maturation of Langerhans cells as dendritic cells able to perform their antigen presentation role to naïve T cells (Wang et al., 1999). In the aforementioned models of skin allergy, the migration of Langerhans cells depends on the local production by skin keratinocytes of IL 1beta, which in turn is dependent on *de novo* production of TNF alpha. In humans, TNF alpha stimulates the activation and migration of Langerhans cells from the dermis, and their subsequent accumulation in human skin-draining lymph nodes (Cumbertbach et al., 1999). This cytokine also promotes the migration of immature Langerhans cells to human lymph nodes involved in chronic skin inflammation (Geissmann et al., 2002). In this regard, the anti-inflammatory property of lactoferrin applied topically to humans and mice has been linked to a decrease in the migration of skin Langerhans cells induced by DPC or oxazolone (Griffiths et al., 2001; Kimber et al., 2002; Cumberbatch et al., 2000). As in the case of DPC or oxazonolone, homolog lactoferrin inhibits the mobilization of Langerhans cells induced by intradermic IL 1beta in humans (Cumberbatch et al., 2003) and mice (Cumberbatch et al., 2000). However, in mice, homolog lactoferrin fails to reduce the migration of Langerhans cells induced by the application of exogenous TNF alpha (Cumberbatch et al., 2000). It seems that the down-regulatory effect of lactoferrin on Langerhans cell migration induced by DPC or oxazolone allergens, occurs after inhibiting *de novo* synthesis of TNF alpha by epidermal keratinocytes.

Another down-regulatory effect of bovine lactoferrin has also been described in the mouse model of zymosan-ear skin inflammation (Hartog et al., 2007). In this model, bovine lactoferrin had an anti-inflammatory effect by suppressing local production of TNF alpha. Furthermore, a combination of lactoferrin and glycine generated a synergistic anti-inflammatory effect (Hartog et al., 2007).

In patients with eczematous dermatitis caused by contacting nickel, recombinant human lactoferrin decreased the inflammatory response by inhibiting type 1 and type 2 T cell responses. In that study lactoferrin suppressed T cell proliferation and inhibited the expression of chemokine receptors CCR10, CXCR3 (expressed on Th1) and CCR4 (expressed on Th2 cells). However, the production of IFN gamma by Th1 and IL 5 by Th2 was partially suppressed by lactoferrin (Moed et al., 2004).

4.4.2 Effect of lactoferrin on cutaneous homeostasis and skin wound healing

4.4.2.1 Stages of skin wound healing

Some of the humoral and cellular components of the inflammatory and immune responses that are modulated by lactoferrin in turn regulate mechanisms with an essential role in cutaneous homeostasis and wound healing. As is known, dermal wound healing is a normal process of repair that involves four continuous, overlapping and precisely programmed stages: i) hemostasis ii) inflammation, iii) fibroplasia, and iv) remodeling (Hardy, 1989; Guo & DiPietro, 2010).

Hemostasis results from vasoconstriction and clotting by fibrin deposition to control bleeding caused by the vascular injury. The clot along with injured surrounding tissue release pro-inflammatory mediators and growth cell factors, such as transforming growth factor (TGF) beta1, fibroblast growth factor (FGF) and epidermal growth factor (EGF) (Guo & DiPietro, 2010).

In the inflammatory phase, sequential infiltration of neutrophils, macrophages and lymphocytes occurs in damaged tissue. The presence of phagocytes is mandatory for bacterial and cellular debris clearance (Hardy, 1989). The pro-inflammatory contribution of lactoferrin in this stage may be linked to its ability to up-regulate the bactericidal activity of neutrophils (Ambruso & Johnston, 1981; Gahr et al., 1991) and macrophages (Lima & Kierszenbaum, 1987) aimed at the control of bacterial growth. During this stage, lactoferrin also modulates the overproduction of ROS released during neutrophil degranulation in order to protect the organism from toxic effects of the same (Britigan el al., 1989).

In the early inflammatory phase, TNF alpha has an essential role in wound healing. However, since its overproduction can cause tissue damage, the fact that lactoferrin decreases TNF released from phagocytes may contribute to preventing the excessive recruitment and activation of phagocytes to sites of inflammation (Crouch et al., 1992). Evidence from *in vitro* cultures of peripheral and bone marrow monocytes of human origin suggest that the down-regulating effects of lactoferrin on inflammation may also be linked to its suppression of the release of IL 1 from monocytes. This in turn decreases GM-CSF production by fibroblasts (Zucali et al., 1989), which may contribute to controlling the mobilization of peripheral blood cells to inflammatory sites.

The fibroplastic phase is characterized by three processes: i) re-epithelialization, ii) wound contraction and iii) production of extracellular matrix components such as collagen (Hardy, 1989). Numerous subtypes of keratinocytes (Patel et al., 2006) and fibroblasts (El Ghalbzouri et al., 2004) play an essential role in scar tissue formation by contributing to wound re-epithelialization. In the early response to injury, re-epithelialization occurs when fibroblasts in the neighborhood of the wound proliferate and then migrate to the wound bed, where they are induced by chemotactic mediators to produce extracellular matrix components (Hardy, 1989). Among these components are proteoglycans (heparan-, chondroitin- and keratan-sulfate), non-proteoglycan polysaccharide (hyalouronic acid) and fibers (collagen, elastin) (Labat-Robert et al., 1990). Dermal healing is accompanied by a process of granulation, which results from the accumulation of fibroblasts and extracellular matrix components along with the formation of new blood vessels to constitute granular tissue (Hardy, 1989).

Generation of granular tissue is a complex process regulated by cytokines such as TGF beta1 produced by keratinocytes, macrophages and fibroblasts (Werner et al., 2007). Transforming growth factor beta1 stimulates the expression of integrins in keratinocytes, which facilitates their migration to perform the re-epithelialization during wound healing (Gailit et al., 1994). Granulation is also dependent on growth factors such as EGF, platelet derived growth factor (PDGF) and basic fibroblast growth factor (bFGF) (Werner et al., 2007). *In vitro* assays show that TGF beta1 and PDGF regulate fibroblast attachment, which represents the step between cell migration and proliferation *in vivo* during wound healing (Ihn et al., 1995). Additionally, TGF beta1, bFGF and other blood derived factors promote cell migration and proliferation leading to the increase of cells in the denuded area, or wound space (Schreier et al., 1993). Other agents that exercise healing effects, by enhancing migration and proliferation of keratinocytes for re-epithelializing of the wound bed, include keratinocyte growth factor 2 (Soler et al., 1999), heparin binding EGF like growth factor (Shirakata et al., 2005), skin beta-defensins (Niyonsaba et al., 2007) and insulin (Liu et al., 2009).

4.4.2.2 Effects of lactoferrin on wound healing

The role of lactoferrin in the fibroplastic phase has been addressed in some *in vitro* cultures of human skin fibroblasts (Tang et al., 2010A) and keratinocytes (Tang et al., 2010B). These assays show that recombinant human lactoferrin sustains the survival of fibroblasts and keratinocytes by protecting them from apoptosis, and in this way enhances re-epithelialization by stimulating the proliferation and migration of these cells.

It has been reported that bovine lactoferrin is also able to enhance collagen gel-contractile activity in human fibroblasts, which is the *in vitro* model for the reorganization of the collagen matrix during the wound healing process. Gel contractile activity induced by bovine lactoferrin is accompanied by the activation of extracellular regulated kinase (ERK) 1/2 and myosin light chain kinase (MLCK), and the subsequent elevation of myosin light chain phosphorylation. The effects of lactoferrin on gel contractile activity and its signaling pathway were mediated by the low density lipoprotein receptor related protein (LRP) (Takayama et al., 2003).

Lactoferrin may contribute to wound healing in the fibroplastic stage by its promotion of the synthesis and secretion of the nerve growth factor, which was observed in one study during the contact of bovine lactoferrin with mouse fibroblasts (Shinoda et al., 1994). The nerve growth factor (NGF) is an angiogenic agent with healing activity on diabetic skin ulcers in humans (Aloe, 2004) and mice (Graiani et al., 2004). Also in the fibroplastic stage, lactoferrin promotes the synthesis of components of extracellular matrix, such as type 1 collagen and hyaluronan, the latter through the activation of the TFG beta1 signaling pathway. This has been shown *in vitro* with assays on human fibroblasts (Saito et al., 2011).

5. Applications of lactoferrin as an adjunctive agent in the treatment of infections associated with diabetic foot ulcers

Whereas the previous discussion demonstrates that lactoferrin possesses pleitotropic properties on cell components involved in the inflammation associated with skin allergy or skin reparation of non-infected surface wounds, what follows is intended to describe potential applications of lactoferrin as an adjunctive agent to control bacterial growth in infected foot ulcers, which can threaten a limb or even the life of diabetic patients. Diabetic foot syndrome encompasses a complex convergence of pathologies, including diabetic neuropathy, peripheral vascular disease, Charcot´s neuroarthropathy, and osteomyelitis and foot ulceration. Diabetic foot ulcers are usually detected at the plantar surface and result from neuropathy, inadequate blood supply (ischemia) (Khanolkar et al., 2008), hypoxia (Tamir, 2007) and disturbances in neutrophil phagocytic function (Bader, 2008). Neuropathy plays a major role in foot ulceration since it underlies the loss of limb sensibility to skin pain caused by dermal abrasions and blisters, owing to disturbances of sensory, motor and autonomic functions (Khanolkar et al., 2008).

At present, the evaluation of lactoferrin as an agent with wound healing properties has been limited to only two studies: an experimental study on diabetic mice (Engelmeyer et al., 2008) and a clinical study on patients (Lyons et al., 2007). In the former, topically applied Talactoferrin, versus the vehicle or becaplermin (a recombinant human platelet-derived growth factor), increased the closure rate. *In vitro* culture assays suggest that the underlying mechanism of the healing effect of Talactoferrin on mouse diabetic ulcers could be linked with its ability to enhance the migration of dermal fibroblasts, THP-1 macrophages, Jurkat T cells and mouse granulocytes. Other activities of Talactoferrin associated with its healing properties include its ability to enhance the production of IL-8, IL-6, MIP-1 alpha and TNF α, all of which have an essential role in the early inflammatory phase of wound healing (Engelmayer et al., 2008).

In the clinical study, Talactoferrin was delivered topically in gel to the non-healing chronic ulcers from fifty five diabetic patients (patients with any sign of osteomyelitis, gangrene o deep tissue infection were excluded). The first phase, an open label, sequential, dose-escalation study, evaluated the safety of Talactoferrin. Groups of patients were treated with 1% (n=3), 2.5% (n=3) or 8.5% (n=3) of Talactoferrin gel applied topically at the ulcer twice daily for 30 days in combination with standard wound care. No adverse effects were detected. The second phase assessed the efficacy of two distinct doses of Talactoferrin. This was a single blind randomized, stratified placebo controlled pilot study of three groups of patients treated with gel containing 2.5% (n=15) and 8.5% (n=15) of Talactoferrin gel or placebo gel (n=16). In combination with standard wound care, Talactoferrin gel was administered topically twice daily to the ulcers for 12 weeks. The results from the second phase showed that Talactoferrin was effective as a healing agent, evidenced by a significant difference ($P<0.01$) between the results in the Tlactoferrin-treated and control groups. The incidence in the reduction of the size of ulcers in the groups treated with 2.5% and 8.5 % Talactoferrin gel was ≥ 75% compared with 45%-25% in the groups treated with placebo gel. Accordingly, Talactoferrin has been shown to be an effective agent with healing properties and seems to be pharmacologically safe and well tolerated. Thus, it may be useful in the treatment of foot ulcers in diabetic patients (Lyons et al., 2007).

Due to the multifactorial characteristic of the diabetic foot syndrome, lactoferrin does not fulfill the therapeutic requirements for use as a single healing agent. However, some standard techniques of un-infected and un-ischemic diabetic ulcers like debridement (i.e., removal of unhealthy tissue from the wound bed) (Tamir, 2007) may be improved by including lactoferrin as an adjunctive therapeutic agent.

Some pharmaceutical formulations of lactoferrin, including liposomes administered intra-articularly in joints (Trif et al., 2001) or by oral route (Ishikado et al., 2005) to control the chronic inflammation of arthritis or other pathologies, as well as bioadhesive tablets administered to treat inflammation associated with oral ulcers (Takahashi et al., 2007; Takeda et al., 2007), may represent systemic or oral delivery formulations for adjunctive treatment of chronic wounds. As is known, a prolonged inflammatory response is a contributing factor of chronic wounds, since it abrogates the normal process of ulcer healing (Pierce, 2001).

Diabetic patients usually suffer skin dryness, which prompts injuries that are highly susceptible to bacterial infections. When foot skin of the plantar surface is injured, microorganisms that are normally retained gain access to underlying layers where bacterial replication leads to local and/or systemic infections (Guo & DiPietro, 2010). Bacterial infections associated with chronic non-healing foot ulcerations, apart from being a common cause of limb amputation, put the life of the diabetic patient at risk (Bader, 2008).

The effectiveness of standard methods of care, including off-loading, debridement, systemic and local antibiotics and topical antiseptics, can be substantially improved when combined with adjunctive techniques. In some cases, adjuncts like wound dressings (Hilton et al., 2004), hyperbaric oxygen and growth factors are needed to provide better conditions for closure. Such conditions include a moist environment to enhance an optimal inflammatory milieu, as well as an adequate supply of oxygen and nutritional factors (Hopf et al., 2001).

Silver wound dressings have been applied to control the formation of biofilms associated with acute and chronic ulcers in diabetic patients (Hilton et al., 2004). However, as the treatment progresses, the single antibacterial effect of the silver is surpassed by the generation of antibacterial resistance caused by the establishment of bacterial biofilms which in turn impede healing of chronic ulcers in diabetic patients. Lactoferrin may be included in the list of adjuncts with a role in the establishment of the proper conditions for the healing of the wound bed, owing to its aforementioned natural antibacterial and wound healing properties. In this regard, a pharmaceutical presentation of lactoferrin and xylitol in hydrogel proved effective in enhancing the antibiofilm efficacy of a commercial silver wound dressing (Ammons et al., 2011B). That study showed that the combination of lactoferrin, xylitol and silver provides significant antimicrobial efficacy against established biofilms formed by methicillin-resistant *Staphylococcus aureus* (MRSA) and *Pseudomonas aeruginosa*. Consequently, lactoferrin in combination with xylitol would be recommended to increase the antibacterial effect of silver wound dressings applied to infected wounds of diabetic patients.

Thus, wound healing and anti-biofilm properties enable lactoferrin, acting as an adjunctive agent, to enhance the efficacy of anti-biofilm targeted techniques for the treatment of infected chronic ulcers like silver wound dressings.

6. Safety measures in the use of Lactoferrin

Toxicological assays on rats chronically treated by the oral route with human recombinant (Cerven et al., 2008; Appel et al, 2006) or native bovine (Yamauchi et al., 2000) lactoferrin show that regardless of their origin, these proteins are pharmacological safe products. In spite of their free toxicity *status*, some concerns have been raised, including bacterial resistance to human lactoferrin, as in the case of *Streptococcus pneumoniae* (Hammerschmidt et al., 1999), and the autoimmune potential of cross reactive anti-lactoferrin antibodies which recognize bacterial antigens like the 65 kDa protein of *Mycobacterium tuberculosis* (Esaguy et al., 1991). Although neither *Streptococcus pneumoniae* or *Mycobacterium tuberculosis* are associated with infections in diabetic foot ulcers, bacterial resistance and the autoimmune potential of cross reactive anti-lactoferrin antibodies warn of the need to be alert to possible problems in the application of lactoferrin as an antibacterial agent. While this requires attention to side effects that could present themselves, it does not in any way undermine all of the positive results of lactoferrin found to date.

The pathological relevance of anti-lactoferrin autoantibodies remains uncertain (Audrain et al., 1996). However, it is possible that in some chronic degenerative diseases such as rheumatoid arthritis (Esaguy et al., 1993), ulcerative colitis, primary sclerosing cholangitis and Crohn´s disease, autoantibodies to lactoferrin may aggravate and sustain the inflammatory condition (Peen et al., 1993).

Host-produced lactoferrin has been associated with some degenerative diseases and therefore the administration of exogenous lactoferrin may aggravate and contribute to the multifunctional pathology of diabetic foot syndrome. In this regard, endogenous lactoferrin has been reported as a major component of amyloid depots in patients with gelatinous drop-like corneal dystrophy (Klinworth et al., 1997), and it has been detected in pathological lesions in a variety of neurodegenerative disorders as Alzheimer´s disease, amyotrophic lateral sclerosis/parkinsonism dementia complex of Guam and sporadic amyotrophic lateral sclerosis, or Pick´s disease (Leveugle et al., 1994).

On the other hand, in some sensitized individuals, lactoferrin from bovine milk can be a strong milk allergen (Gaudin et al., 2008). Therefore in such individuals with diabetic foot, the allergenic potential of bovine lactoferrin should be taken into account before prescribing its oral administration. Additionally, the undesirable pro-inflammatory effects of iron loaded lactoferrin on vascular permeability, as evidenced in the dermis of rats by the increase of albumin extravasation (Erga et al., 2001), could negatively affect the process of skin healing.

7. Conclusion

The antibacterial and wound healing properties of lactoferrin may contribute to enhancing the effectiveness of standard techniques for treatment of infections of diabetic foot ulcers. Futures studies are needed to address the substantive therapeutic contribution of lactoferrin as an adjunctive agent in the treatment of infections associated with diabetic ulcer, including the concerns and limitations of its application.

8. Acknowledgements

We thank Bruce Allan Larsen for reviewing the use of English in this manuscript. This work was supported in part by grants from SEPI-IPN and from COFAA-IPN.

9. References

Actor, J.K.; Hwang, S.A. & Kruzel, M.L. (2009). Lactoferrin as a Natural Immune Modulator. *Current Pharmaceutical Design*, Vol. 15, No. 17, pp. 1956-1973, ISSN 1381-6128

Aloe, L. (2004). Nerve Growth Factor, Human Skin Uulcers and Vascularization. Our experience. *Progress in Brain Research*, Vol. 146, pp. 515-522, ISSN 0079-6123

Ambruso, D.R. & Johnston R.B. (1981). Lactoferrin Enhances Hydroxyl Radical Production by Human Neutrophils, Neutrophil Particulate Fractions, and an Enzymatic Generation System. *The Journal Clinical of Investigation*, Vol. 67, No. 2, (February 1981), pp. 352-360, ISSN 0021-9738

Ammons, M.C.; Ward L.S.; Dowd, S. & James, G.A. (2011A). Combined Treatment of *Pseudomonas aeruginosa* Biofilm with Lactoferrin and Xylitol Inhibits the Ability of Bacteria to Respond to Damage Resulting from Lactoferrin Iron Chelation. *International Journal of Antimicrobial Agents*, Vol. 37, No. 4, (April 2011), pp. 316-326, ISSN 0924-8579

Ammons, M.M.; Ward, L.S. & James, G.A. (2011B). Anti-biofilm Efficacy of a Lactoferrin-Xylitol Wound Hydrogel in Combination with Silver Wound Dressings. *International Wounds Journal*, doi: 10.1111/j.1742-481X.2011.00781.x. (April 2011), ISSN 1742-4801

Ammons, M.C.; Ward, L.S.; Fisher, S.T.; Wolcott, R.D. & James, G.A. (2009). In Vitro Susceptibility of Established Biofilms Composed of Clinical Wound Isolate of *Pseudomonas aeruginosa* Treated with Lactoferrin and Xylitol. *International Journal of Antimicrobial Agents*, Vol. 33, No. 3, (March 2009), pp. 230-236, ISSN 0924-8579

Anderson, B.F.; Baker, H.M.; Dodson, E.J.; Norris, G.E.; Rumball, S.V.; Waters, J.M. & Baker, E.N. (1987). Structure of Human Lactoferrin at 3.2 Å Resolution. *Proceedings of the National Academy of Sciences of the United States of America*, Vol. 84, No. 7, (April 1987), pp. 1769-1773, ISSN 0027-8424

Andrews, S.; Robinson, A. & Rodriguez-Quiñones, F. (2003). Bacterial Iron Homeostasis. *Federation of European Microbiological Societies Microbiology Reviews*, Vol. 27, No. 2-3, (June 2003), pp. 215-237, ISSN 0168-6445

Appel, M,J.; van Veen, H.A.; Vietsch, H.; Salaheddine, M.; Nuijens, J.H.; Ziere, B. & de Loos, F. (2006). Sub-chronic (13 week) Oral Toxicity Study in Rats with Recombinant Human Lactoferrin Produced in the Milk of Transgenic Cows. *Food and Chemical Toxicology*, Vol. 44, No. 7, (July 2006), pp. 964-973, ISSN 0278-6915

Armstrong, D.G. & Lipsky, B.A. (2004). Diabetic Food Infections: Stepwise Medical and Surgical Management. *International Wound Journal*, Vol. 1, No. 2, (June 2004), pp. 123-132, ISSN 1742-4801

Arnold, R.R.; Cole, M.F. & McGhee, J.R. (1977). A Bactericidal Effect for Human Lactoferrin. *Science*, Vol. 197, No. 4300, (July 1977), pp. 263-265, ISSN 0036-8075

Artym, J. & Zimecki, M. (2007). The Effects of Lactoferrin on Myelopoiesis: Can we resolve the Controversy?. *Postępy higieny i medycyny doświadczalnej* (Online), Vol. 61, pp. 129-150, ISSN 1732-2693 (Electronic)

Audrian, M.A.; Gourbil, A.; Muller, J.Y. & Esnault, L.M. (1996). Anti-lactoferrin Autoantibodies: Relation Between Epitopes and Iron Binding Domain. *Journal of Autoimmunity*, Vol. 9, No. 4 (August 1996), pp. 569-574, ISSN 0896-8411

Bader, M.S. (2008). Diabetic Foot Infection. *American Family Physician*, Vol. 78, No. 1, (July 2008), pp. 71-79, ISSN 0002-838X

Baker, E.N. & Baker, H.M. (2009). A Structural Framework for Understanding the Multifunctional Character of Lactoferrin. *Biochimie*, Vol. 91, No. 1, (January 2009), pp. 3-10, ISSN 0300-9084

Baveye, S.; Elass, E.; Fernig, D.G.; Blanquart, C.; Mazurier, J. & Legrand, D. (2000A). Human Lactoferrin Interacts with Soluble CD14 and Inhibits Expression of Endothelial Adhesion Molecules, E-selectin and ICAM-1, Induced by the CD14-Lipopolysaccharide Complex. *Infection and Immunity*. Vol. 68, No. 12, (December 2000), pp. 6519-6525, ISSN 0019-9567

Baveye, S.; Elass. E.; Mazurier, J. & Legrand, D. (2000B). Lactoferrin Inhibits the Binding of Lipopolysaccharides to L-Selectin and Subsequent Production of Reactive Species by Neutrophils. *Federation of European Biochemical Societies Letters*, Vol. 469, No. 1, (March 2000), pp. 5-8, ISSN 0014-5793

Bi, B.Y.; Lefebvre, A.M.; DuÅ, D.; Spik, G. & Mazurier, J. (1997). Effect of Lactoferrin on Proliferation and Differentiation of the Jurkat Human Lymphoblastic T Cell Line. *Archivum Immunologiae et Therapiae Experimentalis*, Vol. 45, No. 4, (August 1997), pp.315-320, ISSN 0004-069X

Bolscher, J.G.; Adão, R.; Nazmi, K.; van den Keybus, P.A.; van 't Hof, W.; Nieuw Amerongen, A.V.; Bastos, M. & Veerman, E.C. (2009). Bactericidal Activity of LFchimera is Stronger and Less Sensitive to Ionic Strength than its Constituent Lactoferricin and Lactoferrampin Peptides. *Biochimie,* Vol. 91, No. 1, (January 2009), pp. 123-132, ISSN 0300-9084

Britigan, B.E.; Serody, J.S.; Hayek, M.B.; Charniga, L.M. & Cohen, M.S. (1991). Uptake of Lactoferrin by Mononuclear Phagocytes Inhibits their Ability to Form Hydroxyl Radical and Protects them from Membrane Autoperoxidation. *Journal of Immunology*, Vol. 147, No. 12, (December 1991), pp. 4271-4277, ISSN 0022-1767

Britigan, B.E.; Hassett, D.J.; Rosen, G.M.; Hamill, D.R. & Cohen M.S. (1989). Neutrophil Degranulation Inhibits Potential Hydroxyl-Radical Formation. *The Biochemical Journal*,Vol. 264, No. 2, (December 1989), pp. 447-455, ISSN 0264-6021

Broxmeyer, H.E.; deSousa, M.; Smithyman, A.; Ralph, P.; Hamilton, J.; Kurland, J.I. & Bognacki, J. (1980). Specificity and Modulation of the Action of Lactoferrin, a Negative Feedback Regulator of Myelopoiesis. *Blood*, Vol. 55, No. 2, (February 1980), pp. 324-333, ISSN 0006-4971

Bullen, J.J.; Rogers, H.J.; Spalding, P.B. & Ward, C.G. (2005). Iron and Infection: The Hearth of the Matter. *Federation of European Microbiological Societies Immunology and Medical Microbiology*, Vol. 43, No. 3, (March 2005), pp. 325-330, ISSN 0928-8244

Bullen, J.J. & Armstrong, J.A. (1979). The Role of Lactoferrin in the Bactericidal Function of Polymorphonuclear Leukocytes. *Immunology*, Vol. 36 No. 4 (April 1979), pp. 781-791, ISSN 0019-2805

Bullen, J.J.; Rogers, H.J. & Leigh, L. (1972). Iron Binding Proteins in Milk and Resistance to *Escherichia coli* Infection in Infants. *British Medical Journal*, Vol. 1, No. 792, (January 1972), pp. 69-75, ISSN 0959-8146

Cerven, D.; DeGeorge, G. & Bethell, D. (2008). 28-Day Repeated Dose Oral Toxicity of Recombinant Human Holo-lactoferrin in rats. *Regulatory Toxicology and Pharmacology*, Vol. 52, No. 2 (November 2008), pp. 174-179, ISSN 0273-2300

Chiancone, E.; Ceci, P.; Ilari, A.; Ribachi, F. & Stefanini, S. (2004). Iron and Protein for Iron Storage and Detoxification. *Biometals,* Vol. 17, No. 3, (June 2004), pp. 197-202, ISSN 0966-0844

Citron, D.M.; Goldstein, E.J.C.; Merriam, C.V.; Lipsky, B.A. & Abramson, M.A. (2007). Bacteriology of Moderate to Severe Diabetic Foot Infections and In Vitro Activity of Antimicrobial Agents. *Journal of Clinical Microbiology,* Vol. 45, No.9, (September 2007), pp. 2819-2828, ISSN 0095-1137

Coddeville, B.; Strecker, G.; Wieruszeski, J.M.; Vliegenhart, J.F.; van Halbeek, H.; Peter-Katalinić J.; Egge, H. & Spik G. (1992). Heterogeneity of Bovine Lactotransferrin Glycans. Characterization of Alpha-D-Galp-(1-->3)-beta-D-Gal- and Alpha-NeuAc-(2-->6)-beta-D-GalpNac-(1-->4)-beta-D-GlcNac-substituted N-linked Glycans. *Carbohydrate Research,* Vol. 236, (December 1992), pp. 145-164, ISSN 0008-6215

Cohen, M.S.; Mao, J.; Rasmussen, G.T.; Serody, J.S. & Britigan B.E. (1992). Interaction of Lactoferrin and Lipopolysaccharide (LPS): Effects on the Antioxidant Property of Lactoferrin and the Ability of LPS to Prime Human Neutrophils for Enhanced Superoxide Production. *The Journal of Infectious Diseases,* Vol. 166, No. 6, (December 1992), pp. 1375-1378, ISSN 0022-1899

Crouch S.P.M.; Slater, K.J. & Fletcher, J. (1992). Regulation of Cytokine Release from Mononuclear Cells by the Iron Binding Protein Lactoferrin. *Blood,* Vol. 80, No. 1, (July 1992), pp. 235-240, ISSN 0006-4971

Cumberbatch, M.; Bhushan, M.; Dearman, R.J.; Kimber, I. & Griffiths,C.E. (2003). IL-1beta-induced Langerhans´Cell Migration and TNF Alpha Production in Human Skin: Regulation by Lactoferrin. *Clinical and Experimental Immunology,* Vol. 132, No. 2, (May 2003), pp. 352-359, ISSN 0009-9104

Cumberbatch, M.; Dearman, R.J.; Uribe-Luna, S.; Headon, D.R.; Ward, P.P.; Conneely, O.M. & Kimber, I. (2000).Regulation of Epidermal Langerhans Cell Migration by Lactoferrin. *Immunology,* Vol. 100, No. 1, (May 2000), pp. 21-28, ISSN 0019-2805

Cumbertbatch, M.; Griffiths, C.E.; Tucker, S.C.; Dearman, R.J.& Kimber, I. (1999). Tumor Necrosis Factor Alpha Induces Langerhans Cell Migration in Humans. *The British Journal of Dermatology,* Vol. 141, No. 2, (August 1999), pp. 192-200, ISSN 0007-0963

De la Rosa, G.; Yang, D.; Tewary, P.; Varadhachary, A.; Oppenheim, J.J. (2008). Lactoferrin Acts as an Alarmin to Promote the Recruitment and Activation of APCs and Antigen Specific Immune Responses. *Journal of Immunology,* Vol. 180, No. 10, (May 2008), pp. 6868-6876, ISSN 0022-1767

Delforge, A.; Stryckmans, P.; Prieels, J.P.; Bieva, C.; Rongè-Collard, E.; Schlusselberg, J. & Efira, A. (1985). Lactoferrin: Its Role as a Regulator of Human Granulopoiesis? *Annals of the New York Academy of Sciences,* Vol. 459, pp. 85-96, ISSN 0077-8923

Dhennin-Duthille, I.; Masson, M.; Damiens, E.; Fillebeen, C.; Spik, G.& Mazurier, J. (2000). Lactoferrin Upregulates the Expression of CD4 Antigen Through the Stimulation of the Mitogen-Activated Protein Kinase in the Human Lymphoblastic T Jurkat Cell Line. *Journal of Cellular Biochemistry,* Vol. 79, No.4, (September 2000), pp. 583-593, ISSN 0730-2312

Diarra, M.S.; Peticlerc, D. & Lacasse, P. (2002). Effect of Lactoferrin in Combination with Penicillin on the Morphology and the Physiology of *Staphylococcus aureus* Isolated from Bovine Mastitis. *Journal of Dairy Science,* Vol. 85, No. 5, (May 2002), pp. 1141-1149, ISSN 0022-0302

Djeha, A. & Brock, J.H. (1992). Effect of Transferrin, Lactoferrin and Chelated Iron on Human T Lymphocytes. *British Journal of Haematology,* Vol. 80, No. 2, (February 1992), pp. 235-241, ISSN 0007-1048

Dobias, L.; Cerna, M.; Rossner, P. & Sram, R. (1994). Genotoxicity and Carcinogenicity of Metronidazole. *Mutation Research,* Vol. 317, No. 3, (June 1994), pp. 177-194, ISSN 0027-5107

Dowd, S.E.; Sun, Y.; Secor, P.R.; Rhoads, D.D.; Wolcott, B.M.; James, G.A.; Wolcott, R.D. (2008). Survey of Bacterial Diversity in Chronic Wounds Using Pyrosequencing, DGGE, and Full Ribosome Shotgun Sequencing. *BMC Microbiology,* Vol. 8, (March 2008), pp. 43-58, ISSN 1471-2180 (online)

Drago-Serrano, M.E. (2007). Lactoferrina: Producción Industrial y Aplicaciones. *Revista Mexicana de Ciencias Farmacéuticas,* Vol. 38, No.3, (Julio-Septiembre 2007), pp. 30-38, ISSN 1870-0195

Edmonds, M. (2006). Diabetic Foot Ulcers. Practical Treatment Recommendations. *Drugs,* Vol. 66, No. 7, pp. 913-929, ISSN 0012-6667

El Ghalbzouri, A. ; Hensbergen, P. ; Gibss, S. ; Kempenaar, J. ; Van der Schors, R. & Ponec, M. (2004).Fibroblasts Facilitate Re-epithelialization in Wounded Human Skin Equivalents. *Laboratory Investigation,* Vol. 84, No. 1, (January 2004), pp. 102-112, ISSN 0023-6837

El-Nahas, A.F. & El-Ashmawy, I.M. (2004). Reproductive and Cytogenetic Toxicity of Metronidazole to Male Mice. *Basic and Clinical Pharmacology and Toxicology,* Vol. 94, No. 5, (May 2005), pp. 226-231, ISSN 1742-7835

Elass, E.; Masson, M.; Mazurier, J. & Legrand, D. (2002). Lactoferrin Inhibits the Lipopolysaccharide Induced Expression and Proteoglycan Binding Ability of Interleukin-8 in Human Endothelial Cells. *Infection and Immunity,* Vol. 70, No. 4, (April 2002), pp. 1860-1866, ISSN 0019-9567

Elbim, C.; Reglier, H.; Fay, M.; Delarche, C.; Andrieu, V.; El Benna, J. & Gougerot-Pocidalo, M.A. (2001). Intracellular Pool of IL-10 Receptors in Specific Granules of Neutrophils: Differential Mobilization by Proinflammatory Mediators. *The Journal of Immunology,* Vol. 166, No. 1, (April 2001), pp. 5201-5207, ISSN 0022-1767

Engelmayer, J.; Blezinger, P. & Varadhachary, A. (2008). Talactoferrin Stimulates Wound Healing with Modulation of Inflammation. *The Journal of Surgical Research,* Vol. 149, No. 2, (October 2008), pp. 278-286, ISSN 0022-4804

Erga, K.S.; Peen, E.; Enestrøm, S. & Reed, R.K. (2001). Effects of Lactoferrin on Rat Dermal Interstitial Fluid Pressure (Pif) and In vitro Endothelial Barrier Function. *Acta Physiologica Scandinavica,* Vol. 171, No. 4, (April 2001), pp. 419-425, ISSN 0001-6772

Esaguy, N.; Freitas, P.M. & Aguas, A.P. (1993). Anti-lactoferrin Auto-antibodies in Rheumatoid Arthritis. *Clinical and Experimental Rheumatology,* Vol. 11, No. 5, (September-October 1993), pp. 581-582, ISSN 0392-856X

Esaguy, N.; Aguas, A.P.; van Embden, J.D. & Silva, M.T. (1991). Mycobacteria and Human Autoinmune Disease: Direct Evidence of Cross Reactivity Between Human Lactoferrin and the 65 Kilodalton Protein of Tubercle and Leprosy Bacilli. *Infection and Immunity,* Vol. 59, No. 3, (March 1991), pp. 1117-1125, ISSN 0019-9567

Farnaud, S. & Evans, R.W. (2003). Lactoferrin –A Multifunctional Protein with Antimicrobial Properties. *Molecular Immunology* Vol. 40, No. 7, (November 2003), pp. 395-405, ISSN 0161-5890

Flores-Villaseñor, H.; Canizalez-Román, A.; Reyes-Lopez, M.; Nazmi, K.; de la Garza, M.; Zazueta-Beltrán, J.; León-Sicairos, N. & Bolscher, J.G. (2010). Bactericidal Effect of Bovine Lactoferrin, LFcin, LFampin and LFchimera on Antibiotic-Resistant *Staphylococcus aureus* and *Escherichia coli*. *Biometals*, Vol. 23, No. 3, (June 2010), pp. 569-578, ISSN 0966-0844

Gahr, M.; Speer, C.P.; Damerau, B. & Sawatzki, G. (1991). Influence of Lactoferrin on the Function of Human Polymorphonuclear Leukocytes and Monocytes. *Journal of Leukocyte Biology*, Vol. 49, No.5, (May 1991), pp. 427-433, ISSN 0741-5400

Gailit, J. ; Welch, M.P. & Clark, R.A. (1994). TGF-beta 1 Stimulates Expression of Keratinocyte Integrins During Re-epithelialization of Cutaneous Wounds. *The Journal of Investigative Dermatology*, Vol. 103, No. 2, (August 1994), pp. 221-227, ISSN 0022-202X

Gaudin, J.C.; Rabesona, H.; Choiset, Y.; Yeretssian, G.; Chobert, J.M.; Sakanyan, V.; Drouet, M. & Haertlé, T. (2008). Assessment of the Immunoglobulin E-Mediated Immune Response to Milk-Specific Proteins in Allergic Patients Using Microarrays. *Clinical and Experimental Allergy*, Vol. 38, No. 4, (April 2008), pp. 686-693, ISSN 0954-7894

Geissmann, F.; Dieu-Nosjean, M.C.; Dezutter, C.; Valladeau, J.; Kayal, S.; Leborgne, M.; Brousse, N.; Saeland, S. & Davoust, J. (2002). Accumulation of Immature Langerhans Cells in Human Lymph Nodes Draining Chronically Inflamed Skin. *The Journal of Experimental Medicine*, Vol. 196, No. 4, (August 2002), pp. 417-430, ISSN 0022-1007

Gentile, P. & Broxmeyer, H.E. (1983). Suppression of Mouse Myelopoiesis byAdministration of Human Lactoferrin In Vivo and Comparative Action of Human Transferring. *Blood*, Vol. 61, No. 5, (May 1983), pp. 982-993,ISSN 0006-4971

Gifford, J,L.; Hunter, H.N. & Vogel, H.J. (2005). Lactoferricin: a Lactoferrin Derived Peptide with Antimicrobial, Antiviral, Antitumor and Immunological properties. *Cellular and Molecular Life Sciences*, Vol. 62, No. 22, (November 2005), pp. 2588-2598, ISSN1420-682X

Gómez, H.F.; Ochoa, T.J.; Herrera-Insua, I.; Carlin, L.G. & Cleary, T.G. (2002). Lactoferrin Protects Rabbits from *Shigella flexneri* Induced Inflammatory Enteritis. *Infection and Immunity*, Vol. 70, No. 12, (December 2002), pp.7050-7053, ISSN 0019-9567

Graiani, G.; Emanueli, C.; Desortes, E.; Van Linthout, S.; Pinna, A.; Figueroa, C.D.; Manni, L. & Madeddu, P. (2004). Nerve Growth Factor Promotes Reparative Angiogenesis and Inhibits Endothelial Apoptosis in Cutaneous Wounds of Type 1 Diabetic Mice. *Diabetologia*, Vol. 47, No. 6, (June 2004), pp. 1047-1054, ISSN 0012-186X

Griffiths. C.E.; Cumberbatch, M.; Tucker, S.C.; Dearman, R.J.; Andrew, S.; Headon, D.R. & Kimber, I. (2001). Exogenous Topical Lactoferrin Inhibits Allegen Induced Langerhans Cell Migration and Cutaneous Inflammation in Humans. *The British Journal of Dermatology*, Vol. 144, No. 4, (April 2001), pp. 715-725, ISSN 0007-0963

Guillén, C.; McInnes, I.B.; Vaughan, D.M.; Kommajosyula, S.; Van Berkel, P.H.C.; Leung, B.P.; Aguila, A. & Brock, J.H. (2002). Enhanced Th1 Response to *Staphylococcus aureus* Infection in Human Lactoferrin Transgenic Mice. *Journal of Immunology*, Vol. 168, No. 8, (April 2002), pp. 3950-3957, ISSN 0022-1767

Guo, S. & DiPietro, M.L. (2010). Factors Affecting Wound Healing, *Journal of Dental Research*, Vol. 89, No. 3, (March 2010), pp. 219-229, ISSN 0022-0345

Gutteridge, J.M.; Paterson, S.K.; Segal, A.W. & Halliwell, B. (1981). Inhibition of Lipid Peroxidation by the Iron Binding Protein Lactoferrin. *The Biochemical Journal*, Vol. 199, No. 1, (October 1981), pp. 259-261, ISSN 0264-6021

Hammerschmidt, S., Bethe, G.; Remane, P.H. & Chhatwal, G.S. (1999). Identification of Pneumococcal Surface Protein A as a Lactoferrin-binding Protein of *Streptococcus pneumoniae*. *Infection and Immunity*, Vol. 67, No. 4, (April 1999), pp. 1683-1687, ISSN 0019-9567

Hampton, M.B.; Kettle, A.J. & Winterbourn, C.C. (1998). Inside the Neutrophil Phagosome: Oxidants, Myeloperoxidase and Bacterial Killing. *Blood*, Vol. 92, No.9, (November 1998), pp. 3007-3017, ISSN 0006-4971

Hardy, M.A. (1989). The Biology of Scar Formation. *Physical Theraphy*, Vol. 69, No. 12, (December 1989), pp. 1014-1024, ISSN 0031-9023

Hartog, A.; Leenders, I.; Van Der Kraan, P.M. & Garssen, J. (2007). Anti-inflammatory Effects of Orally Ingested Lactoferrin and Glycine in Different Zymosan Induced Inflammation Models: Evidence for Synergistic Activity. *International Immunopharmacology*, Vol. 7, No. 13, (December 2007), pp. 1784-1792, ISSN 1567-5769

Håversen, L.A.; Baltzer, L.; Dolphin, G.; Hanson, L.Å. & Mattsby-Baltzer, I. (2003A). Anti-Inflammatory Activities of Human Lactoferrin in Acute Dextran Sulphate Induced Colitis in Mice. *Scandinavian Journal of Immunology*, Vol. 57, No. 1, (January 2003), pp. 2-10, ISSN 0300-9475

Håversen, L.A.; Engberg, I.; Baltzer, L.; Dolphin, G.; Hanson, L.Å. & Mattsby-Baltzer, I. (2003B).Human Lactoferrin and Peptides Derived from a Surface Exposed Helical Region Reduce Experimental *Escherichia coli* Urinary Tract Infection in Mice. *Infection and Immunity*, Vol. 68, No. 10, (October 2003), pp. 5816-5823, ISSN 0019-9567

Håversen, L.; Ohlsson, B.G.; Hahn-Zoric, M.; Hanson, L.A. & Mattsby-Baltzer, I. (2002). Lactoferrin Down Regulates the LPS Induced Ccytokine Production in Monocytic Cells Via NF-kappa B. *Cellular Immunology*, Vol. 220, No. 2, (December 2002), pp. 83-95, ISSN 0008-8749

Hill, K.E.; Malic, S.; McKee, R.; Rennison, T.; Harding, K.G.; Williams, D.W. & Thomas, D.W. (2010). An In Vitro Model of Chronic Wound Biofilms to Test Wound Dressings and Assess Antimicrobial Susceptibilities. *Journal of Antimicrobial Chemotherapy*, Vol. 65, No. 6, (June 2010), pp. 1195-1206, ISSN 0305-7453

Hilton, J.R.; Williams, D.T.; Beuker, B.; Miller, D.R. & Harding, K.G. (2004). Wound Dressing in Diabetic Foot Disease. (2004). *Clinical Infectious Diseases*, Vol. 39, Suppl 2, (August 2004), pp. S100-S103, ISSN 1058-4838

Hopf, H.W.; Humphrey, L.M.; Puzziferri, N.; West, J.M.; Attinger, C.E. & Hunt, T.K. (2001). Adjuncts to Preparing Wounds for Closure: Hyperbaric Oxygen, Growth Factors, Skin Substitutes, Negative Pressure Wound Therapy (Vacuum Assisted Closure). *Foot and Ankle Clinics*, Vol. 6, No. 4, (December 2001), pp. 661-682, ISSN 1083-7515

Hwang, S.A.; Wilk, K.M.; Budnicka, M.; Olsen, M.; Bangale Y.A.; Hunter, R.L.; Kruzel, M.L. & Actor, J.K. (2007). Lactoferrin Enhanced Efficacy of the BCG Vaccine to Generate Host Protective Responses Against Challenge with Virulent *Mycobacterium tuberculosis*. *Vaccine*, Vol. 25, No. 37-38, (September 2007), pp. 6730-6743, ISSN 0264-410X

Ihn, H. ; Kikuchi, K. ; Soma, Y. ; Sato, S. ; Fujimoto, M. ; Tamaki, T. ; Igarashi, A. & Takehara, K. (1995). The Stimulatory Effects of PDGF and TGF-beta 1 on Dermal Fibroblast Attachment. *Acta Dermato Venereologica*, Vol. 75, No. 5, (September 1995), pp. 367-371, ISSN 0001-5555

Ishikado, A.; Imanaka, H.; Takeuchi, T.; Harada, E. & Makino, T. (2005). Liposomalization of Lactoferrin Enhanced it´s Anti-Inflammatory Effects Via Oral Administration. *Biological and Pharmaceutical Bulletin*, Vol. 28, No. 9, (September 2005), pp. 1717-1721, ISSN 0918-6158

Jenssen, H. & Hancock R.E.W. (2009). Antimicrobial Properties of Lactoferrin. *Biochimie*, Vol. 91, No. 1, (January 2009), pp. 19-29, ISSN 0300-9084

Kanitakis, J. (2002). Anatomy, Hystology and Immunochemistry of Normal Human Skin. *European Journal of Dermatology*, Vol. 12, No. 4, (July-August 2002), pp. 390-399, ISSN 1167-1122

Kapoor, K.; Chandra, M.; Nag, D.; Paliwal, J.K.; Gupta, R.C. & Saxena, R.C. (1999). Evaluation of Metronidazole Toxicity: a Prospective Study. *International Journal of Clinical Pharmacology Research*, Vol. 19, No. 3, pp. 83-88, ISSN 0251-1649

Khanolkar, M.P.; Bain, S.C. & Stephens, J.W. (2008). The Diabetic Foot. *Quartely Journal of Medicine*, Vol. 101, No. 9, (September 2008), pp. 685-695, ISSN 1460-2725

Kimber, I.; Cumberbatch, M.; Dearman, R.J.; Headon, D.R.; Bhushan, M. & Griffithis C.E.M. (2002). Lactoferrin: Influences on Langerhans Cells, Epidermal Cytokines, and Cutaneous Inflammation. *Biochemistry and Cell Biology*, Vol. 80, No. 1, (January 2002), pp. 103-107, ISSN 0829-8211

Klinworth, G.K.; Valnickova, Z.; Kielar, R.A.; Baratz, K.H.; Campbell, R.J. & Enghild, J.J. (1997). Familial Subepithelial Corneal Amyloidosis a Lactoferrin-Related Amyloidosis. *Investigative Ophthalmology and Visual Science*, Vol. 38, No. 13, (December 1997), pp. 2756-2763, ISSN 0146-0404

Komine, Y.; Komine, K.; Kai, K.; Itagaki, M.; Kuroishi, T.; Aso, H.; Obara, Y. & Kumagai, K. (2006). Effect of Combination Therapy with Lactoferrin and Antibiotics against Staphylococcal Mastitis on Dying Cows. *Journal of Veterinary Medical Sciences*, Vol. 68, No. 3, (March 2006), pp. 205-211, ISSN 0916-7250

Kruzel, M.L.; Bacsi, A.; Choudhury, B.; Sur, S. & Boldogh, I. (2006). Lactoferrin Decreases Pollen Antigen Induced Allergic Airway Inflammation in a Murine Model of Asthma. *Immunology*, Vol. 119, No. 2, (October 2006), pp. 159-166, ISSN 0019-2805

Labat-Robert, J.; Bihari-Varga, M. & Robert, L. (1990). Extracellular Matrix. *Federation of European Biochemical Societies, Letters*, Vol. 268, No. 2, (August 1990), pp. 386-393, ISSN 0014-5793

Lee, H.Y.; Park, J.H.; Seok, S.H.; Baek, M.W.; Kim, D.J.; Lee, B.H:, Kang, P.D.; Kim, Y.S. & Park, J.H. (2005). Potential Antimicrobial Effects of Human Lactoferrin against Oral Infection with *Listeria monocytogenes*. *Journal of Medical Microbiology*, Vol. 54, Pt. 11, (November 2005), pp. 1049-1054, ISSN 0022-2615

Leffell, M. & Spitznagel, J.K. (1974). Intracellular and Extracellular Degranulation of Human Polymorphonuclear Azurophil and Specific Granules Induced by Immune Complexes. *Infection and Immunity*, Vol. 10, No.6, (December 1974), pp. 1241-1249, ISSN 0019-9567

Legrand, D. & Mazurier, J. (2010). A critical Review of the Roles of Host Lactoferrin in Immunity. *Biometals*, Vol. 23, No. 3, (June 2010), pp. 365-376, ISSN 0966-0844

Legrand, D.; Elass. E.; Pierce, A. & Mazurier, J. (2004). Lactoferrin and Host Defense: an Overview of its Immuno-modulating and Anti-inflammatory Properties. *Biometals*, Vol. 17, No. 3, (June 2004), pp. 225-229, ISSN 0966-0844

Leid, J.G.; Kerr, M.; Selgado, C.; Johnson, C.; Moreno, G.; Smith, A.; Shirtliff, M.E.; O´Toole, G.A. & Cope E.K. (2009). Flagellum mediated Biofilm Defense Mechanism of *Pseudomonas aeruginosa* against Host Derived Lactoferrin. *Infection and Immunity*, Vol. 77, No. 10, (October 2009), pp. 4559-4566, ISSN 0019-9567

Leitch, E.C. & Willcox, M.D. (1999A). Elucidation of he Antistaphylococcal Action of Lactoferrin and Lysozyme. *Journal of Medical Microbiology*, Vol. 48, No. 9, (September 1999), pp.867-871, ISSN 0022-2615

Leitch, E.C. & Willcox, M.D. (1999B). Lactoferrin Increases the Susceptibility of *S. epidermidis* Biofilms to Lysozyme and Vancomicin. *Current Eye Research*, Vol. 19, No. 1, (July 1999), pp. 12-19, ISSN 0271-3683

Leitch, E.C. & Willcox, M.D. (1998). Synergic Antistaphylococcal Properties of Lactoferrin and Lysozyme. *Journal of Medical Microbiology*, Vol. 47, No. 9, (September 1998), pp. 837-842, ISSN 0022-2615

León-Sicairos, N.; Reyes-López, M.; Ordaz-Pichardo, C. & de la Garza, M. (2006). Microbicidal Action of Lactoferrin and Lactoferricin and Their Synergistic Effect with Metronidazole in *Entamoeba histolytica*. *Biochemistry and Cell Biology*, Vol. 84, No. 3, (June 2006), pp. 327-336, ISSN 0829-8211

Levay, P.F. & Viljoen, M. (1995). Lactoferrin: A General Review. *Haematologica*. Vol. 80, No. 3, (May-June 1995), pp. 252-267, ISSN 0390-6078

Leveugle, B.; Spik, G.; Perl, D.P.; Bouras, C.; Fillit, H.M. & Hof, P.R. (1994). The Iron-Binding Protein Lactotransferrin is Present in Pathological Lesions in a Variety of Neurodegenerative Disorders: A comparative Immunohistochemical Analysis. *Brain Research*, Vol. 650, No. 1, (July 1994), pp. 20-31, ISSN 0006-8993

Li, K.J.; Lu, M.C.; Hsieh, S.C.; Wu, C.H.; Yu, H.S.; Tsai, C.Y. & Yu, C.L. (2006). Release of Surface-Expression Lactoferrin from Polymorphonuclear Neutrophils after Contact with CD4+ T Cells and Its Modulation on Th1/Th2 cytokine production. *Journal of Leukocyte Biology*, Vol. 80, No. 2, (August 2006), pp. 350-358, ISSN 0741-5400

Lima, M.F. & Kierszenbaum, F. (1987). Lactoferrin Effects of Phagocytic Cell Function. II: The Presence of Iron is Required for the Lactoferrin Molecule to Stimulate Intracellular Killing by Macrophages but not to Enhance the Uptake of Particles and Microorganisms. *Journal of Immunology*, Vol. 139, No 5, (September 1987), pp. 1647-1651, ISSN 0022-1767

Ling, J.M. & Schryvers, A. (2006). Perspectives on Interactions between Lactoferrin and Bacteria. *Biochemistry and Cell Biology*, Vol. 84, No. 3, (June 2006), pp. 275-281, ISSN 0829-8211

Liu, Y. ; Petreaca, M. ; Yao, M. & Martins-Green, M. (2009).Cell and Molecular Mechanisms of Keratinocyte Function Stimulated by Insulin During Wound Healing. *BMC Cell Biology*, Vol. 10, (January 2009), pp. 1-15, ISSN 1471-2121 (electronic)

Lopez-Novoa, J.M.; Quiros, Y.; Vicente-Vicente, L.; Morales, A.I. & López-Hernández, F.J. (2011). New Insights into the Mechanism of Aminoglycoside Nephrotoxicity: an Integrative Point of View. *Kidney International*, Vol. 79, No. 1, (January 2010), pp. 33-45, ISSN 0085-2538

Lyons, T.E.; Miller, M.S.; Serena, T.; Sheehan, P.; Lavery, L.; Kirsner, R.S.; Armstrong, D.G.; Reese, A.; Yankee, E.W. & Veves A. (2007). Talactoferrin Alfa, a Recombinant Human Lactoferrin Promotes Healing of Diabetic Neuropathic Ulcers: A Phase 1/2 Clinical Study. *The American Journal of Surgery* Vol. 193, No. 1, (January 2007), pp. 49-54, ISSN 0002-9610

Malhotra, R.; Priest, R. & Bird, M.I. (1996). Role for L-selectin in Lipopolysaccharide Induced Activation of Neutrophils. *The Biochemical Journal*, Vol. 320, Pt. 2, (December 1996), pp. 589-593, ISSN 0264-6021

Masson, P.L. & Heremans J.F. (1971). Lactoferrin in Milk from Different Species. *Comparative Biochemistry and Physiology B*, Vol. 39, No. 1, (May 1971), pp. 119-129, ISSN 0305-0491

Miller, M.B. & Bassler, B.L. (2001). Quorum Sensing in Bacteria. *Annual Review of Microbiology*, Vol. 55, No. 10, pp.165-199, ISSN 0066-4227.

Miyauchi, H.; Hashimoto, S.; Nakajima, M.; Shinoda, I.; Fukuwatari, Y. & Hayasawa, H. (1998). Bovine Lactoferrin Stimulates the Phagocytic Activity of Human Neutrophils: Identification of its Active Domain. *Cellular Immunology*, Vol. 187, No. 1, (July 1998), pp. 34-37, ISSN 0008-8749

Moed, H.; Stoof, T.J.; Boorsma, D.M.; vonBlomberg, B.M.; Gibbs, S.; Bruynzeel, D.P.; Scheper, R.J. & Rustmeyer, T. (2004). Identification of Anti-inflammatory Drugs According to Their Capacity to Suppress Type-1 and Type-2 Cell Profiles. *Clinical and Experimental Allergy*, Vol. 34, No. 12, (December 2004), pp. 1868-1875, ISSN 0954-7894

Moore, S.A.; Anderson, B.F.; Groom, C.R.; Haridas, M. & Baker, E.N. (1997). Three Dimensional Structure of Diferric Bovine Lactoferrin at 2.8Å Resolution. *Journal of Molecular Biology*, Vol. 274, No. 2, (November 1997), pp. 222-236, ISSN 0022-2836

Mosquito, S.; Ochoa, T.J.; Cok, J. & Cleary, T.G. (2010). Effect of Bovine Lactoferrin in *Salmonella* ser. Typhimurium Infection in Mice. *Biometals*, Vol. 23, No. 3, (June 2010), pp. 515-521, ISSN 0966-0844

Mudry, M.D.; Carballo, M.; Labal de Vinuesa, M.; Gonzalez-Cid, M. & Larripa, I. (1994). Mutagenic Bioassay of Certain Pharmacologycal Drugs: Metronidazole (MTZ). *Mutation Research*, Vol. 305, No. 2, (March 1994), pp. 127-132, ISSN 0027-5107

Na, Y.J.; Han, S.B.; Kang, J.S.; Yoon, Y.D.; Park, S.K.; Kim, H.M.; Yan, K.H. & Joe, C.O.(2004). Lactoferrin Works as a New LPS Binding Protein in Inflammatory Activation of Macrophages. *International Immunopharmacology*, Vol. 4, No. 9, (September 2004), pp. 1187-1199, ISSN 1567-5769

Nairz, M.; Schroll, A.; Sonnweber, T. & Weiss G. (2010). The Struggle for Iron – a Metal at the Host-Pathogen Interface. *Cellular Microbiology*, Vol. 12, No. 12, (December 2010), pp. 1691-1702, ISSN 1462-5814

Niyonsaba, F. ; Ushio, H. ; Nakano, N. ; Ng, W. ; Sayama, K. ; Hashimoto, K. ; Nagoaka, I. ; Okumura, K. & Ogawa, H. (2007). Antimicrobial Peptides Human Beta Defensins Stimulate Epidermal Keratinocyte Migration, Proliferation and Production of Pro-inflammatory Cytokines and Chemokines. *The Journal of Investigative Dermatology*, Vol. 127, No. 3, (March 2007), pp. 594-604, ISSN 0022-202X

O´Meara, S.; Cullum, N.; Majid, M. & Sheldon, T. (2000). Systematic Reviews of Wound Care Management: (3) Antimicrobial Agents for Chronic Wounds; (4) Diabetic Foot Ulceration. *Health Technology Assessment*, Vol. 4, No. 21, pp. 1-237, ISSN 1366-5278

Oo, T.Z.; Cole, N.; Garthwaite, L.; Willcox, M.D.; Zhu, H. (2010). Evaluation of Synergistic Activity of Bovine Lactoferrin with Antibiotics in Corneal Infection.*The Journal of Antimicrobial Chemotherapy*, Vol. 65, No. 6, (June 2010), pp, 1243-1251, ISSN0305-7453

Patel, G.K.; Wilson, C.H.; Harding, K.G.; Finlay, A.Y. & Bowden, P.E. (2006). Numerous Keratinocytes Subtypes Involved in Wound Re-epithelialization, *The Journal of Investigative Dermatology*, Vol, 126, No. 2, (February 2006), ISSN 0022-202X

Peen, E.; Almer, S.; Bodemar, G.; Rydén, B.D.; Sjölin, C.; Tejle, K. & Skogh, T. (1993). Anti-Lactoferrin Antibodies and other Types of ANCA in Ulcerative Colitis, Primary Sclerosing Cholangitis, and Crohn´s Disease. *Gut*, Vol. 34, No. 1, (January 1993), pp. 56-62, ISSN 0017-5749

Pierce, G.F. (2001). Inflammation in Non-healing Diabetic Wounds. The Space-Time Continuum Does Matter.*The American Journal of Pathology*, Vol. 159, No. 2, (August 2001), pp. 399-403, ISSN 0002-9440

Powlson, A.S. & Coll, A.P. (2010). The Treatment of Diabetic Foot Infections. *Journal of Antimicrobial Chemotherapy* Vol. 65, Suppl 3, (November 2010), pp. 3-9, ISSN 0305-7453

Puddu, P.; Latorre, D.; Valenti, P. & Gessani, S. (2010). Immunoregulatory Role of Lactoferrin-Lipopolysaccharide interactions. *Biometals*, Vol. 23, No. 3, (June 2010), pp. 387-397, ISSN 0966-0844

Roe, F. (1983) Toxicologic Evaluation of Metronidazole with Particular Reference to Carcinogenic, Mutagenic and Teratogenic Potential. *Surgery*, Vol. 93, No. 1 Pt 2, (January 1983), pp. 158-164, ISSN 0039-6060

Russell, M.W.; Bobek, L.A.; Brock, J.H.; Hajishengallis, G. & Tenovuo. J. (2005). Innate Humoral Defense Factors. In: *Mucosal Immunology*, Mestecky, J.; Bienenstock, J.; Lamm, M.E.; Mayer, L.; McGhee, J.R. & Strober, W. (Eds), 73-110, ISBN 0-12-491544-2 (v.1), Elsevier, San Diego California, USA

Saito, S.; Takayama, Y.; Mizumachi, K. & Suzuki, C.(2011). Lactoferrin Promotes Hyaluronan Synthesis in Human Dermal Fibroblast. *Biotechnology Letters*, Vol. 33, No. 1, (January 2011), pp. 33-39, ISSN 0141-5492

Sanchez, M.S. & Watts, J. (1999). Enhancement of the Activity of Novobiocin against *Escherichia coli* by Lactoferrin. *Journal of Dairy Science,* Vol. 82, No. 3, (March 1999), pp. 494-499, ISSN 0022-0302.

Sawatzki, G. & Rich, I.N. (1989). Lactoferrin Stimulates Colony Stimulating Factor Production In Vitro and In Vivo. *Blood Cells*, Vol. 15, No. 2, (August 1989), pp. 371-385, ISSN 0340-4684

Schreier, T. ; Degen, E. & Baschong, W. (1993). Fibroblast Migration and Proliferation During In vitro Wound Healing. A Quantitative Comparison Between Various Growth Factors and a Low Molecular Weight Blood Dialysate Used in the Clinic to Normalize Wound Healing. *Research in Experimental Medicine*, Vol. 193, No. 4, (July-August 1993), pp. 195-205, ISSN 0300-9130

Shinoda, I.; Takase, M.; Fukuwatari, Y.; Shimamura, S.; Köller, M. & König, W. (1996). Effects of Lactoferrin and Lactoferricin on the Release of Interleukin 8 from Human Polymorphonuclear Leukocytes. *Bioscience, Biotechnology and Biochemistry*, Vol. 60, No. 3, (March 1996), pp. 521-523, ISSN 0916-8451

Shinoda, I.; Takase, M.; Fukuwatari, Y.; Shimamura, S. (1994). Lactoferrin Promotes Nerve Growth Factor Synthesis/Secretion in Mouse Fibroblast L-M Cells. *Advances in Experimental Medicine and Biology*, Vol. 357, pp. 279-285, ISSN 0065-2598

Shirakata, Y.; Kimura, R.; Nanba, D.; Iwamoto, R.; Tokumaru, S.; Morimoto, C.; Yokota, K.; Nakamura, M.; Sayama, K.; Mekada, E.; Higashiyama, S. & Hashimoto, K. (2005). Heparin Binding EGF Like Growth Factor Accelerates Keratinocyte Migration and Skin Wound Healing. *Journal of Cell Science*, Vol. 118, Pt. 11, (June 2005), pp. 2363-2370, ISSN 0021-9533

Singh, P.K.; Parsek, M.R.; Greenberg, E. P. & Welsh, M.J. (2002). A Component of Innate Immunity Prevents Bacterial Biofilm Development. *Nature*,Vol. 417, No. 6888, (May 2002), pp. 552-555, ISSN 0028-0836

Skaar, E.P. (2010). The Battle for Iron between Bacterial Pathogens and their Vertebrates Hosts. *PLoS Pathogens*, Vol. 6, No. 8, (August 2010), pp. e1000949 ISSN 1553-7366

Soler, P.M. ; Wright, T.E. ; Smith, P.D. ; Maggi, S.P. ; Hill, P.D. ; Ko, F. ; Jimenez, P.A. & Robson, M.C. (1999). In Vivo Characterization of Keratinocyte Growth Factor 2 as a Potential Wound Healing Agent. *Wound Repair and Regeneration*, Vol. 7, No. 3, (May-June 1999), pp. 172-178, ISSN 1067-1927

Sorimachi, K.; Akimoto, K.; Hattori, Y.; Teiri, T. & Niwa, A. (1997). Activation of Macrophages by Lactoferrin: Secretion of TNF-alfa, IL-8 and NO. *Biochemistry and Molecular Biology International*, Vol. 43, No. 1, (September 1997), pp. 79-87, ISSN 1039-9712

Spadaro, M.; Caorsi, C.; Cerutti, P.; Varadhachary, A.; Forni, G.; Pericle, P.& Giovarelli, M. (2008). Lactoferin, a Major Defense Protein of Innate Immunity, Is a Novel Maturation Factor for Human Dendritic Cells. *The FASEB Journal*, Vol. 22, No. 8, (August 2008), pp. 2747-2757, ISSN 0892-6638

Spik, G.; Strecker, G.; Fournet, B.; Bouquelet, S.; Montreuil, J.; Dorland, L.; van Halbeek, H.& Vliegenhart, J.F. (1982). Primary Structure of the Glycans from Human Lactotransferrin. *European Journal of Biochemistry*, Vol. 121, No. 2 (January 1982), pp. 413-419, ISSN 0014-2956

Takahashi, Y.; Takeda, C.; Seto, I.; Kawano, G. & Machida, Y. (2007). Formulation and Evaluation of Lactoferrin Bioadhesive Tablets. *International Journal of Pharmaceutics*, Vol. 343, No. 1-2, (October 2007), pp. 220-227, ISSN 0378-5173

Takayama, Y. & Takezawa T. (2006).Lactoferrin Promotes Collagen Gel Contractile Activity of Fibroblast Mediated by Lipoprotein Receptors. *Biochemistry and Cell Biology*, Vol. 84, No. 6, (June 2006), pp. 268-274, ISSN 0829-8211

Takayama, Y.; Takahashi, H.; Mizumachi, K. & Takezawa, T. (2003). Low Density Lipoprotein Receptor-Related Protein (LRP) is Required for Lactoferrin-Enhanced Collagen Contractile activity of Human Fibroblasts. *The Journal of Biological Chemistry*. Vol. 278, No. 24, (June 2003), pp. 22112-22118, ISSN 0021-9258

Takeda, C.; Takahashi, Y.; Seto, I.; Kawano, G.; Takayama, K.; Onishi, H. & Machida, Y. (2007). Influence of Pectins on Preparation Characteristics of Lactoferrin Bioadhesive Tablets. *Chemical and Pharmaceutical Bulletin*, Vol. 55, No. 8, (August 2007), pp. 1164-1168, ISSN 0009-2363

Tamir, E. (2007). Treating the Diabetic Foot Ulcer: Practical Approach and General Concepts. *Israel Medical Association Journal*, Vol. 9, No. 8, (August 2007), pp. 610-615, ISSN 1565-1088

Tang, L.; Cui, T.; Wu, J.J.; Liu-Mares, W. ; Huang, N. & Li, J. (2010A). A Rice Derived Recombinant Human Lactoferrin Stimulates Fibroblast Proliferation, Migration, and Sustains Cell Survival. *Wound Repair and Regeneration*, Vol. 18, No. 1, (January-February 2010), pp. 123-131, ISSN 1067-1927

Tang, L.; Wu, J.J.; Ma, Q.; Cui, T. ; Andreopoulos, F.M. ; Gil, J. ; Valdes, J. ; Davis, S.C. & Li, J. (2010B). Human Lactoferrin Stimulates Skin Keratinocyte Function and Wound Re-epithelialization. *The British Journal of Dermatology*, Vol. 163, No. 1, (July 2010), pp. 38-47, ISSN 0007-0963

Togawa, J.; Nagase, H.; Tanaka, K.; Inamori, M.; Nakajima, A.; Ueno, N.; Saito, T. & Sekihara, H. (2002). Oral Administration of Lactoferrin Reduces Colitis in Rats Via Modulation of the Immune System and Correction of Cytokine Imbalance. *Journal of Gastroenterology and Hepatology*. Vol. 17, No. 12, (December 2002), pp. 1291-1298, ISSN 0815-9319

Tomita, M.; Wakabayashi, H.; Shin, K.; Yamauchi, K.; Yaeshima, T. & Iwatsuki K. (2009). Twenty-Five Years of Research on Bovine Lactoferrin Applications. *Biochimie*, Vol. 91, No. 1, (January 2009), pp. 52-57, ISSN 0300-9084

Trif, M.; Guillen, C.; Vaughan, D.M.; Telffer, J.M.; Brewer, J.M.; Roseanu, A.& Brock, J.H. (2001). Liposomes as Possible Carriers for Lactoferrin in the Local Treatment of Inflammatory Diseases. *Experimental Biology and Medicine*, Vol. 226, No. 6, (June 2001), pp. 559-564, ISSN 1535-3702

Vaerman, J.P. (1984). Effector Mechanisms of IgA. *Annales de Biologie Clinique* (Paris), Vol. 42, No. 1, pp. 61-70, ISSN 0003-3898

Van Amersfoort, E.S.; van Berkel, T.J.C. & Kuiper, J. (2003). Receptors, Mediators, and Mechanisms Involved in Bacterial Sepsis and Septic Shock. *Clinical Microbiology Reviews*, Vol. 16, No. 3, (July 2003), pp. 379-414, ISSN 0893-8512

Viani, R.M.; Gutteberg, T.J.; Lathey, J.L. & Spector, S.A. (1999). Lactoferrin Inhibits HIV-1 Replication In Vitro and Exhibits Synergy when Combined with Zidovudine. *Acquired Immune Deficiency Syndrome*, Vol. 13, No. 10, pp. 1273-1274, ISSN 0269-9370

Wang, B.; Amerio, P. & Sauder, D.N. (1999). Role of Cytokines in Epidermal Langerhans Cell Migration. *Journal of Leukocyte Biology*, Vol. 66, No. 1, (July 1999), pp. 33-39, ISSN 0741-5400

Wang, D.; Pabst, K.M.; Aida, Y. & Pabst, M.J. (1995). Lipopolysaccharide Inactivating Activity of Neutrophils is Due to Lactoferrin. *Journal of Leukocyte Biology*, Vol. 57, No. 6, (June 1995), pp. 865-874, ISSN 0741-5400

Weber-Dabrowska, B.; Zimecki, M.; Kruzel, M.; Kochanowska, I. & Lusiak-Szelachowska, M. (2006). Alternative Therapies in Antibiotic-Resistant Infection. *Advances in Medical Science*, Vol. 51, pp.242-244, ISSN 1896-1126

Weinberg, E.D. (2009). Iron Availability and Infection. *Biochimica et Biophysica Acta*, Vol. 1790, No. 7, (July 2009), pp. 600-605, ISSN 0304-4165

Weinberg, E.D. (2001). Human Lactoferrin: a Novel Therapeutic with Broad Spectrum Potential. *Journal of Pharmacy and Pharmacology*, Vol. 53, No. 10, (October 2001), pp. 1303-1310, ISSN 0022-3573

Werner, S.; Krieg, T. & Smola, H. (2007). Keratinocyte-Fibroblast Interactions in Wound Healing. *The Journal of Investigative Dermatology*, Vol. 127, No. 5, (May 2007), pp. 998-1008, ISSN 0022-202X

Wilk, K.M.; Hwang, S.A. & Actor J.K. (2007). Lactoferrin Modulation of Antigen Presenting Cell Response to BCG Infection. *Postepy higieny i medycyny doświadczalnej* (online Journal), Vol. 61, (May 2007), pp. 277-282, ISSN 1732-2693 (electronic)

Winton, E.F.; Kinkade, J.M.; Vogler, W.R.; Parker, M.B.& Barnes, K,C. (1981). In Vitro Studies of Lactoferrin and Murine Granulopoiesis. *Blood*, Vol. 57, No. 3, (March 1981), pp. 574-578, ISSN 0006-4971

Xu, G.; Xiong, W.; Hu, Q.; Zuo, P.; Shao, B.; Lan, F.; Lu, X.; Xu, Y. & Xiong, S. (2010). Lactoferrin-derived Peptides and Lactoferricin Chimera Inhibit Virulence Factor Production and Biofilm Formation in *Pseudomonas aeruginosa*. *Journal of Applied Microbiology*, Vol. 109, No. 4, (October 2010), pp.1311-1318, ISSN 1364-5072.

Yamauchi, K.; Wakabayashi, H.; Shin, K. & Takase, M. (2006). Bovine Lactoferrin: Benefits and Mechanisms of Action against Infections. *Biochemistry and Cell Biology*, Vol. 84, No. 3, (June 2006), pp. 291-296, ISSN 0829-8211

Yamauchi, K.; Toida, T.; Nishimura, S.; Nagano, E.; Kusuoka, O.; Teraguchi, S.; Hayasawa, H.; Shimamura, S. & Tomita M. (2000). 13-week Oral Repeated Administration Toxicity Study of Bovine Lactoferrin in Rats. *Food and Chemical Toxicology*, Vol. 38, No. 6, (June 2000), pp. 503-512, ISSN 0278-6915

Zimecki, M.; Mazurier, J.; Spik, G. & Kapp, JA. (1995). Human Lactoferrin Induces Phenotypic and Functional Changes in Murine Splenic B cells. *Immunology*, Vol. 86, No.1, (September 1995), pp. 122-127, ISSN 0019-2805

Zimecki, M.; Mazurier, J.; Machnicki, M.; Wieczorek, Z; Montreuil, J. & Spik, G. (1991). Immunostimulatory Activity of Lactotransferrin and Maturation of CD4-CD8- Thymocytes. *Immunology Letters*, Vol. 30, No. 1, (September 1991), pp. 119-123, ISSN 0165-2478

Zimecki, M.; Mazurier, J.; Spik, G. & Kapp, J.A. (1996). Lactoferrin Inhibits Proliferative Response and Cytokine Production of Th1 but not Th2 Cell Lines. *Archivum Immunologiae et Therapiae Experimentalis*, Vol. 44, No. 1, (January 1996), pp. 51-56, ISSN 0004-069X

Zimecki, M.; Miedzybrodzki, R.; Mazurier, J.; Spik, G. (1999A). Regulatory Effects of Lactoferrin and Lipopolysaccharide on LFA-1 Expression on Human Peripheral Blood Mononuclear Cells. *Archivum Immunologiae et Therapiae Experimentalis*, Vol. 47, No. 4, (August 1999), pp. 257-264, ISSN 0004-069X

Zimecki, M.; Miedzybrodzki, R. & Szymaniec, S. (1998). Oral Treatment of Rats with Bovine Lactoferrin Inhibits Carrageenan Induced Inflammation; Correlation with

Decreased Cytokine Production. *Archivum Immunologiae et Therapiae Experimentalis*, Vol. 46, No. 6, (December 1998), pp. 361-365, ISSN 0004-069X

Zimecki, M.; Artym, J.; Chodaczek, G.; Kocieba, M. & Kruzel, ML. (2004). Protective Effects of Lactoferrin in *Escherichia coli* Induced Bacteremia in Mice: Relationship to Reduced Serum TNF Alpha Level and Increased Turnover of Neutrophils. *Inflammation Research*, Vol. 53, No. 7, (July 2004), pp. 292-296, ISSN 1023-3830

Zimecki, M.; Spiegel, K.; Właszczyk, A.; Kübler, A. & Kruzel, M.L. (1999B). Lactoferrin Increases the Output of Neutrophil Precursors and Attenuates the Spontaneous Production of TNF-α and IL-6 by Peripheral Blood Cells. *Archivium Immunologiae et Theraphiae Experimentalis*, Vol. 47, No. 2, (April 1999), pp.113-118, ISSN 0004-069X

Zucali, J.R.; Broxmeyer, H.E.; Levy, D. & Morse, C. (1989). Lactoferrin Decreases Monocyte-Induced Fibroblast Production of Myeloid Colony Stimulating Activity by Suppressing Monocyte Release of Interleukin-1. *Blood*, Vol. 74, No. 5, (October 1989), pp. 1531-1536, ISSN 0006-4971

14

Charcot Neuro-Osteoarthropathy

A.C. van Bon
Internal Medicine, Academic Medical Center Amsterdam, Amsterdam
The Netherlands

1. Introduction

Charcot neuro-osteoarthropathy (CN) is most often seen in patients with diabetes although it has been associated with syringomyelia, tabes dorsalis, leprosy and hereditary sensory neuropathy. It is defined by painful or relatively painless bone and joint destruction and deformity in limbs that have lost sensory innervation, it commonly develops in the mid-foot but also in the forefoot and hind foot [1]. The estimated prevalence in diabetic population is between 0,1% and 7,5% [2]. Due to the rapid severe and irreversible foot deformity, recognition of acute CN is extremely important. The clinical presentation between type 1 and type 2 diabetes is not different, but on epidemiological level the age of presentation of an acute CN is at an earlier age and longer disease duration [3].

2. Risk factors and pathophysiology

Trauma, previous ulcer, infection or surgery of the foot are predisposing factors for CN as well as neuropathy, osteopenia and renal impairment, although the exact pathogenesis is still unknown [3].

In peripheral blood monocytes isolated from Charcot patients, the osteoclast formation was significant increased compared to diabetic patients and healthy controls. The osteoclastic resorption increased after addition of receptor activator of NFκB ligand (RANKL). So in the acute stage of CN, the osteoclast activity is increased probably by increased expression of receptor activator of NFκB ligand (RANKL) via release of proinflammatory cytokines as TNF-alfa [4,5]. Central role in this process of local inflammation is trauma. Patients with diabetes do not notice most traumas due to the peripheral neuropathy. Trauma will induce pro-inflammatory cytokines like TNF-alfa and RANKL will be expressed. Due to loss in pain perception by the distal neuropathy, the TNF-alfa release will persist and the RANKL pathway is persistently stimulated [6].

3. Clinical presentation

The acute stage is characterized by unilateral erythema and oedema of the affected foot. The temperature is at least 2° Celsius higher than the non-affected foot, which can be measured with an infrared skin thermometer. Mostly the mid foot is affected, followed by the fore foot and hind foot.

The differential diagnosis of a red, hot swollen foot is: severe infection (osteomyelitis) in case of a concurrent foot ulcer, cellulitis, bone fracture, gout or septic arthritis. Most difficult is to differentiate between an acute CN and osteomyelitis if a foot ulcer is present. Clinical directions in favour for osteomyelitis are a positive probe to the bone test and radiological abnormalities in relation to the ulcer, that is mostly located on pressure points like metatarsal heads or rocker-bottom. Radiological abnormalities in favour of CN are radiological abnormalities in the mid foot. The chronic not active Charcot foot is characterized with joint deformity, and or (sub) luxation of the metatarsals leading to rocker-bottom. These deformities cause elevated plantar pressure leading to abundant callus formation and an increased risk for foot ulcers.

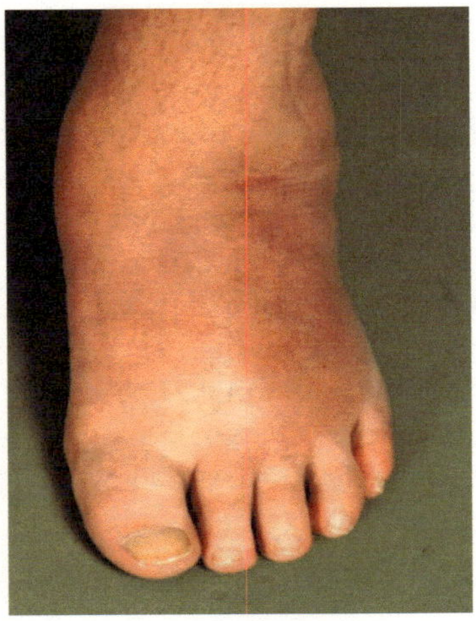

Fig. 1. Red hot swollen foot.

4. Diagnosis

Although in a very early stage of an acute CN the plain X-ray can be false negative, the initial screening tool for an acute CN is still a plain X-ray in three directions: dorsoplantar, lateral and pronated oblique). The radiological description is according to the five D's: bone density, joint distention, bony debris, joint disorganization and dislocation of the joint [2].

The density of the bone is usually normal, except in elderly or type 1 diabetic patients. Large joint effusions cause distention. The most frequent dislocation is the tarsometatarsal subluxation: Lisfranc's dislocation. Less frequent are dislocations of the talonavicular joint (Chopart) or subtalar or intertarsal joints. Sella and Barrette introduced five stage of Charcot deformity based on clinical and radiological features [7].

Stage 0: clinical stage of warm red swollen foot

Stage 1: localized osteoporosis, subchondral cysts, erossions and diastasis

Stage 2: joint subluxations

Stage 3: joint dislocations

Stage 4: sclerosis fusion

Therefore has a plain X-ray an important role in diagnosis and follow up of CN.

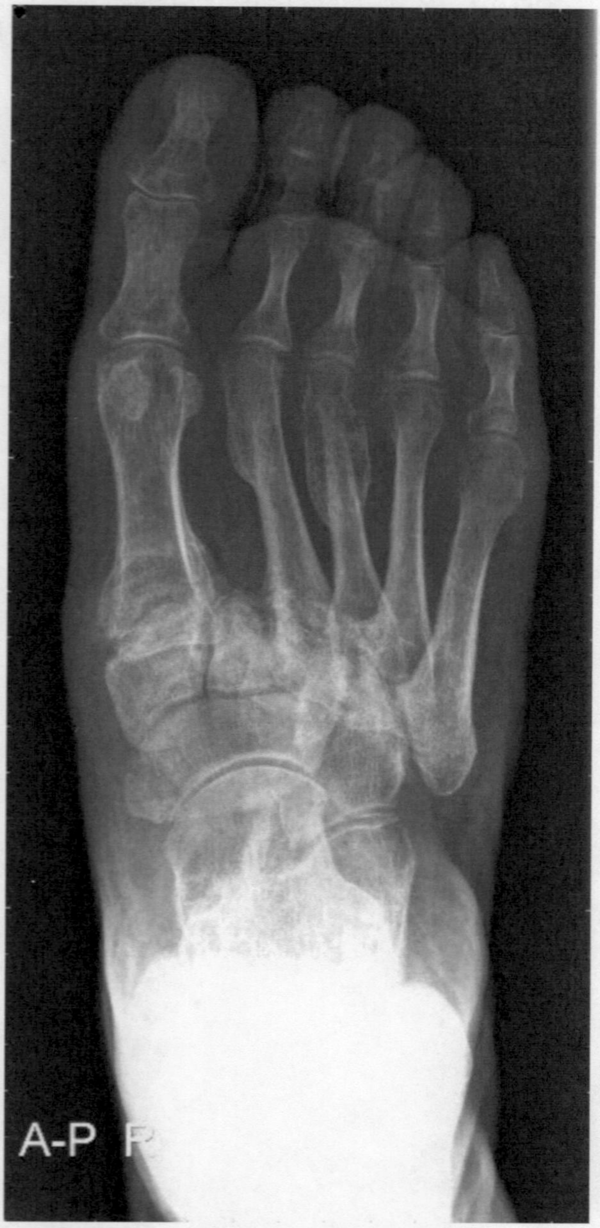

Fig. 2. Dislocation in tarsometatarsal joints: Lisfranc's dislocation

Magnetic resonance imaging (MRI) is the second step in the diagnosis the CN foot. Especially in Sella and Barrette stage 0, the early phase of the acute CN, MRI will show subchondral bone marrow oedema and or microfractures. The images should included T1 and short tau inversion recovery (STIR) or T2 fat saturated sequences. The use of computed tomography (CT) is not well investigated. The five D's as mentioned above can be adapted to CT images. Bone scintigraphy (technetium) is the most often used nuclear method. Focal hyperperfusion and or focal bony uptake are seen on the scintigraphy but are not specific for CN. Also in osteomyelitis these characteristics are seen.

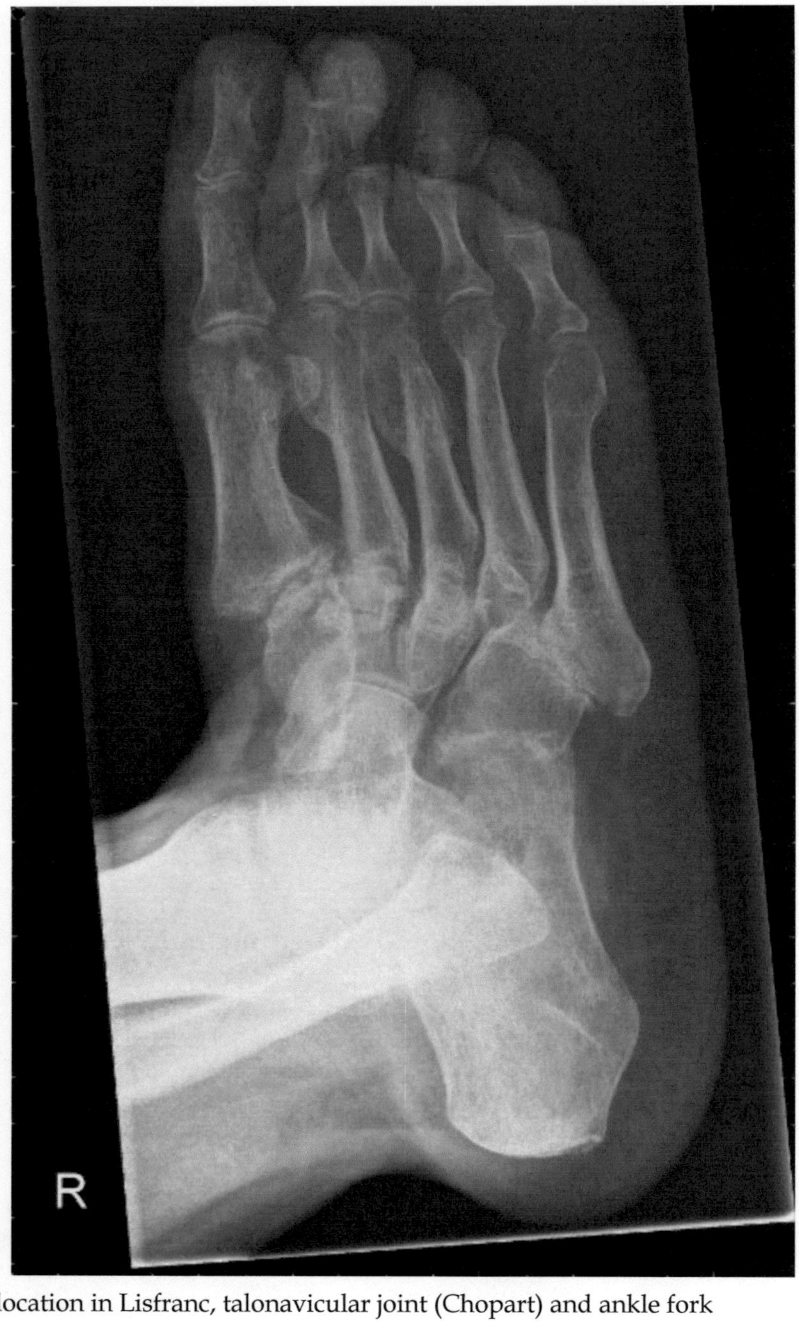

Fig. 3. Dislocation in Lisfranc, talonavicular joint (Chopart) and ankle fork

5. Treatment

Acute CN

The current standard treatment is off-loading the affected foot with a total contact cast or a prefabricated walking cast. Off-loading will prevent extensive bone damage, which can lead to sub-luxation and dislocation leading to severe foot deformity. Off-loading is continued until clinical signs of activity (temperature differential) are resolved and there is no longer evidence on X-ray of continuing bone destruction. Median time of off-loading treatment is 9 (7-12) months [8].

Chronic CN

If the CN is inactive, the patients have to be rehabilitated. This process has to be gradually to prevent recurrence for CN leading to further bone destruction. Patients need orthopaedic shoes during this process and the walking distance is extended slowly, first with two crutches followed with one and finally without.

Operative orthopaedic treatment is indicated for chronic recurrent ulcers on pressure points like rocker-bottom or joint instability. Operative procedures in acute CN are strongly not recommended: the bone structure is too instable for internal of external fixation and every orthopaedic intervention is a risk factor for increase in activity of CN. Osteotomy is possible in inactive CN in combination with bony prominence that cause recurrent ulcers. Obvious, arterial insufficiency is ruled out or has been treated before elective surgery.

6. Additional treatment with bisphosphonates?

To shorten the time of CN activity, intervention at the level of osteoclasts and or osteoblasts might be useful. Because bisphosphonates induce osteoclast apoptosis [9], several trials with bisphosphonates were performed. In the acute setting of CN the use of oral alendronate 70 mg once weekly on top of standard care (total contact cast immobilisation) was studied in a small double blind placebo controlled trial [10]. After 6 months, a reduction in bone turnover markers was demonstrated, but not in skin temperature. In another double blind placebo controlled trial studied the additional effect of one single infusion of intravenous pamidronate in patients with acute CN [11]. The intervention group had a faster fall in temperature of the affected foot at four weeks, a greater reduction in bone turnover markers and significant reduction in Charcot related symptoms during the study. In one not-randomized study confirmed the effect of pamidronate on temperature reduction and fall in bone turnover markers in acute CN [12]. However, all three studies did not report reduction in immobilisation time, as a clinical marker for the activity of CN.

Risk of bisphosphonates

Minor side effects of oral bisphosphonates are gastrointestinal symptoms, hypocalcaemia, skin reactions, acute phase reactions like malaise or fever or skin. These side effects have biological plausibility and causality has been proven.

No causality is proven for some severe adverse effects of bisphosphonates: osteonecrosis of jaw, atypical hip fractures, possible oesophagus cancer, atrial fibrillation and musculoskeletal pain. But clinical correlations were seen and reported in literature, for example osteonecrosis of the jaw [13]. Risk factors for developing osteonecrosis of the jaw are intravenous administration of bisphosphonates, history of inflammatory dental disease, glucocorticoids use and long duration of bisphosphonates use [14]. Of note, all severe events were seen if the bisphosphonates were used for several years. Furthermore, the reported data are conflicting and sometimes incomplete.

In conclusion, there is no indication for bisphosphonates in the treatment of an acute CN if no data are known about reduction is immobilisation time.

7. Possible candidates for additional treatment in acute CN

Strontium ranelate

Another potential intervention is strontium ranelate that is successfully used in the treatment of osteoporosis [15-17]. This drug has a direct inhibitive action on both osteoclast activity and differentiation. In addition, strontium ranelate stimulates the osteoprogenitor cells and collagen in osteoblasts [18,19]. Recent evidence has shown that strontium ranelate induced osteoprotegerin- (OPG) mRNA expression and suppressed RANKL mRNA in human osteoblasts [20]. Furthermore strontium ranelate induced osteoblast replication and differentiation [20]. Strontium ranelate is to date it has not yet been used as treatment in the acute stage of CN.

Denosumab

Denosumab is a fully human monoclonal antibody to the receptor activator of nuclear factor-κB ligand (RANKL) that blocks its binding to RANK, inhibiting the development and activity of osteoclasts, decreasing bone resorption, and increasing bone density. Given its unique actions, denosumab may be useful in the treatment of osteoporosis and bone metastatic disease. Some clinical trials have been performed and show favourable results [21,22]. In acute CN, no studies have been performed so far.

8. Summary

Charcot neuro-osteoarthropathy is most often seen in patients with diabetes and is characterized as red, hot swollen foot. In the presence of a foot ulcer, the differential diagnosis with osteomyelitis is very difficult. In the early stage of acute CN, X ray can be false negative in contrast to MRI or CT. The latter investigations can be useful to differentiate between osteomyelitis and acute CN. The treatment of acute CN is offloading in plaster cast until the active CN is clinical and radiological inactive.

9. References

[1] Edmonds ME. Progress in care of the diabetic foot. Lancet 1999; 354(9175): 270-272.

[2] Schoots IG, Slim FJ, Busch-Westbroek TE, Maas M. Neuro-osteoarthropathy of the foot-radiologist: friend or foe? Semin Musculoskelet Radiol 2010; 14(3): 365-376.

[3] Petrova NL, Edmonds ME. Charcot neuro-osteoarthropathy-current standards. Diabetes Metab Res Rev 2008; 24 Suppl 1: S58-S61.

[4] Mabilleau G, Petrova NL, Edmonds ME, Sabokbar A. Increased osteoclastic activity in acute Charcot's osteoarthropathy: the role of receptor activator of nuclear factor-kappaB ligand. Diabetologia 2008; 51(6): 1035-1040.
[5] Piaggesi A , arcocci C, olioa F, i GregorioS, accetti F, avalesi R. Markers for charcot's neurogenic osteoarthropathy in diabetic patients. Diabetes 2000; 49(Suppl 1): A32.
[6] Jeffcoate WJ. Charcot neuro-osteoarthropathy. Diabetes Metab Res Rev 2008; 24 Suppl 1: S62-S65.
[7] Sella EJ, Barrette C. Staging of Charcot neuroarthropathy along the medial column of the foot in the diabetic patient. J Foot Ankle Surg 1999; 38(1): 34-40.
[8] Bates M, Petrova NL, Edmonds ME. How long does it take to progress from cast to shoes in the management of Charcot osteoarthropathy. Diabetic Medicine 23[Supll 2], 27 -A100. 2006.
[9] Reszka AA, Rodan GA. Mechanism of action of bisphosphonates. Curr Osteoporos Rep 2003; 1(2): 45-52.
[10] Pitocco D, Ruotolo V, Caputo S, Mancini L, Collina CM, Manto A *et al.* Six-month treatment with alendronate in acute Charcot neuroarthropathy: a randomized controlled trial. Diabetes Care 2005; 28(5): 1214-1215.
[11] Jude EB, Selby PL, Burgess J, Lilleystone P, Mawer EB, Page SR *et al.* Bisphosphonates in the treatment of Charcot neuroarthropathy: a double-blind randomised controlled trial. Diabetologia 2001; 44(11): 2032-2037.
[12] Anderson JJ, Woelffer KE, Holtzman JJ, Jacobs AM. Bisphosphonates for the treatment of Charcot neuroarthropathy. J Foot Ankle Surg 2004; 43(5): 285-289.
[13] Lewiecki EM. Safety of long-term bisphosphonate therapy for the management of osteoporosis. Drugs 2011; 71(6): 791-814.
[14] Ruggiero SL, Mehrotra B. Bisphosphonate-related osteonecrosis of the jaw: diagnosis, prevention, and management. Annu Rev Med 2009; 60: 85-96.
[15] Meunier et al. Effects of long-term strontium ranelate treatment on vertebral fracture risk in postmenopausal women with osteoporosis. Osteoporos Int 2009; 20: 1663-1673
[16] Reginster J et al. Effects of long-term strontium ranelate treatment on the risk of nonvertebral and vertebral fractures in postmenopausal osteoporosis.. Artritis and Rheumatism 2008; 58: 1687-1695
[17] O'Donnell S et al. Strontium ranelate for preventing and treating postmenopausal osteoporosis (review). Cochrane database of systematic reviews 2006; 4
[18] Hamdy NAT. Strontium ranelate improves bone microarchitecture in osteoporosis. Rheumatology 2009; 48: iv9-iv13
[19] Brennan TC, Rybchyn MS, Green W, Atwa S, Conigrave AD, Mason RS. Osteoblasts play key role in the mechanisms of action of strontium ranelate. BJP 2009; 157: 1291-1300
[20] Brennan et al. Osteoblasts play key role in the mechanisms of action of strontium ranelate. British Journal of pharmacology 2009; 157: 1291-1300
[21] SR. Cummings, J San Martin, MR. McClung, ES. Siris, R Eastell, et al, FREEDOM Trial Denosumab for Prevention of Fractures in Postmenopausal Women with Osteoporosis. N Engl J Med 2009; 361:756-765

[22] Smith MR, Egerdie B, Hernandez Toriz N, Feldman R, Tannela TL et al HALT Prostate study group. Denosumab in men receiving androgen-deprivation therapy for prostate cancer. N Engl J Med 2009; 361: 745-55